Current Concepts in Soft Tissue Pathology

Guest Editor

ELIZABETH A. MONTGOMERY, MD

SURGICAL PATHOLOGY CLINICS

surgpath.theclinics.com

Consulting Editor
JOHN R. GOLDBLUM, MD

September 2011 • Volume 4 • Number 3

SAUNDERS an imprint of ELSEVIER, Inc.

W.B. SAUNDERS COMPANY
A Division of Elsevier Inc.

1600 John F. Kennedy Boulevard • Suite 1800 • Philadelphia, Pennsylvania 19103-2899

http://www.surgpath.theclinics.com

SURGICAL PATHOLOGY CLINICS Volume 4, Number 3
September 2011 ISSN 1875-9181, ISBN-13: 978-1-4557-2899-2

Editor: Joanne Husovski

Surgical Pathology Clinics (ISSN 1875-9181) is published quarterly by Elsevier Inc., 360 Park Avenue South, New York, NY 10010. Months of issue are March, June, September, and December. Business and Editorial Office: Elsevier Inc., 1600 John F. Kennedy Blvd., Ste. 1800, Philadelphia, PA 19103-2899. Accounting and Circulation Offices: Elsevier Inc., 3251 Riverport Lane, Maryland Heights, MO 63043. Periodicals postage paid at New York, NY and at additional mailing offices. Subscription prices are $170.00 per year (US individuals), $199.00 per year (US institutions), $84.00 per year (US students/residents), $213.00 per year (Canadian individuals), $225.00 per year (Canadian Institutions), $213.00 per year (foreign individuals), $225.00 per year (foreign institutions), and $104.00 per year (international & Canadian students/residents). Foreign air speed delivery is included in all *Clinics'* subscription prices. All prices are subject to change without notice. **POSTMASTER:** Send address changes to *Surgical Pathology Clinics*, Elsevier, 3251 Riverport Lane, Maryland Heights, MO 63043. Customer Service: 1-800-654-2452 (US). From outside the United States, call 1-314-447-8871. Fax: 1-314-447-8029. E-mail: JournalsCustomerServiceusa@elsevier.com (for print support) and JournalsOnlineSupport-usa@elsevier.com (for online support).

Reprints. For copies of 100 or more, of articles in this publication, please contact the Commercial Reprints Department, Elsevier Inc., 360 Park Avenue South, New York, NY 10010-1710. Tel. (212) 633-3812; Fax: (212) 462-1935; E-mail: reprints@elsevier.com.

Printed and bound by CPI Group (UK) Ltd, Croydon, CR0 4YY

Transferred to Digital Print 2011

Contributors

CONSULTING EDITOR

JOHN R. GOLDBLUM, MD
Chairman, Department of Anatomic Pathology;
Professor of Pathology, Cleveland Clinics,
Lerner College of Medicine, Cleveland Clinic,
Cleveland, Ohio

GUEST EDITOR

ELIZABETH A. MONTGOMERY, MD
Professor of Pathology and Oncology,
Department of Pathology, The Johns Hopkins
Medical Institutions, Baltimore, Maryland

AUTHORS

AARON AUERBACH, MD, MPH
Department of Pathology, Joint Pathology
Center, Silver Spring, Maryland

JUSTIN A. BISHOP, MD
Assistant Professor, Department of Pathology,
The Johns Hopkins Hospital, Baltimore,
Maryland

DAVID S. CASSARINO, MD, PhD
Department of Pathology, Sunset Medical
Center, Southern California Permanente
Medical Group, Los Angeles, California

ASHLEY M. CIMINO-MATHEWS, MD
Resident Pathologist, Department of
Pathology, The Johns Hopkins Hospital,
Baltimore, Maryland

ANDREA T. DEYRUP, MD, PhD
Associate Professor of Clinical Pathology,
Department of Orthopaedic Surgery, University
of South Carolina School of Medicine;
Pathology Consultants of Greenville,
Greenville, South Carolina

HILLARY ELWOOD, MD
Resident, Department of Pathology, The Johns
Hopkins Hospital, Baltimore, Maryland

CYRIL FISHER, MA, MD, DSc, FRCPath
Department of Histopathology, The Royal
Marsden Hospital, London, United Kingdom

DORA LAM-HIMLIN, MD
Assistant Professor and Senior Associate
Consultant of Pathology and Laboratory
Medicine, Mayo Clinic Arizona, Scottsdale,
Arizona

ROBERT E. LEBLANC, MD
Department of Pathology, The Johns Hopkins
Hospital, Baltimore, Maryland

ELIZABETH A. MONTGOMERY, MD
Professor of Pathology and Oncology,
Department of Pathology, The Johns Hopkins
Medical Institutions, Baltimore, Maryland

KAROKH H. SALIH, MBChB, FICPath
Program Director, Department of Pathology,
College of Medicine, University of Sulaimani,
As-Sulaimaniyah, Iraq

UMER N. SHEIKH, MD
Department of Pathology, St. John Hospital
and Medical Center, Detroit, Michigan

AATUR D. SINGHI, MD, PhD
Department of Pathology, The Johns Hopkins
Medical Institutions, Baltimore, Maryland

JANIS TAUBE, MD, MSc
Assistant Professor, Departments of
Dermatology and Pathology, The Johns
Hopkins Hospital, Baltimore, Maryland

KHIN THWAY, FRCPath
Department of Histopathology, Royal Marsden
Hospital, The Royal Marsden NHS Foundation
Trust, London, United Kingdom

MUHAMMAD I. ZULFIQAR, MD
Department of Pathology, St. John Hospital
and Medical Center, Detroit, Michigan

Contents

tumors, clear cell fibrous papule, and distinctive dermal clear cell mesenchymal tumor; malignant tumors include clear cell sarcoma, liposarcoma, and rare malignant perivascular epithelioid cell tumors. Clear cell variants of other benign and malignant soft tissue tumors include fibrous histiocytoma, atypical fibroxanthoma, myoepithelioma, leiomyoma and leiomyosarcoma, and rhabdomyosarcoma. Metastatic clear cell tumors, including renal cell carcinoma and adrenal cortical carcinoma, should be considered in the differential diagnosis and excluded through clinical history, imaging studies, and immunohistochemical stains.

Primitive round cell neoplasms (small round cell tumors) of soft tissue are a diverse group of malignant tumors composed of monotonous undifferentiated cells with high nuclear-cytoplasmic ratio. Many occur more frequently, although not exclusively, in childhood. As tumors with primitive round cell morphology are seen in virtually every basic tumor category, the diagnosis of small round cell neoplasms requires the use of ancillary diagnostic techniques: immunohistochemistry and often molecular genetics. The principal tumors in this group include Ewing sarcoma/primitive neuroectodermal tumor, desmoplastic small round cell tumor, alveolar rhabdomyosarcoma, poorly differentiated synovial sarcoma, neuroblastoma, and ganglioneuroblastoma.

This article presents an overview of soft tissue tumors that have a plexiform histomorphology. The more commonly encountered entities, including plexiform fibrohistiocytic tumor, cellular neurothekeoma, dermal nerve sheath myxoma, plexiform schwannoma, and plexiform neurofibroma, are discussed in detail, and other tumors are noted. Information on clinical features, microscopic findings, ancillary studies, differential diagnosis, and prognosis is provided for each entity.

Myxoid tumors of soft tissue constitute a heterogeneous group of neoplasms characterized by the presence of a myxoid stromal matrix, which appears on H&E as an amorphous material and may be confused with edema. Superficial myxoid lesions in general are benign and deep ones are malignant. Grossly, they have a variable gelatinous quality and overlapping histologic features that may present diagnostic difficulties for pathologists. Most are sporadic neoplasms, with only a small percentage arising in patients with hereditary disorders. Discussed are key features of classic myxoid lesions, histologic features, characteristic clinical presentations, immunohistochemical patterns, cytogenetic analysis, and differential diagnosis.

Epithelioid variants have been described for most mesenchymal tumors, including leiomyosarcoma, pleomorphic liposarcoma, epithelioid fibrous histiocytoma, and myxofibrosarcoma. Soft tissue tumors that commonly show epithelioid morphology include epithelioid vascular lesions, epithelioid sarcoma, sclerosing epithelioid fibrosarcoma, and epithelioid malignant peripheral nerve sheath tumor. Many of the entities described in this review were originally described as "simulating carcinoma" or "often mistaken for carcinoma" and this pitfall should be considered when evaluating epithelioid lesions in soft tissue. Many epithelioid soft tissue tumors express epithelial antigens to a varying degree and an immunohistochemical panel is essential for correct classification.

Surgical Pathology Clinics

THE CLINICS ARE NOW AVAILABLE ONLINE!

Access your subscription at:
www.theclinics.com

Pattern Approach to Soft Tissue Tumors

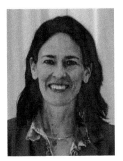

Elizabeth A. Montgomery, MD
Guest Editor

Over 150 types of soft tissue tumors are well-described in the medical literature. They are classified according to lines of differentiation by the World Health Organization and can be confusing to separate. Most authors offer material categorized by line of differentiation, whereas pathologists tend to diagnose based on histologic pattern. As such, in daily practice, we tend to note whether a tumor is, for example, myxoid or spindled as its key morphologic characteristic, and then form our differential diagnosis accordingly. Thus, we would consider intramuscular myxoma and myxoid liposarcoma for a deep myxoid lesion even though one is formally classified as an adipose tissue tumor, whereas the other is not known to have a certain line of differentiation. Although Drs Fisher, Thway, and I have previously published a book offering this approach, we are so enthusiastic about this pattern approach that it seems reasonable to also offer it as part of the *Surgical Pathology Clinics* series. Thus, in this issue, we cover several common soft tissue topics using a pattern approach with the exception of a section on myofibroma, myoepithelioma, and myopericytoma since these three entities are easily confused based on their overlapping names. It is hoped that the readers will enjoy, learn, and benefit from this approach.

Elizabeth A. Montgomery, MD
Department of Pathology
The Johns Hopkins Medical Institutions
401 North Broadway, Weinberg 2242
Baltimore, MD 21231-2410, USA

E-mail address:
emontgom@jhmi.edu

Surgical Pathology 4 (2011) ix
doi:10.1016/j.path.2011.08.013
1875-9181/11/$ – see front matter © 2011 Elsevier Inc. All rights reserved.

SOFT TISSUE PSEUDOSARCOMAS

Justin A. Bishop, MD

KEYWORDS

- Pseudosarcomas • Spindle cell melanoma • Sarcomatoid carcinoma • Cellular schwannoma
- Ancient schwannoma • Spindle cell/pleomorphic lipoma • Nodular fasciitis
- Proliferative fasciitis/myositis • Atypical decubital fibroplasia • Massive localized lymphedema
- Papillary endothelial hyperplasia • Atypical stromal cells

ABSTRACT

Soft tissue pathology is one of the most challenging areas of diagnostic pathology, not only because of the morphologic diversity of such lesions, but also because of their rarity and pathologists' subsequent lack of exposure to these tumors. Many lesions mimic malignant mesenchymal neoplasms, collectively referred to as "pseudosarcomas." The list of proliferations that can simulate a sarcoma is extensive and heterogeneous. This review addresses malignant, nonmesenchymal neoplasms; mesenchymal neoplasms that histologically mimic sarcomas but are benign; and benign reactive soft tissue lesions that are neither neoplastic nor malignant, but have worrisome clinical and/or morphologic features.

MALIGNANT, NONMESENCHYMAL PSEUDOSARCOMAS

MELANOMA

Overview

Melanoma is a malignant neoplasm derived from melanosomes that can have a variety of histologic appearances. It is the spindle cell variant of melanoma that most mimics sarcomas.[1–3] When associated with a fibrous stroma, spindle cell melanoma may be referred to as desmoplastic melanoma.[4]

Gross/Clinical Features

Spindle cell melanomas are uncommon.[5] They most commonly present as plaques on the skin of the head and neck in the form of desmoplastic melanoma.[6] Patients with desmoplastic melanoma are about 10 years older on average than those with conventional melanoma,[6,7] and there is a slight male predominance.[6,8]

Microscopic Features

Most often, but not always, spindle cell melanomas arise in the setting of an overlying in situ melanoma of the skin, usually of the lentigo maligna type.[7] Spindle cell melanomas generally are amelanotic, a fact that adds to the potential diagnostic confusion. The spindled cells are infiltrative, invading the dermis as single cells or short fascicles (Fig. 1). Spindle cell melanomas characteristically display neurotropism. There is classically a lymphocytic reaction to the tumor (see Fig. 1).[7] Melanoma is notorious for being a great mimicker in diagnostic pathology.[3] Accordingly, the cytologic appearance may range from deceptively bland to wildly pleomorphic.[4] Spindle cell melanomas have a disorganized architecture, usually without the well-formed fascicles or storiform patterns typical of many true sarcomas (Fig. 2). That being said, melanomas can rarely show heterologous differentiation in the form of cartilage or bone formation, further mimicking true sarcomas (Fig. 3).[9–11] Spindle cell melanomas consistently express S-100 diffusely (see Fig. 2), whereas other melanocytic markers, such as HMB-45, Melan-A, and MiTF, are or negative.[4] Two newer nuclear melanocytic markers, MiTF and SOX10, have, however, shown promise in staining desmoplastic melanomas.[12,13]

Department of Pathology, The Johns Hopkins Hospital, 401 North Broadway, Weinberg 2242, Baltimore, MD 21231, USA
E-mail address: jbishop@jhmi.edu

Surgical Pathology 4 (2011) 699–719
doi:10.1016/j.path.2011.08.001
1875-9181/11/$ – see front matter © 2011 Elsevier Inc. All rights reserved.

surgpath.theclinics.com

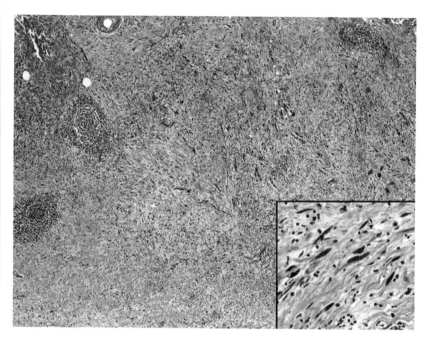

Fig. 1. Desmoplastic melanoma. There is an increase in dermal cellularity and lymphoid follicles at low power. At higher power, the spindled cells are hyperchromatic and separated by collagen fibers (inset) (hematoxylin-eosin [H&E], original magnification ×40 [inset ×200]).

Differential Diagnosis

Spindle cell melanomas can mimic virtually any soft tissue lesion. When a desmoplastic melanoma is cytologically bland, it can be misinterpreted as a scar or a benign neurofibroma. Usually, close inspection of a spindled melanoma reveals some atypia in the form of nuclear enlargement and hyperchromasia (see **Fig. 1**). When spindle cell melanomas are more pleomorphic, they may mimic sarcomas, such as malignant peripheral nerve sheath tumor, leiomyosarcoma, or pleomorphic undifferentiated sarcoma. If present, an overlying in situ component is very helpful in confirming melanoma. Melanomas often display a nested

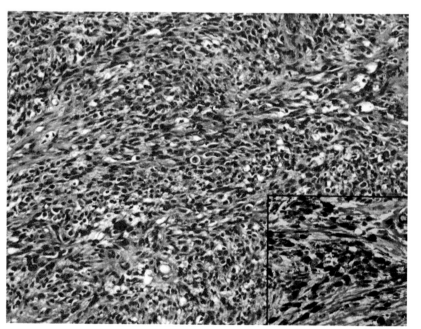

Fig. 2. Spindle cell melanoma. This melanoma, with spindled cells and a vaguely fascicular architecture, closely mimics a sarcoma. Strong, diffuse immunoreactivity with S-100 is very suggestive of melanoma (inset) (H&E, original magnification ×200 [inset S00 immunostain, ×200]).

Fig. 3. Spindle cell melanoma. Melanoma can closely resemble sarcomas, even demonstrating cartilaginous differentiation (H&E, original magnification ×200).

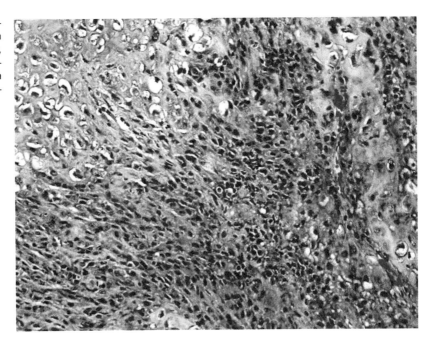

pattern of growth.[3] Prominent neurotropism, a lymphocytic reaction, and intranulcear inclusions are also important clues to the melanocytic nature of spindled melanomas. Diffuse, strong S-100 positivity supports the diagnosis of melanoma.

Prognosis

Although desmoplastic melanoma has a higher rate of local recurrence (likely because of the tumor's high rate of neural invasion), it metastasizes to lymph nodes less frequently than conventional melanoma.[4,14,15] Overall, when pure (ie, not associated with a significant conventional melanoma

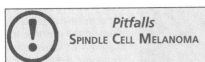

Pitfalls
SPINDLE CELL MELANOMA

! Can mimic virtually any soft tissue lesion from a scar to undifferentiated sarcoma.

! Presence of a more epithelioid component is suggestive, and finding an intraepidermal component is diagnostic. Thorough sampling is key!

! For the desmoplastic variant, a lymphoid reaction and neurotropism are diagnostic clues.

! HMB45 and Melan-A are often negative, but S-100 is strongly positive.

component) the prognosis of desmoplastic melanoma is actually better than that of melanoma overall.[4,14,15]

CARCINOMA

Overview

Carcinomas are malignant epithelial neoplasms that may have a spindled and/or pleomorphic giant cell morphology that mimics a true soft tissue sarcoma.[3] In the past, there was controversy regarding the histogenesis of sarcomatoid carcinomas with some belief that they represented collision tumors; however, recent evidence strongly supports the notion that these are true epithelial neoplasms that have undergone mesenchymal metaplasia.[16–20]

Gross/Clinical Features

Sarcomatoid carcinomas can occur in virtually any organ, and the terminology of these tumors varies on location (eg, anaplastic carcinoma in the thyroid, malignant mixed Müllerian tumor in the gynecologic tract). There are no unifying clinical or gross characteristics common to all sarcomatoid carcinomas from various organs.

Microscopic Features

All sarcomatoid carcinomas share, by definition, either a spindled or pleomorphic/giant cell histologic appearance. Although any architectural

Key Features
SARCOMATOID CARCINOMA

- Most important feature is presence of a conventional carcinomatous component, present either as nests within the tumor or dysplasia of the overlying epithelium.

- Striking mesenchymal appearance, and may even exhibit heterologous elements (eg, bone formation).

- Typically "pink" at low power.

- Despite its mesenchymal appearance, sarcomatous architecture is not usually well developed.

- Immunohistochemistry for cytokeratins and p63 may be helpful in confirming the epithelial nature of the malignant spindled cells, but negative results do not rule it out.

power, spindled carcinomas are often more "pink" than sarcomas because they are composed of plump cells with eosinophilic cytoplasm.[3] Most sarcomatoid carcinomas contain areas of epithelial differentiation at the histologic level, either in the form of foci of differentiated carcinoma within the tumor or foci of dysplasia/carcinoma in situ of the overlying epithelium (see **Fig. 4**). Occasionally the spindle cell proliferation undergoes heterologous differentiation (eg, bone formation), further mimicking a true mesenchymal neoplasm (**Fig. 5**). Expression of "mesenchymal" immunohistochemical markers (eg, vimentin, actin) is common and should not be taken as evidence of a mesenchymal origin.

Differential Diagnosis

Distinguishing sarcomatoid carcinoma from a true sarcoma can be difficult. In most cases, the distinction requires evidence of epithelial differentiation. Thorough sampling usually reveals areas of overt epithelial differentiation. In the absence of a carcinomatous component or overlying dysplasia, immunohistochemical studies can be of value. Most sarcomatoid carcinomas express cytokeratins, but the lack of expression does not exclude the diagnosis, as approximately 30% of spindled carcinomas are cytokeratin negative.[3] P63 can be helpful, as it is often expressed in sarcomatoid carcinomas,[21–24] but positivity has also been reported in sarcomas.[25,26] The expression of organ-specific markers can be helpful in

pattern may be seen, sarcomatoid carcinomas generally have a more haphazard growth than true sarcomas, without a well-formed architecture typical of most sarcomas (**Fig. 4**).[3] Sarcomatoid carcinomas are usually highly cellular and overtly malignant at the cytologic level, with nuclear enlargement, pleomorphism, and atypical mitoses; however, these neoplasms can occasionally be deceptively bland, masquerading as a benign reactive process like granulation tissue. At low

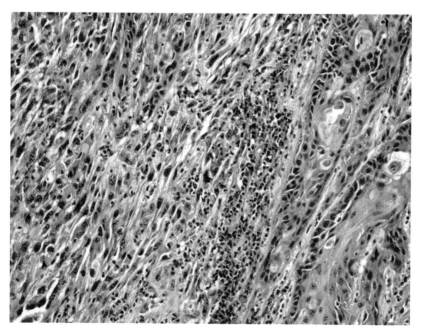

Fig. 4. Sarcomatoid carcinoma. Although much of this laryngeal tumor displays mesenchymal differentiation (*left*), the focal presence of conventional squamous cell carcinoma (*right*) confirms the diagnosis of sarcomatoid carcinoma (H&E, original magnification ×100).

Fig. 5. Sarcomatoid carcinoma. This example of spindle cell carcinoma shows heterologous osteoid differentiation, mimicking an osteosarcoma (*left*) (H&E, original magnification ×200).

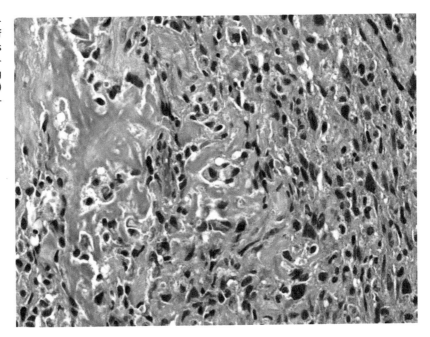

confirming epithelial differentiation, even in the absence of cytokeratin positivity (eg, PAX8 in anaplastic thyroid carcinoma[27] or sarcomatoid renal cell carcinoma[28]).

Practically speaking, in many instances, the location of the tumor makes the diagnosis of sarcomatoid carcinoma much more likely. In the thyroid, for example, any mesenchymal-appearing malignancy (except angiosarcoma) is presumed to be anaplastic carcinoma, even in the absence of epithelial differentiation.[29] In effect, a malignant spindle cell tumor arising in an organ (ie, not soft tissue) should be considered a carcinoma until proven otherwise.[3]

Prognosis

The prognosis of sarcomatoid carcinoma depends on the organ from which it arises. For example, in the lung, sarcomatoid carcinomas have a worse prognosis than conventional non–small cell carcinomas,[20] whereas in the head and neck, the prognosis can actually be better because tumor growth is often exophytic and more easily excised.[30]

BENIGN, NEOPLASTIC PSEUDOSARCOMAS

SCHWANNOMA

Overview

Schwannoma is an encapsulated, benign nerve sheath tumor that can occasionally have histologic features that are worrisome for malignancy.[31]

Gross/Clinical Features

Schwannomas can occur at any age, but are most common in patients 20 to 50 years old.[31] They are slow growing, and most often located in the head and neck or extremities.[31] Although some are associated with familial tumor syndromes, the vast majority of schwannomas are sporadic.[32] Schwannomas are usually well-circumscribed, encapsulated tumors; however, in the sinonasal tract, they are unencapsulated and can even erode bone (**Fig. 6**).[33,34]

Microscopic Features

The diagnosis of schwannoma is usually straightforward. They typically contain cellular ("Antoni A") areas admixed with less cellular, myxoid ("Antoni B") zones. The tumor cells are arranged in short fascicles or whorls. The tumor nuclei are long, twisted, and frequently line up, sometimes in a palisading fashion (ie, the Verocay body). A lymphoid cuff and hyalinized vessels are also characteristic. Diagnostic difficulty can arise when Antoni B areas and Verocay bodies are rare or absent in the so-called "cellular schwannoma." Cellular schwannomas can have an alarmingly hypercellular appearance (see **Fig. 6**) that may be coupled with occasional mitotic figures or, rarely, focal necrosis.[35–39] In addition, in long-standing schwannomas, so-called "ancient change" may be seen (**Fig. 7**). These degenerative changes include nuclear atypia, cystic change,

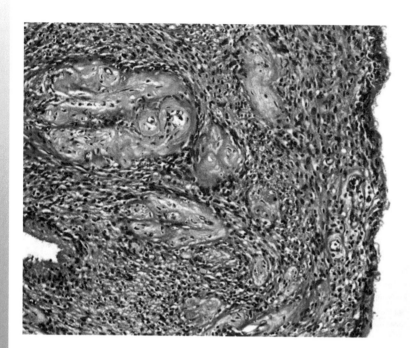

Fig. 6. Cellular schwannoma. In the sinonasal tract, schwannomas are unencapsulated. In this example, the tumor abuts the surface epithelium (*right*). Although the high cellularity and lack of circumscription are worrisome, the presence of hyalinized vessels is very suggestive of schwannoma (H&E, original magnification ×200).

hyalinization, hemorrhage, and calcification.[40] Schwannomas are strongly and diffusely immunoreactive for S-100.

Differential Diagnosis

Cellular schwannomas may be confused with true sarcomas, such as fibrosarcoma, leiomyosarcoma, or malignant peripheral nerve sheath tumor. It is important to recognize that despite its high cellularity, the tumor nuclei are bland, and although mitoses can be seen, they are usually not plentiful, particularly in proportion to the high cellularity. Unlike most true sarcomas, cellular schwannomas are usually well circumscribed or encapsulated (except in the sinonasal tract, where knowledge of this quirk is necessary[33,34]). Identification of other features typical for schwannomas, such as a focal Antoni B pattern or hyalinized vessels, can be helpful (see **Figs. 6** and **7**). Finally, diffuse, strong S-100 expression is very reassuring; whereas malignant peripheral nerve sheath tumors are also often S-100 positive, the expression is focal.

The nuclear atypia seen in ancient schwannoma can cause the unwary pathologist to consider the diagnosis of a sarcoma, such as pleomorphic undifferentiated sarcoma. Although the atypia seen in ancient schwannomas can be striking, and may include hyperchromatic and multilobulated nuclei, the changes have a smudgy,

degenerative quality. In addition, mitoses are rare, far out of proportion with the degree of atypia seen. As for the cellular variant, recognizing other supporting features of schwannoma (eg, hyalinized vessels) and other degenerative features (eg, cystic change, hemorrhage) is helpful for placing the atypia in its appropriate context.[31]

Prognosis

All schwannomas, even those with cellular or ancient features, are benign, with only rare recurrences and no metastatic potential following resection.[31]

Pitfalls
SCHWANNOMA

! The cellular variant of schwannoma has no (or rare) Antoni B areas, and can be alarmingly hypercellular.

! Bizarre atypia may be seen in scwhannomas with ancient change.

! In the sinonasal tract, schwannomas are usually not encapsulated.

Fig. 7. Ancient schwannoma. This schwannoma has "ancient" changes, including cystic degeneration, hyalinization, and hemosiderin. The thick-walled vessels are characteristic of schwannoma. Degenerative cytologic atypia is typical (inset) (H&E, original magnification ×40 [inset ×200]).

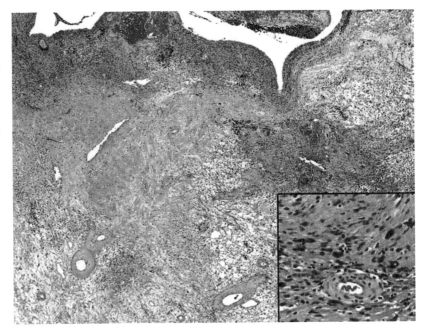

SPINDLE CELL/PLEOMORPHIC LIPOMA

Overview

Spindle cell lipoma and pleomorphic lipoma are ends of a spectrum that are best considered a single entity: spindle cell/pleomorphic lipoma (SCPL). SCPL is a benign tumor with a characteristic clinical presentation that has histologic features that may mimic a sarcoma.[41,42]

Gross/Clinical Features

SCPL is classically encountered in the subcutaneous tissue of the posterior neck, back, and shoulder.[43–46] There is a marked male predominance, and patients are usually 45 to 60 years old. SCPL is slow growing and painless. Most are well circumscribed, small at 3 to 5 cm, and have the gross appearance of fat, possibly with myxoid change.[43–46]

Microscopic Features

The features of spindle cell lipoma and pleomorphic lipoma overlap, and are often seen together in the same tumor. The amount of fat present in SCPL is quite variable, and ranges from abundant to not present at all. The small, uniform spindle cells contain cytologically bland, elongated nuclei with tapered ends (**Fig. 8**). Nucleoli are inconspicuous and mitotic figures are generally absent. The spindled cells are characteristically set in a myxoid stroma, and separated by bundles of ropy collagen. As with most tumors with a myxoid component, mast cells are easily found. The characteristic histologic feature of pleomorphic lipoma is the "floretlike" giant cell. The giant cell has eosinophilic cytoplasm and multiple, hyperchromatic nuclei in a wreathlike arrangement (**Fig. 9**). SCPL is strongly CD34-positive. S-100 is positive in the mature adipocytes, but not the spindled or giant cells.

Differential Diagnosis

The differential diagnosis of SCPL is broad. It may closely resemble solitary fibrous tumor or myofibroblastoma, so much so that many experts believe that all of these CD34-positive tumors exist in the same family.[41,47] The collagen of SCPL is reminiscent of that seen in neurofibroma, but the spindled cells of SCPL are consistently S100-negative.[41] Because of the presence of fat and myxoid stroma, SCPL can cause confusion with myxoid liposarcoma. When giant cells are abundant in SCPL, it may closely mimic atypical lipomatous tumor/well-differentiated liposarcoma. However, SCPL does not have the characteristic plexiform, "chicken-wire" vascular pattern of myxoid liposarcoma. Unlike liposarcoma, SCPL is well

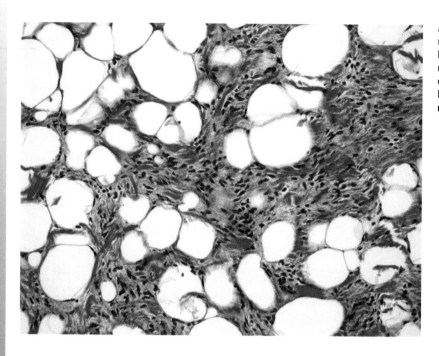

Fig. 8. Spindle cell/pleomorphic lipoma. Dispersed between fat lobules are monomorphous spindled cells and pink, ropey collagen (H&E, original magnification ×200).

circumscribed, superficial, and lacks lipoblasts. The classic clinical location of SCPL is another helpful clue. The ropey collagen and diffuse CD34 staining of SCPL are not seen in myxoid liposarcoma or atypical lipomatous tumor/well-differentiated liposarcoma. Finally, MDM2 and CDK4 can be useful immunohistochemical adjuncts, as they are usually negative in SCPL, but positive in atypical lipomatous tumor/well-differentiated liposarcoma.[48,49]

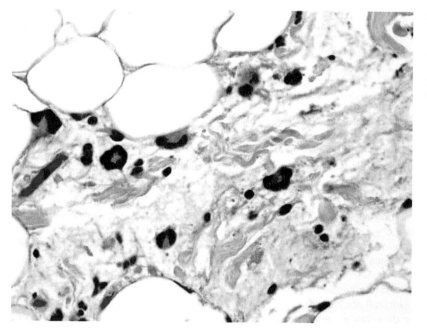

Fig. 9. Spindle cell/pleomorphic lipoma. Floret-like giant cells with a wreathlike arrangement of nuclei characterize pleomorphic lipomas (H&E, original magnification ×400).

Differential Diagnosis
SPINDLE CELL/PLEOMORPHIC LIPOMA

- Myofibroblastoma
- Solitary fibrous tumor
- Neurofibroma
- Dermatofibrosarcoma protuberans
- Well-differentiated liposarcoma/Atypical lipomatous tumor
- Myxoid liposarcoma

FIBROBLASTIC/MYOFIBROBLASTIC PSEUDOSARCOMAS

NODULAR FASCIITIS

Overview

Nodular fasciitis (NF) is the most common soft tissue pseudosarcoma.[42,50] It is a benign lesion that is thought to be a reactive proliferation of fibroblasts and myofibroblasts.

Gross/Clinical Features

NF occurs most often in adults in their third to fourth decades, with no sex predilection.[51–54] Although it can occur in virtually any site, NF is most commonly encountered in the upper extremities (especially forearm) and the head and neck.[51–53] Clinically, NF is a solitary mass that can be painful and is often worrisome because of its typically rapid growth over a period of weeks.[50] Although thought by most to be a reactive, non-neoplastic lesion, only 10% to 15% of affected patients report a history of trauma,[52,55] and recent data indicate that there is a consistent fusion of the nonmuscle myosin (*MYH9*) gene with the *USP6* oncogene in NF, suggesting that it is a benign self-limiting neoplasm.[56] Grossly, NF is well circumscribed but unencapsulated, and usually small (ie, smaller than 2–3 cm). Its cut surface varies from firm and fibrous to myxoid and gelatinous.[42,50–52]

Microscopic Features

At low power, NF is typically in the fibrous septa of subcutaneous tissue, is well circumscribed, and architecturally displays a haphazard, vaguely storiform, or "S-shaped" pattern of growth (**Fig. 10**). NF consists of irregular, short fascicles of plump myofibroblasts with an appearance similar to those of granulation tissue (ie, "tissue culture"–like) (**Fig. 11**). Cytologically, the myofibroblasts are bland and lack pleomorphism. The nuclei are hypochromatic and vesicular, with smooth nuclear contours and delicate nucleoli (see **Fig. 11**). The mitotic rate in NF is typically high, a potentially alarming feature, but atypical mitoses are not seen. Lymphocytes, giant cells, and especially extravasated red blood cells are often intermixed with the spindled cells (see

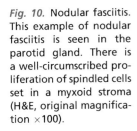

Fig. 10. Nodular fasciitis. This example of nodular fasciitis is seen in the parotid gland. There is a well-circumscribed proliferation of spindled cells set in a myxoid stroma (H&E, original magnification ×100).

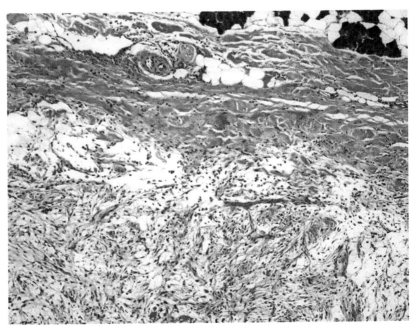

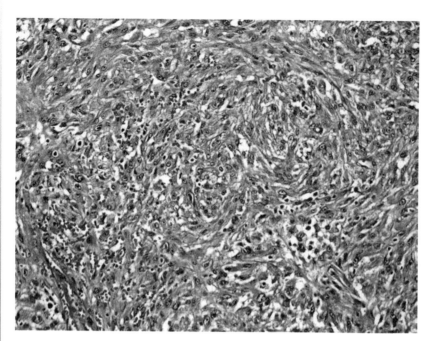

Fig. 11. Nodular fasciitis. Tissue culture–like fibroblasts in a vaguely stori-form architecture are seen. Note the extravasated red blood cells (H&E, original magnification ×200).

Fig. 11). Microcysts and microscopic areas of hemorrhage are common. Depending on the age of the lesion, NF varies from myxoid to fibrotic; the stages of evolution often coexist in the same lesion, imparting a "zoned" pattern. Variants of NF include ossifying fasciitis, in which metaplastic bone is seen,[57] intravascular fasciitis, in which the proliferation is in small to medium-sized vessels,[58] and cranial fasciitis, which involves the scalp and skull of infants.[59]

Immunohistochemical results are typical for a myofibroblastic proliferation: positive for smooth muscle actin and calponin, but negative for desmin or caldesmon.[42,51]

Differential Diagnosis

As a pseudosarcoma, the most important entity to consider in the differential diagnosis of NF is a true soft tissue sarcoma. True sarcomas typically arise deeper in the soft tissue, and are often larger and more infiltrative than NF. At the microscopic level, true sarcomas usually have a more organized architectural pattern than NF, and display overtly malignant cytologic features (eg, nuclear pleomorphism, hyperchromasia, atypical mitotic figures, necrosis) without a tissue culture–like appearance.

A benign entity to consider in the differential diagnosis is fibromatosis. Like NF, fibromatosis consists of spindled cells with very bland nuclei; however, fibromatosis is more deep seated and infiltrative, and grows in broad fascicles with prominent-appearing vessels. If there is doubt,

---

Key Features
NODULAR FASCIITIS

- Solitary mass, often painful and rapidly growing.
- Typically involves the upper extremities or head and neck.
- Well circumscribed and usually situated in the subcutaneous tissue.
- Plump, tissue culture–like myofibroblasts in short fascicles.
- Inflammatory cells and extravasated red blood cells.
- Mitotic figures numerous, but no atypical forms.

Variants of nodular fasciitis: ossifying fasciitis, Intravascular fasciitis, Cranial fasciitis.

nuclear expression of beta-catenin confirms the diagnosis of fibromatosis.[60]

Prognosis

NF is benign, and excision is curative. Recurrences are rare.[50,52,54]

PROLIFERATIVE FASCIITIS/PROLIFERATIVE MYOSITIS

Overview

Proliferative fasciitis (PF) and proliferative myositis (PM) are benign fibroblastic proliferations of the subcutaneous fascia and muscle, respectively.[42,50]

Gross/Clinical Features

PF and PM are less common than nodular fasciitis, and affect slightly older patients, with an average age of approximately 50 years.[61–63] Like nodular fasciitis, PF and PM present as rapidly growing, solitary, and sometimes painful and mobile masses.[42,55] There is no sex predilection. PF occurs most often in the upper extremities and trunk, whereas PM affects the muscles of the trunk and limb girdles.[62,63] Grossly, PF is a poorly circumscribed, elongated mass that extends along preexisting fibrous septa of the subcutis.[50] Similarly, PM is an infiltrative, scarlike process of the muscle and overlying fascia.[50]

Microscopic Features

The histologic features of PF and PM are similar to those of nodular fasciitis. In PM, the fibroblastic proliferation may alternate with atrophic skeletal muscle fibers, imparting a "checkerboardlike" pattern (**Fig. 12**).[42] The unique microscopic feature of PF/PM is clusters of cells that resemble ganglion cells (**Fig. 13**).[61–63] These ganglionlike cells are rounded to polygonal modified fibroblasts with abundant amphophilic to basophilic cytoplasm, 1 or 2 nuclei with vesicular chromatin and prominent nucleoli, and occasional cytoplasmic inclusions. Pediatric cases are rare, but tend to be more alarming microscopically, with increased cellularity, an elevated mitotic rate, and even necrosis.[64] Both the background spindled cells and ganglionlike cells label as myofibroblastic, although the expression of actin in the ganglionlike cells is often weak and can be absent.[50,64]

Differential Diagnosis

The large, ganglionlike cells of PF and PM can cause considerable diagnostic confusion. Indeed, in Chung and Enzinger's[62] series of PF, 16 of 53 cases were originally diagnosed as sarcomas, whereas in Enzinger and Dulcey's[63] series of PM, 14 of 33 cases were similarly misdiagnosed. One consideration is ganglioneuroblastoma, a tumor with true ganglion cells; however, aside from the ganglionlike cells, ganglioneuroblastoma bears

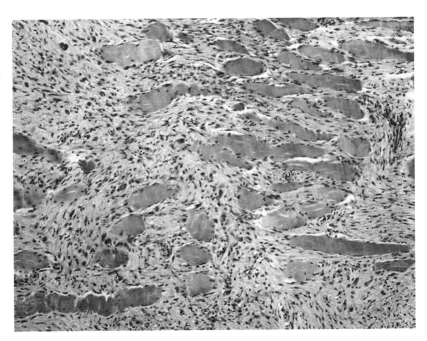

Fig. 12. Proliferative myositis. The presence of a spindled proliferation mingling between atrophic skeletal muscle fibers imparts a "checkerboard"-like pattern (H&E, original magnification ×100).

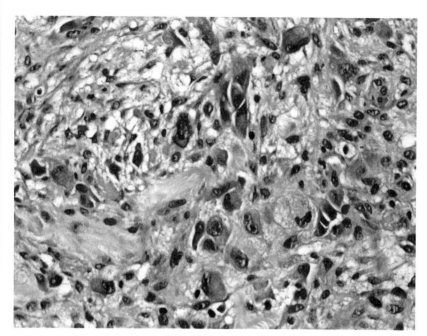

Fig. 13. Proliferative fasciitis. Large ganglionlike cells in clusters are seen in a background that otherwise resembles nodular fasciitis (H&E, original magnification ×400).

little resemblance to PF/PM at the clinical or histologic level. If in doubt, the lack of neuroendocrine immunohistochemical marker (eg, synaptophysin or chromogranin) expression in PF/PM confirms that the large cells are not actual ganglion cells. Another consideration in the differential diagnosis of PF/PM is a true soft tissue sarcoma with a giant cell component (eg, undifferentiated pleomorphic sarcoma); however, the giant cells of most sarcomas are pleomorphic and not like ganglion cells, and are associated with overtly malignant cellular features. The ganglionlike cells of PF/PM can be mistaken for the rhabdomyoblasts of rhabdomyosarcoma, especially in rare pediatric cases[64]; however, rhabdomyosarcomas are typically large and deeply situated. This differential is easily resolved by immunohistochemistry, as rhabdomyoblasts are positive for desmin and myogenin.[42]

△△ Differential Diagnosis
PROLIFERATIVE FASCIITIS/
PROLIFERATIVE MYOSITIS

- Nodular fasciitis
- Ganglioneuroblastoma
- Undifferentiated pleomorphic sarcoma
- Rhabdomyosarcoma

Prognosis

As for nodular fasciitis, complete excision is curative of PF/PM.[50,55]

ATYPICAL DECUBITAL FIBROPLASIA (ISCHEMIC FASCIITIS)

Overview

Atypical decubital fibroplasia (ADF), first described by Montgomery and colleagues[65] in 1992, is a benign degenerative/reparative soft tissue proliferation that results from chronic pressure-induced ischemia.

Gross/Clinical Features

ADF typically presents as a painless mass overlying a bony protuberance, classically,[65,66] but not always,[67] in patients who are debilitated or wheelchair bound. Most patients with ADF are elderly, and there is a slight female predominance.[65–67] Grossly, ADF is poorly circumscribed and involves the subcutaneous tissue.[65–67] It is usually 3 to 4 cm in diameter, and its cut surface often has a myxoid quality.[50]

Microscopic Features

Microscopically, ADF is characterized by a lobular and zonal pattern at low power. In the center of the zones is an area of fibrinoid fat necrosis and myxoid stroma, surrounded by a rim of proliferating, ectatic, granulation tissue–like vessels (**Fig. 14**).[65–67] The vessels contain plump endothelial cells, and many have fibrin thrombi. Around the vessels are a proliferation of fibroblasts, some of which are giant cells with abundant basophilic cytoplasm, large nuclei, and prominent nucleoli (**Fig. 15**). These large cells are hyperchromatic, but have a smudgy chromatin pattern typical of degenerative processes. As in nodular fasciitis, the fibroblastic cells may have an elevated mitotic rate, but atypical forms are absent.

Differential Diagnosis

The large, atypical fibroblasts strongly resemble the ganglionlike cells of proliferative fasciitis/myositis; however, proliferative fasciitis/myositis occurs in younger patients and is not associated with chronic pressure. In addition, unlike proliferative fasciitis/myositis, ADF is characterized by a zonated pattern with central necrosis and a rim of granulation tissue. The presence of necrosis and atypical cells, understandably, is quite alarming to pathologists and can result in a misdiagnosis of a sarcoma. In fact, in Montgomery and colleagues'[65] original report, a malignant diagnosis was considered in almost half of cases. The presence of atypical cells, fat, and myxoid change can be misinterpreted as a liposarcoma, especially the myxoid type. Myxoid malignant fibrous histiocytoma (myxofibrosarcoma) is another consideration. However, ADF lacks the

Pitfalls
ATYPICAL DECUBITAL FIBROPLASIA

! Necrosis common.

! Atypical cells at the periphery of necrotic zones.

! Mitotic rate may be high.

! Recognition of clinical scenario, along with zonated pattern, overall low cellularity, and background inflammatory changes are helpful in avoiding misdiagnosis.

characteristic "chicken wire" vascular pattern of myxoid liposarcoma, it is generally paucicellular, and the atypia of ADF is more smudgy and degenerative appearing than in liposarcoma or myxoid malignant fibrous histiocytoma. The zonated pattern is also a helpful finding not seen in true sarcomas.

Prognosis

ADF is benign, and treated with local excision. Local recurrence of ADF is uncommon, but more frequent than in the other reactive pseudosarcomas,

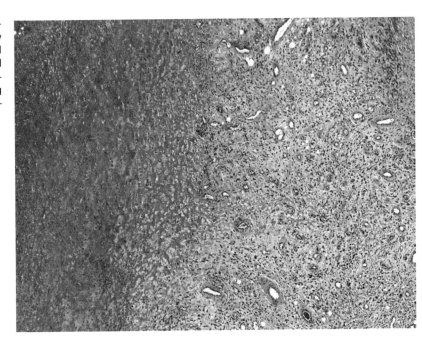

Fig. 14. Atypical decubital fibroplasia. At low power, there is a zonal pattern with fibrinoid necrosis on the left rimmed by proliferating blood vessels (H&E, original magnification ×40).

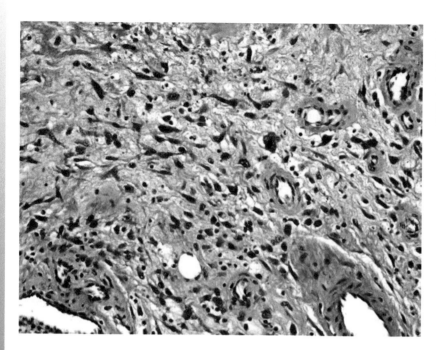

Fig. 15. Atypical decubital fibroplasia. At the edge of the necrotic zone, there are atypical fibroblasts with hyperchromatic, smudgy nuclei (H&E, original magnification ×400).

presumably because of the persistence of the underlying ischemic insult.[65–67]

MASSIVE LOCALIZED LYMPHEDEMA

Overview

Massive localized lymphedema (MLL) is a benign, masslike process that is thought to arise from the obstruction of lymphatic channels by folds of fat.[55]

Gross/Clinical Features

Massive lymphedema typically involves patients who are morbidly obese. It presents as a unilateral medial extremity mass, most commonly involving the thigh.[68,69] Grossly, the lesions are pendulous

Key Features
MASSIVE LOCALIZED LYMPHEDEMA

- Occurs as pendulous masses in the morbidly obese.

- Thickened overlying skin with a "cobblestone" or "peau d'orange" gross appearance.

- Overall normal architecture maintained, but fat separated by thickened septae with fibrosis, edema, and mildly atypical stromal cells.

and very large (mean size 33 cm in the original series[68]), and the overlying skin is thickened with a "cobblestone" or "peau d'orange" appearance. The cut surface reveals exaggerated fibrous septae, separate lobules of fat, and serous fluid may seep from cystic structures.[68,69]

Microscopic Features

At the histologic level, MLL is characterized by marked dermal fibrosis, dilated lymphatic channels, and expansion of the fibrous septae that separate subcutaneous fat by edema, collagen, and increased numbers of stromal fibroblasts that are mildly atypical (**Fig. 16**). The overlying epidermis may display acanthosis and hyperkeratosis (**Fig. 17**). Proliferative capillaries are occasionally seen at the interface of the fat and the fibrous septae.[68,69]

Differential Diagnosis

The expanded interlobular septae with mildly atypical stromal fibroblasts seen in MLL, along with its large size, can mimic atypical lipomatous tumor/well-differentiated liposarcoma; however, lipoblasts or significant atypia are not seen in MLL, and atypical lipomatous tumor/well-differentiated liposarcoma is not situated in the subcutaneous tissue. In addition, the overall architecture of the normal subcutaneous adipose tissue is preserved in MLL. Recognition of the background changes

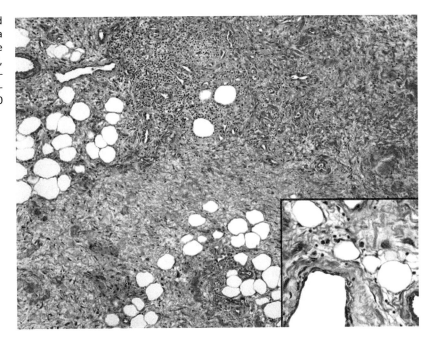

Fig. 16. Massive localized lymphedema. The septa between fat lobules are expanded and fibrotic, with mildly atypical stromal cells (inset) (H&E, original magnification ×100 [inset ×200]).

of lymphedema is helpful, as is the rim of reactive vessels at the interface of the adipose and fibrous tissue. Finally, simply inquiring about the weight of the patient can simplify the diagnosis considerably.

Prognosis

MLL is benign, although it may recur after surgical excision.[68,69] In addition, as with other settings of chronic lymphedema (ie, Stuart Treves syndrome),

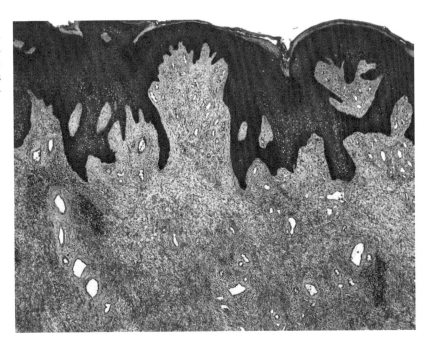

Fig. 17. Massive localized lymphedema. The overlying skin shows acanthosis, hyperkeratosis, and dilated lymphatic channels (H&E, original magnification ×40).

angiosarcomas can rarely arise in the setting of MLL.[70]

PAPILLARY ENDOTHELIAL HYPERPLASIA

Overview

First described by Masson (and therefore sometimes dubbed "Masson tumor"),[71] papillary endothelial hyperplasia (PEH) is a benign but exuberant endothelial proliferation that represents a form of organizing thrombus.[42]

Gross/Clinical Features

Classically, PEH presents clinically as a solitary red-blue mass of the fingers, head and neck, or trunk.[42] However, PEH can be seen in essentially any vessel, including those of a vascular neoplasm or malformation.[42] Patients of any age or sex may be affected.[42]

Microscopic Features

PEH consists microscopically of papillary fronds of fibrin or collagen, lined by a single layer of endothelial cells (Fig. 18). The process is typically confined to a vessel lumen, although limited extravascular extension may be seen. The lining endothelial cells are often plump, but do not have significant atypia or mitotic activity. The endothelial nature of the cells can be confirmed by immunohistochemistry (eg, CD31, CD34, Factor VIII).

Pitfalls
PAPILLARY ENDOTHELIAL
HYPERPLASIA

! Architecture mimics that of angiosarcoma.

! No cytologic atypia.

! Usually occurs within a vessel.

! Low mitotic rate.

Differential Diagnosis

The importance of recognizing PEH lies predominantly in distinguishing it from angiosarcoma. The most helpful features in making this distinction are the lack of nuclear pleomorphism or necrosis, a low mitotic rate, the intravascular location, and the lack of multilayered tufted structures in PEH.[42]

Prognosis

PEH is entirely benign, and almost always cured by simple excision.[72]

BENIGN NASAL POLYPS WITH ATYPICAL STROMAL CELLS

Overview

Occasionally, non-neoplastic polyps of the sinonasal tract can contain worrisome stromal cells with cytologic atypia.[73–77] Interestingly, similar

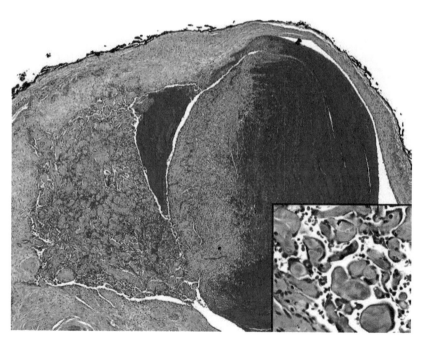

Fig. 18. Papillary endothelial hyperplasia. At low power it is evident that the proliferation is occurring within a vessel and in the setting of an organizing thrombus. At higher power, a single layer of endothelial cells without atypia surround cores of fibrin (inset) (H&E, original magnification ×40 [inset ×200]).

atypical cells have been reported in benign polyps of the larynx,[78] female genital tract,[79] and bladder,[80,81] and in benign polyps and ulcers of the gastrointestinal tract.[82,83]

Gross/Clinical Features

The most common sinonasal polyp is inflammatory, and is typically associated with allergy symptoms, such as rhinitis. They are often bilateral. The polyps are 2 to 4 cm, and gray-yellow with a gelatinous and semitranslucent quality. Rarely, inflammatory polyps can have an alarming clinical appearance, including large size, rapid growth, hemorrhage, visual disturbances, and bone erosion.[84–86]

Microscopic Features

Sinonasal inflammatory polyps are one of the most common entities in head and neck pathology, and usually cause no diagnostic difficulty. They consist of polypoid fragments of respiratory epithelium with a very edematous stroma and abundant chronic inflammatory cells, especially eosinophils (**Fig. 19**). The basement membrane is characteristically thickened. In some cases, there are cells with varying degrees of atypia scattered throughout the stroma. These cells are stellate or spindled, distributed singly, and their nuclei may be hyperchromatic, often with a prominent nucleolus. Mitotic activity is sparse, and atypical mitoses are not seen. Immunohistochemical studies have shown that these cells are most likely myofibroblasts, and they express vimentin and actin. Interestingly, most of these cells also express cytokeratins (AE1/AE3).[73]

Differential Diagnosis

When atypical stromal cells are prominent, sinonasal polyps may be confused with true sarcomas, especially rhabdomyosarcoma. Another consideration in the differential diagnosis of a benign nasal polyp with atypical stromal cells is sarcomatoid carcinoma. Reactive epithelial atypia overlying the polyp and aberrant cytokeratin expression in the stromal cells may cause further confusion with a spindled carcinoma. In benign polyps, however, the atypical stromal cells are without mitoses and the overall cellularity is low, because the atypical cells are distributed randomly throughout the stroma. The "cambium layer" of subepithelial tumor cell condensation that is characteristic for botryoid embryonal rhabdomyosarcoma is not seen in benign nasal polyps, and the atypical cells are negative for desmin and myogenin.

Prognosis

The presence of atypical stromal cells has no bearing on the excellent prognosis of the underlying benign sinonasal polyp.[73]

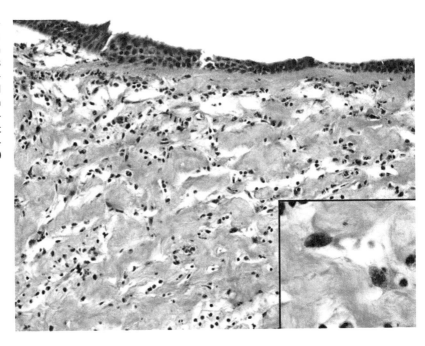

Fig. 19. Sinonasal inflammatory polyp. Beneath the respiratory epithelium (*top*), there are numerous inflammatory cells including eosinophils. Scattered throughout the stroma are mildly atypical spindled cells with prominent nucleoli (inset) (H&E, original magnification ×200 [inset ×600]).

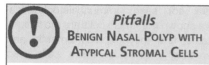

Pitfalls
BENIGN NASAL POLYP WITH ATYPICAL STROMAL CELLS

! Clinically can be worrisome, with rapid growth, visual disturbances, and bone erosion.

! Atypical stromal cells are stellate or spindled, with prominent nucleoli and hyperchromasia.

! Minimal mitotic figures.

! Atypical cells scattered throughout singly, without condensation beneath the epithelium

SUMMARY

The term "pseudosarcomas" encompasses a large group of diverse lesions that share the ability to simulate a soft tissue malignancy. Although there are certainly no absolute truths, a few themes common among the pseudosarcomas are apparent. A "tissue culture"–like appearance of lesional cells favors a pseudosarcoma. The lack of a well-formed architecture casts doubt on the diagnosis of a sarcoma, although the process may of course still be malignant (eg, melanoma, carcinoma). A soft tissue tumor that is well circumscribed or encapsulated should be considered benign until proven otherwise. Finally, a zonated pattern at low power favors a reactive process. Awareness of the pitfalls, attention to characteristic clinical scenarios and pathologic features, and judicious use of immunohistochemistry can help prevent misdiagnosing these pseudosarcomas.

REFERENCES

1. Zelger BG, Steiner H, Wambacher B, et al. Malignant melanomas simulating various types of soft tissue tumors. Dermatol Surg 1997;23(11):1047–54.

2. Lodding P, Kindblom LG, Angervall L. Metastases of malignant melanoma simulating soft tissue sarcoma. A clinico-pathological, light- and electron microscopic and immunohistochemical study of 21 cases. Virchows Arch A Pathol Anat Histopathol 1990; 417(5):377–88.

3. Brooks JSJ. Disorders of soft tissue. In: Mills SE, Carter D, Greenson JK, et al, editors. Sternberg's diagnostic surgical pathology, vol. 1. 5th edition. Philadelphia: Lippincott Williams & Wilkins; 2010. p. 124–97.

4. Busam KJ. Melanocytic proliferations. In: Dermatopathology. Philadelphia: Saunders; 2010. p. 437–98.

5. Quinn MJ, Crotty KA, Thompson JF, et al. Desmoplastic and desmoplastic neurotropic melanoma: experience with 280 patients. Cancer 1998;83(6): 1128–35.

6. Busam KJ. Desmoplastic melanoma. Clin Lab Med 2011;31(2):321–30.

7. Weiss SW, Goldblum JR. Malignant tumors of peripheral nerves. In: Weiss SW, Goldblum JR, editors. Enzinger & Weiss's soft tissue tumors. 5th edition. Philadelphia: Mosby; 2008. p. 903–44.

8. Fisher C, Montgomery EA, Thway K. Cutaneous spindle cell lesions. In: Biopsy interpretation of soft tissue tumors. Philadelphia: Lippincott Williams & Wilkins; 2011. p. 67–90.

9. Banerjee SS, Coyne JD, Menasce LP, et al. Diagnostic lessons of mucosal melanoma with osteocartilaginous differentiation. Histopathology 1998;33(3): 255–60.

10. Cachia AR, Kedziora AM. Subungual malignant melanoma with cartilaginous differentiation. Am J Dermatopathol 1999;21(2):165–9.

11. Giele H, Hollowood K, Gibbons CL, et al. Subungual melanoma with osteocartilaginous differentiation. Skeletal Radiol 2003;32(12):724–7.

12. Ramos-Herberth FI, Karamchandani J, Kim J, et al. SOX10 immunostaining distinguishes desmoplastic melanoma from excision scar. J Cutan Pathol 2010; 37(9):944–52.

13. Koch MB, Shih IM, Weiss SW, et al. Microphthalmia transcription factor and melanoma cell adhesion molecule expression distinguish desmoplastic/ spindle cell melanoma from morphologic mimics. Am J Surg Pathol 2001;25(1):58–64.

14. Busam KJ, Mujumdar U, Hummer AJ, et al. Cutaneous desmoplastic melanoma: reappraisal of morphologic heterogeneity and prognostic factors. Am J Surg Pathol 2004;28(11):1518–25.

15. George E, McClain SE, Slingluff CL, et al. Subclassification of desmoplastic melanoma: pure and mixed variants have significantly different capacities for lymph node metastasis. J Cutan Pathol 2009;36(4): 425–32.

16. Ansari-Lari MA, Hoque MO, Califano J, et al. Immunohistochemical p53 expression patterns in sarcomatoid carcinomas of the upper respiratory tract. Am J Surg Pathol 2002;26(8):1024–31.

17. Armstrong AB, Wang M, Eble JN, et al. TP53 mutational analysis supports monoclonal origin of biphasic sarcomatoid urothelial carcinoma (carcinosarcoma) of the urinary bladder. Mod Pathol 2009;22(1):113–8.

18. Sung MT, Wang M, MacLennan GT, et al. Histogenesis of sarcomatoid urothelial carcinoma of the urinary bladder: evidence for a common clonal origin with divergent differentiation. J Pathol 2007; 211(4):420–30.

19. Torenbeek R, Hermsen MA, Meijer GA, et al. Analysis by comparative genomic hybridization of

epithelial and spindle cell components in sarcomatoid carcinoma and carcinosarcoma: histogenetic aspects. J Pathol 1999;189(3):338–43.

20. Corrin B, Chang YL, Rossi G, et al. Sarcomatoid carcinoma. In: Travis WD, Brambilla E, Muller-Hermelink HK, et al, editors. World Health Organization classification of tumours. Pathology and genetics of tumours of the lung, pleura, thymus and heart. Lyon (France): IARC Press; 2004. p. 53–8.

21. Lewis JS, Ritter JH, El-Mofty S. Alternative epithelial markers in sarcomatoid carcinomas of the head and neck, lung, and bladder-p63, MOC-31, and TTF-1. Mod Pathol 2005;18(11):1471–81.

22. Dotto JE, Glusac EJ. P63 is a useful marker for cutaneous spindle cell squamous cell carcinoma. J Cutan Pathol 2006;33(6):413–7.

23. Reis-Filho JS, Schmitt FC. P63 expression in sarcomatoid/metaplastic carcinomas of the breast. Histopathology 2003;42(1):94–5.

24. Romanelli P, Miteva M, Schwartzfarb E, et al. P63 is a helpful tool in the diagnosis of a primary cutaneous carcinosarcoma. J Cutan Pathol 2009;36(2):280–2.

25. Kallen ME, Nunes Rosado FG, Gonzalez AL, et al. Occasional staining for p63 in malignant vascular tumors: a potential diagnostic pitfall. Pathol Oncol Res 2011 [Epub ahead of print].

26. Lee CH, Espinosa I, Jensen KC, et al. Gene expression profiling identifies p63 as a diagnostic marker for giant cell tumor of the bone. Mod Pathol 2008;21(5):531–9.

27. Bishop JA, Sharma R, Westra WH. PAX8 immunostaining of anaplastic thyroid carcinoma: a reliable means of discerning thyroid origin for undifferentiated tumors of the head and neck. Hum Pathol 2011. [Epub ahead of print].

28. Chang A, Montgomery E, Epstein JI. Immunohistochemical profile of sarcomatoid renal cell carcinoma. Mod Pathol 2010;23(Suppl 1):183A.

29. Rosai J, Carcangiu ML, DeLellis RA. Undifferentiated (anaplastic) carcinoma. In: Tumors of the thyroid gland. Washington, DC: ARP Press; 1992. p. 135–59.

30. Batsakis JG, Suarez P. Sarcomatoid carcinomas of the upper aerodigestive tracts. Adv Anat Pathol 2000;7(5):282–93.

31. Weiss SW, Goldblum JR. Benign tumors of peripheral nerves. In: Weiss SW, Goldblum JR, editors. Enzinger & Weiss's soft tissue tumors. 5th edition. Philadelphia: Mosby; 2008. p. 825–96.

32. Antinheimo J, Sankila R, Carpen O, et al. Population-based analysis of sporadic and type 2 neurofibromatosis-associated meningiomas and schwannomas. Neurology 2000;54(1):71–6.

33. Hasegawa SL, Mentzel T, Fletcher CD. Schwannomas of the sinonasal tract and nasopharynx. Mod Pathol 1997;10(8):777–84.

34. Buob D, Wacrenier A, Chevalier D, et al. Schwannoma of the sinonasal tract: a clinicopathologic and immunohistochemical study of 5 cases. Arch Pathol Lab Med 2003;127(9):1196–9.

35. White W, Shiu MH, Rosenblum MK, et al. Cellular schwannoma. A clinicopathologic study of 57 patients and 58 tumors. Cancer 1990;66(6):1266–75.

36. Lodding P, Kindblom LG, Angervall L, et al. Cellular schwannoma. A clinicopathologic study of 29 cases. Virchows Arch A Pathol Anat Histopathol 1990;416(3):237–48.

37. Fletcher CD, Davies SE, McKee PH. Cellular schwannoma: a distinct pseudosarcomatous entity. Histopathology 1987;11(1):21–35.

38. Casadei GP, Scheithauer BW, Hirose T, et al. Cellular schwannoma. A clinicopathologic, DNA flow cytometric, and proliferation marker study of 70 patients. Cancer 1995;75(5):1109–19.

39. Woodruff JM, Godwin TA, Erlandson RA, et al. Cellular schwannoma: a variety of schwannoma sometimes mistaken for a malignant tumor. Am J Surg Pathol 1981;5(8):733–44.

40. Dahl I. Ancient neurilemmoma (schwannoma). Acta Pathol Microbiol Scand A 1977;85(6):812–8.

41. Weiss SW, Goldblum JR. Benign lipomatous tumors. In: Weiss SW, Goldblum JR, editors. Enzinger & Weiss's soft tissue tumors. 5th edition. Philadelphia: Mosby; 2008. p. 429–70.

42. Montgomery E. Soft tissue tumors. In: Silverberg SG, DeLellis R, Frable WJ, et al, editors. Silverberg's principles and practice of surgical pathology and cytopathology, vol. 1. 4th edition. Philadelphia: Churchill Livingstone; 2006. p. 307–418.

43. Enzinger FM, Harvey DA. Spindle cell lipoma. Cancer 1975;36(5):1852–9.

44. Azzopardi JG, Iocco J, Salm R. Pleomorphic lipoma: a tumour simulating liposarcoma. Histopathology 1983;7(4):511–23.

45. Bolen JW, Thorning D. Spindle-cell lipoma. A clinical, light- and electron-microscopical study. Am J Surg Pathol 1981;5(5):435–41.

46. Shmookler BM, Enzinger FM. Pleomorphic lipoma: a benign tumor simulating liposarcoma. A clinicopathologic analysis of 48 cases. Cancer 1981;47(1):126–33.

47. McMenamin ME, Fletcher CD. Mammary-type myofibroblastoma of soft tissue: a tumor closely related to spindle cell lipoma. Am J Surg Pathol 2001;25(8):1022–9.

48. Aleixo PB, Hartmann AA, Menezes IC, et al. Can MDM2 and CDK4 make the diagnosis of well differentiated/dedifferentiated liposarcoma? An immunohistochemical study on 129 soft tissue tumours. J Clin Pathol 2009;62(12):1127–35.

49. Binh MB, Sastre-Garau X, Guillou L, et al. MDM2 and CDK4 immunostainings are useful adjuncts in

diagnosing well-differentiated and dedifferentiated liposarcoma subtypes: a comparative analysis of 559 soft tissue neoplasms with genetic data. Am J Surg Pathol 2005;29(10):1340–7.

50. Weiss SW, Goldblum JR. Benign fibroblastic/myofibroblastic proliferations. In: Weiss SW, Goldblum JR, editors. Enzinger & Weiss's soft tissue tumors. 5th edition. Philadelphia: Mosby; 2008. p. 175–256.

51. Montgomery EA, Meis JM. Nodular fasciitis. Its morphologic spectrum and immunohistochemical profile. Am J Surg Pathol 1991;15(10):942–8.

52. Bernstein KE, Lattes R. Nodular (pseudosarcomatous) fasciitis, a nonrecurrent lesion: clinicopathologic study of 134 cases. Cancer 1982;49(8): 1668–78.

53. Shimizu S, Hashimoto H, Enjoji M. Nodular fasciitis: an analysis of 250 patients. Pathology 1984;16(2): 161–6.

54. Allen PW. Nodular fasciitis. Pathology 1972;4(1): 9–26.

55. Rosenberg AE. Pseudosarcomas of soft tissue. Arch Pathol Lab Med 2008;132(4):579–86.

56. Erickson-Johnson MR, Chou MM, Evers BR, et al. Fusion of non-muscle myosin MYH9 to the USP6 oncogene in nodular fasciitis. Mod Pathol 2011; 24(Suppl 1):13A.

57. Daroca PJ Jr, Pulitzer DR, LoCicero J 3rd. Ossifying fasciitis. Arch Pathol Lab Med 1982;106(13):682–5.

58. Patchefsky AS, Enzinger FM. Intravascular fasciitis: a report of 17 cases. Am J Surg Pathol 1981;5(1): 29–36.

59. Lauer DH, Enzinger FM. Cranial fasciitis of childhood. Cancer 1980;45(2):401–6.

60. Montgomery E, Lee JH, Abraham SC, et al. Superficial fibromatoses are genetically distinct from deep fibromatoses. Mod Pathol 2001;14(7):695–701.

61. Kern WH. Proliferative myositis: a pseudosarcomatous reaction to injury: a report of seven cases. Arch Pathol 1960;69:209–16.

62. Chung EB, Enzinger FM. Proliferative fasciitis. Cancer 1975;36(4):1450–8.

63. Enzinger FM, Dulcey F. Proliferative myositis. Report of thirty-three cases. Cancer 1967;20(12):2213–23.

64. Meis JM, Enzinger FM. Proliferative fasciitis and myositis of childhood. Am J Surg Pathol 1992; 16(4):364–72.

65. Montgomery EA, Meis JM, Mitchell MS, et al. Atypical decubital fibroplasia. A distinctive fibroblastic pseudotumor occurring in debilitated patients. Am J Surg Pathol 1992;16(7):708–15.

66. Perosio PM, Weiss SW. Ischemic fasciitis: a juxtaskeletal fibroblastic proliferation with a predilection for elderly patients. Mod Pathol 1993;6(1):69–72.

67. Liegl B, Fletcher CD. Ischemic fasciitis: analysis of 44 cases indicating an inconsistent association with immobility or debilitation. Am J Surg Pathol 2008;32(10):1546–52.

68. Farshid G, Weiss SW. Massive localized lymphedema in the morbidly obese: a histologically distinct reactive lesion simulating liposarcoma. Am J Surg Pathol 1998;22(10):1277–83.

69. Wu D, Gibbs J, Corral D, et al. Massive localized lymphedema: additional locations and association with hypothyroidism. Hum Pathol 2000;31(9): 1162–8.

70. Shon W, Ida CM, Boland-Froemming JM, et al. Cutaneous angiosarcoma arising in massive localized lymphedema of the morbidly obese: a report of five cases and review of the literature. J Cutan Pathol 2011;38(7):560–4.

71. Steffen C. The man behind the eponym: C. L. Pierre Masson. Am J Dermatopathol 2003;25(1):71–6.

72. Weiss SW, Goldblum JR. Reactive vascular proliferations. In: Weiss SW, Goldblum JR, editors. Enzinger & Weiss's soft tissue tumors. 5th edition. Philadelphia: Mosby; 2008. p. 668–76.

73. Nakayama M, Wenig BM, Heffner DK. Atypical stromal cells in inflammatory nasal polyps: immunohistochemical and ultrastructural analysis in defining histogenesis. Laryngoscope 1995;105(2):127–34.

74. Klenoff BH, Goodman ML. Mesenchymal cell atypicality in inflammatory polyps. J Laryngol Otol 1977; 91(9):751–6.

75. Kindblom LG, Angervall L. Nasal polyps with atypical stroma cells: a pseudosarcomatous lesion. A light and electron-microscopic and immunohistochemical investigation with implications on the type and nature of the mesenchymal cells. Acta Pathol Microbiol Immunol Scand A 1984;92(1):65–72.

76. Compagno J, Hyams VJ, Lepore ML. Nasal polyposis with stromal atypia. Review of follow-up study of 14 cases. Arch Pathol Lab Med 1976;100(4):224–6.

77. Tuziak T, Kram A, Woyke S. Edematous nasal polyp with atypical stromal cells misdiagnosed cytologically as rhabdomyosarcoma. A case report. Acta Cytol 1995;39(3):521–4.

78. Lewis JS Jr. Spindle cell lesions—neoplastic or non-neoplastic? Spindle cell carcinoma and other atypical spindle cell lesions of the head and neck. Head Neck Pathol 2008;2(2):103–10.

79. Nucci MR, Young RH, Fletcher CD. Cellular pseudosarcomatous fibroepithelial stromal polyps of the lower female genital tract: an underrecognized lesion often misdiagnosed as sarcoma. Am J Surg Pathol 2000;24(2):231–40.

80. Tsuzuki T, Epstein JI. Fibroepithelial polyp of the lower urinary tract in adults. Am J Surg Pathol 2005;29(4):460–6.

81. Young RH. Fibroepithelial polyp of the bladder with atypical stromal cells. Arch Pathol Lab Med 1986; 110(3):241–2.

82. Berry GJ, Pitts WC, Weiss LM. Pseudomalignant ulcerative change of the gastrointestinal tract. Hum Pathol 1991;22(1):59–62.

83. Shekitka KM, Helwig EB. Deceptive bizarre stromal cells in polyps and ulcers of the gastrointestinal tract. Cancer 1991;67(8):2111–7.

84. Yfantis HG, Drachenberg CB, Gray W, et al. Angiectatic nasal polyps that clinically simulate a malignant process: report of 2 cases and review of the literature. Arch Pathol Lab Med 2000;124(3):406–10.

85. Rejowski JE, Caldarelli DD, Campanella RS, et al. Nasal polyps causing bone destruction and blindness. Otolaryngol Head Neck Surg 1982;90(4):505–6.

86. Winestock DP, Bartlett PC, Sondheimer FK. Benign nasal polyps causing bone destruction in the nasal cavity and paranasal sinuses. Laryngoscope 1978; 88(4):675–9.

SPINDLE CELL SARCOMAS

Cyril Fisher, MA, MD, DSc, FRCPath

KEYWORDS

- Synovial sarcoma • Malignant peripheral nerve sheath tumor • Fibrosarcoma
- Inflammatory myofibroblastic tumor • Myofibrosarcoma • Leiomyosarcoma
- Spindle cell rhabdomyosarcoma • Endothelial neoplasms

ABSTRACT

Information is presented on the pathology of spindle cell sarcomas. Synovial sarcoma, malignant peripheral nerve sheath tumor, fibrosarcoma, inflammatory myofibroblastic tumor, low-grade myofibrosarcoma, leiomyosarcoma, spindle cell rhabdomyosarcoma, and endothelial neoplasms are discussed in terms of an overview of the tumor, microscopic and gross features, diagnostic techniques, genetic markers, differential diagnosis, clinical details, and prognosis.

leiomyosarcoma, fibrosarcoma, rhabdomyosarcoma, inflammatory myofibroblastic tumor, and angiosarcoma. In the abdomen, gastrointestinal stromal tumor, dedifferentiated liposarcoma, and follicular dendritic cell sarcoma enter the differential diagnosis. It should also be remembered that spindle cell tumors of nonmesenchymal lineage can occur in many anatomic locations and mimic sarcomas. These include carcinoma, especially in relation to epithelial structures, and viscera, melanoma, and some lymphoreticular tumors, notably follicular dendritic cell sarcoma.

OVERVIEW

Spindle cell sarcomas constitute a large and diverse morphologic category of tumors composed of elongated cells with rounded, ovoid, or tapered nuclei and variable amounts of cytoplasm, disposed in a variety of patterns with a range of appearances modified by stromal fibrosis or myxoid accumulation. They occur in soft tissue, bone, or viscera; represent a variety of cell lineages; and exhibit a range of behavior so that accurate diagnosis and grading are essential for correct clinical management. Because of their common cell morphology and limited patterns, they can be difficult to distinguish from each other and from some reactive lesions.

The clinical history is frequently contributory, and subtle morphologic clues are present in most cases. Their identification and interpretation, however, require experience as well as familiarity with the application of ancillary diagnostic methods, including immunohistochemistry and, increasingly, molecular genetic techniques.

Spindle cell sarcomas include synovial sarcoma, malignant peripheral nerve sheath tumor,

SYNOVIAL SARCOMA

OVERVIEW

Synovial sarcoma was first described in detail, as a "primitive sarcoma of synovial joints," more than a century ago by Lejars and Rubens-Duval, who illustrated both glandular and spindle cell components.[1] The successive introduction of diagnostic techniques has established synovial sarcoma as a translocation-associated sarcoma with variable epithelial differentiation that is not related to synovium and only very rarely arises in any joint. The most common presentation is in a young adult as a deep soft tissue mass around or adjacent to a large joint, usually the knee, but it can occur at any anatomic site,[2] including superficial soft tissues, viscera, and head and neck. It can be initially indolent with the patient describing gradual enlargement for many years, but very small examples (smaller than 1 cm) are sometimes encountered, especially in the distal extremities.[3] Radiologic techniques reveal variably sized foci

The author has nothing to disclose.
Department of Histopathology, The Royal Marsden Hospital, 203 Fulham Road, London SW3 6JJ, UK
E-mail address: cyrilfisher@gmail.com

Surgical Pathology 4 (2011) 721–744
doi:10.1016/j.path.2011.08.002

of calcification in many cases. Rarely, synovial sarcoma arises following radiation therapy.[4–6]

GROSS FEATURES

Synovial sarcoma is typically circumscribed but not encapsulated, with a soft, white-tan cut surface. Cyst formation and hemorrhage are sometimes seen, with focal necrosis in poorly differentiated examples. Spontaneous total infarction is a rare phenomenon.

MICROSCOPIC FEATURES

Biphasic synovial sarcoma has an epithelial and a spindle cell component. The epithelial component can be glandular or adenopapillary (with neoplastic spindle cells rather than collagen in the papillary core), or form solid nodules or cords of cuboidal cells with oval vesicular nuclei, moderate amounts of cytoplasm, and distinct cell membranes. Rare variations include large, dilated glands with scanty spindle cell component, and widespread keratinizing squamous metaplasia.

The spindled component can be sparse, predominant, or occur alone as monophasic spindle cell synovial sarcoma (which is encountered more frequently than typical biphasic synovial sarcoma). The spindle cells (**Fig. 1**) have typically uniform, relatively small, short spindle or oval pale-staining nuclei, the edges of which can appear to overlap

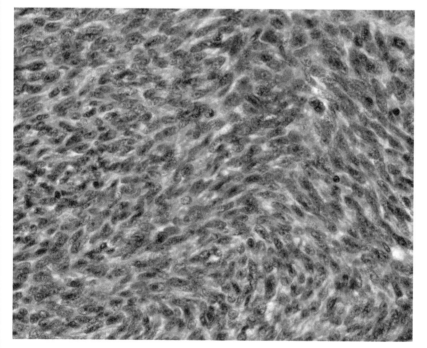

Fig. 1. Synovial sarcoma. The monophasic spindle variant is composed of fascicles of uniform short spindle cells, with nuclei that appear to overlap. Note the mast cells (hematoxylin-eosin [H&E], original magnification ×100).

each other slightly because cytoplasm is minimal and cell membranes not distinct. Mitotic figures are often hard to find except in poorly differentiated synovial sarcoma. The cells form highly cellular fascicles or patternless sheets with minimal stroma, although a variable degree of myxoid change can be seen, and a pericytomatous pattern is present in many cases. Other features include numerous focal nuclear palisading, mast cells, cyst formation, and rarely fibrosis with amianthoid fibers. More than 30% of synovial sarcomas show stromal microcalcification and occasionally there is osteochondroid metaplasia. Rarely, biphasic or monophasic tumors with widespread calcification (calcifying synovial sarcoma) or extensive osteoid or bone formation (ossifying synovial sarcoma) occur, mostly in the lower leg or foot. These have a more favorable outcome. Poorly differentiated synovial sarcoma is commonly a small, round-cell tumor that resembles Ewing sarcoma or lymphoma, and occurs more proximally. Rare examples have rhabdoid cells with abundant eccentric cytoplasm. As might be expected, poorly differentiated areas of synovial sarcoma (Fig. 2) have focal necrosis, and increased mitotic activity and proliferation index (Ki67).[7]

OTHER DIAGNOSTIC TECHNIQUES

More than 90% of synovial sarcomas of all types express epithelial membrane antigen (EMA) and cytokeratins, including AE1/AE3, Cam 5.2, CK7, and CK19. Essentially all cases show nuclear positivity for TLE1 (Fig. 3).[8] This is not wholly specific, as examples of nerve sheath tumors, solitary fibrous tumors, and mesothelioma can display positivity.[9,10] The sensitivity of this marker means that it is valuable in excluding synovial sarcoma when the result is negative. Synovial sarcomas also show diffuse staining for bcl-2,[11] and a variable proportion express S100 protein,[12] CD99,[13] CD56,[14] and calponin. CD34 is essentially always negative, and reduced (but not absent) expression of INI1 has been shown in synovial sarcoma.[15] An antibody derived from the SYT fusion gene[16] is of limited diagnostic use. Genetically, the most synovial sarcomas have a reciprocal balanced chromosomal translocation t(X;18)(p11.2:q11.2), in which the SS18 (formerly SYT) gene on chromosome 18 fuses with the SSX gene The latter has 5 variants, of which only SSX1 and SSX2 are found in the rearranged genes,[17] with SSX4 present in very rare cases.[18] Expression of CD133, a stemlike cell marker, in synovial sarcoma cells and cell lines has supported the suggestion that synovial sarcoma is of a primitive progenitor or stem cell origin.[19]

All the histologic subtypes have similar molecular genetic changes[5,18,19]; however, most biphasic tumors have the SYT-SSX1 fusion,[20,21] whereas monophasic synovial sarcomas display either fusion. Poorly differentiated synovial sarcoma has

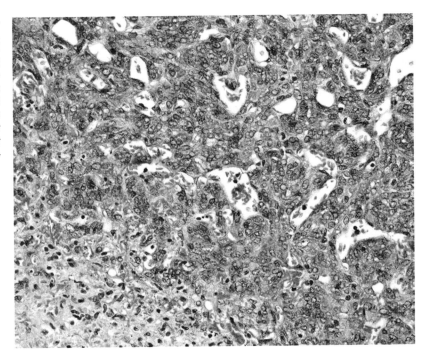

Fig. 2. Poorly differentiated synovial sarcoma. This is a small round-cell tumor resembling Ewing sarcoma. There is a prominent hemangiopericytic pattern. More typical spindle cell areas can often be found by further sampling of the tumor (H&E, original magnification ×100).

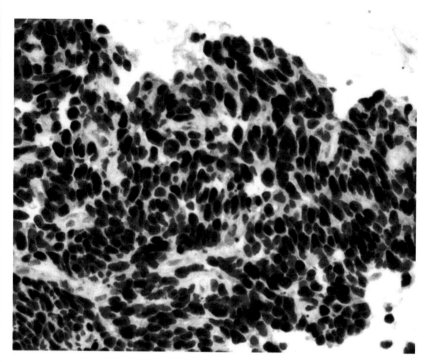

Fig. 3. Immunostaining for TLE1 is diffusely positive in nuclei of synovial sarcoma of all morphologic types (immunoperoxidase, original magnification ×100).

been found to have a distinct gene expression profile.[22–24] Other findings from gene expression profiling studies of synovial sarcoma include up-regulation of ERBB2, IGFBP2, and IGF2,[25] and a possible genetic signature related to development of metastases.[26] These observations lead to potential targeted therapy using "small molecules," small interfering RNAs, or monoclonal antibodies.[27,28]

DIAGNOSIS AND DIFFERENTIAL DIAGNOSIS

Synovial sarcoma can be distinguished from malignant peripheral nerve sheath tumor by its more rounded and uniform nuclei, and by expression of TLE1 (strong and diffuse), bcl-2, CK7, and CK19. Demonstration of the translocation or fusion gene transcripts is of diagnostic use in distinguishing synovial sarcoma from other morphologically similar neoplasms, including malignant peripheral nerve sheath tumor and Ewing sarcoma/primitive neuroectodermal tumor (PNET). Solitary fibrous tumor has a hemangiopericytic pattern and expresses bcl-2 and CD56, but has more fibrosis and is CD34 positive, unlike in synovial sarcoma, and lacks the specific translocation. Adult-type fibrosarcoma has longer sweeping fascicles and a more evident herringbone pattern, and lacks epithelial and other markers as well as the relevant genetic features. Infantile fibrosarcoma is a fibroblastic-myofibroblastic tumor of variable

morphology with smooth muscle actin (SMA) positivity and a different translocation (t[12;15] [p13;q25] with fusion of ETV6 and NTRK3). Spindle cell carcinoma tends to be more pleomorphic and has more widespread cytokeratin positivity. A primary carcinoma elsewhere is often found when the tumor presents in a nonvisceral location, and

---

△△ ***Differential Diagnosis***
SYNOVIAL SARCOMA

- Malignant peripheral nerve sheath tumor
- Solitary fibrous tumor
- Adult type fibrosarcoma
- Leiomyosarcoma
- Carcinosarcoma
- Ewing sarcoma/PNET
- Small cell carcinoma
- Endometrial stromal sarcoma
- Teratoma
- Ectopic hamartomatous thymoma
- Spindle epithelial tumor with thymuslike elements (thyroid)

Pitfalls
SYNOVIAL SARCOMA

! Synovial sarcoma can occur in almost any anatomic site, including viscera. It should be considered in the diagnosis of a uniform spindle cell tumor with fascicular architecture that does not resemble any of the neoplasms usually encountered in that organ or site.

! The hemangiopericytomatous pattern and diffuse positivity for bcl2 can lead to misinterpretation as solitary fibrous tumor, which can also express TLE1 focally; however, solitary fibrous tumor is usually CD34 positive and synovial sarcoma is negative.

! The calcifying and ossifying variants can be mistaken for a benign lesion, such as juvenile aponeurotic fibroma, but the spindle cells in synovial sarcoma display focal cytokeratin positivity.

! Poorly differentiated synovial sarcoma can be mistaken for Ewing sarcoma or small cell carcinoma, as both can express cytokeratins focally and the former is also CD99 positive. Use of TLE1, FLI1, TTF1, and genetic analysis can assist diagnosis.

there is often an in situ component overlying a tumor apparently arising in submucosa or wall of a viscus.

PROGNOSIS

Synovial sarcoma is generally an aggressive tumor that metastasizes to lung, bone, and occasionally lymph node in up to 50% of cases.[29] The 5-year survival is 36% to 76% and 10-year survival is 20% to 63%.[30] Adverse prognostic factors include high disease stage and grade, male sex, age older than 40 years, tumor size larger than 5 cm, poorly differentiated histology, and proximal location. Favorable parameters include young age (childhood), very small size, distal location, and extensive ossification. It has been proposed that synovial sarcoma with the SSX2 gene rearrangement has a better outcome,[29] but this not been confirmed as a predictive factor independent of grade.

MALIGNANT PERIPHERAL NERVE SHEATH TUMOR

OVERVIEW

Malignant peripheral nerve sheath tumor (MPNST) can arise in patients with neurofibromatosis type 1

(NF-1), in which the incidence of malignant change is about 5%,[31] or sporadically. Genetic factors include inactivation of the tumor suppressor gene *NF1* in both sporadic cases and those arising in NF-1,[32] p53 gene mutations, deletion of *INK4A* gene (encoding p16) on chromosome 9p21,[33] and abnormalities in 17p. The commonest sites of MPNST are proximal limbs, trunk, or head and neck. The tumor presents as a painful mass with associated neurologic clinical features. Tumors in patients with NF-1 arise at a younger age than sporadic ones (with a peak in the fourth decade), and are more frequent in men and in axial locations. They also behave more aggressively and more frequently show divergent differentiation. Many tumors arise in a preexisting typical or plexiform neurofibroma or in a nerve trunk.

MACROSCOPIC FEATURES

The tumor forms a mass within or attached to nerve trunk or plexiform neurofibroma, and can extend within a nerve. The cut surface is solid and can display focal necrosis, hemorrhage, or myxoid change.

MICROSCOPIC FEATURES

MPNST can have spindled, epithelioid, pleomorphic, or rarely small round-cell cytomorphology, and can also show foci of divergent differentiation. Commonly, spindled MPNST displays a fibrosarcomalike, herringbone fascicular pattern (**Figs. 4–6**). The cells are elongated, with scanty cytoplasm

Key Features
MALIGNANT PERIPHERAL NERVE SHEATH TUMOR

- Many cases are related to nerve trunk or neurofibroma, especially plexiform neurofibroma.

- Increased incidence in neurofibromatosis type 1.

- Alternating myxoid and cellular zones.

- Wavy, buckled, or arrowhead-shaped nuclei.

- Nuclear palisading, neuroid whorls.

- Subendothelial infiltration into vessel walls.

- No specific immunohistochemical marker.

- S100 protein is positive in about two-thirds of cases.

- Nestin might be contributory for diagnosis in some cases.

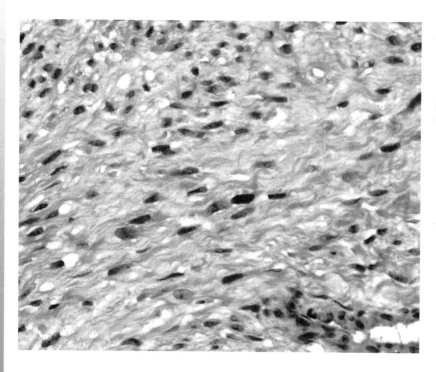

Fig. 4. MPNST, well differentiated. Wavy spindle cells with mildly pleomorphic hyperchromatic nuclei are irregularly dispersed within a fibrillary stroma (H&E, original magnification ×150).

and nuclei that are wavy, serpiginous, buckled, or lanceolate, with one end pointed and the other blunt; in its extreme form the nucleus can appear triangular. Characteristic features include alternating cellular and myxoid zones, ill-defined nuclear palisading, neuroid whorls, and infiltration of tumor cells into vessel walls (**Fig. 7**). Pleomorphic or small round-cell areas can occur, and mitoses and

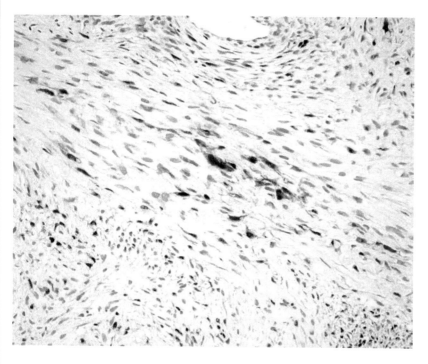

Fig. 5. MPNST, well differentiated. Immunostaining for S100 protein is typically nuclear and focal rather than diffuse (immunoperoxidase, original magnification ×75).

Fig. 6. MPNST, poorly differentiated. This is a cellular spindle cell sarcoma with mitotic activity. The nuclear features of nerve sheath cells can, however, be discerned (H&E, original magnification ×150).

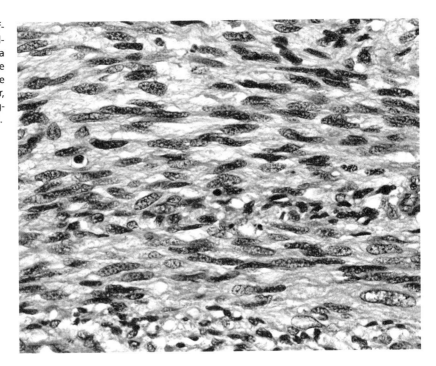

necrosis are usual. Some MPNSTs are histologically low grade (neurofibromalike) and resemble cellular neurofibroma but with more widespread nuclear atypia and mitotic activity. In the stroma, hyaline nodules are sometimes seen, and can suggest low-grade fibromyxoid sarcoma.

Divergent differentiation, most commonly seen in NF-1–associated MPNST, especially in head and neck or trunk, is usually mesenchymal (osteochondroid or skeletal muscle or rarely angiosarcoma) or, very rarely, epithelial as glandular structures (often with focal neuroendocrine differentiation). MPNST

Fig. 7. MPNST. Involvement of vessel wall by subendothelial infiltration of tumor cells is a characteristic feature of this neoplasm (H&E, original magnification ×150).

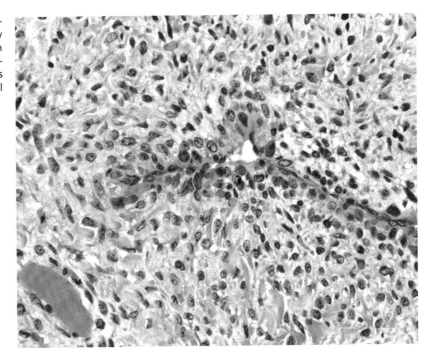

with divergent rhabdomyosarcomatous differentiation is termed malignant Triton tumor. Malignant perineurioma is a very rare high-grade malignant neoplasm that displays focal positivity for EMA and ultrastructural evidence of perineurial cell differentiation.[34]

OTHER DIAGNOSTIC TECHNIQUES

About two-thirds of all spindled MPNSTs express S100 protein, usually focally or in single cells (see **Fig. 5**). Other antigens, such as glial fibrillary acidic protein, are inconsistently expressed, or nonspecific (eg, NSE). Pancytokeratin is occasionally focally positive, but CK7 and CK19, seen in most monophasic synovial sarcomas, are negative. Unlike in synovial sarcoma, CD34 is positive in about 25% of MPNSTs, and bcl-2 is negative or only focally positive. There are no diagnostic genetic features.

DIAGNOSIS AND DIFFERENTIAL DIAGNOSIS

Diagnosis of spindled MPNST depends on demonstration of nerve sheath differentiation, which usually means positivity for S100 protein. Because Schwannian differentiation is variable and often incomplete, this is usually focal in spindle cell MPNST (unlike in epithelioid PNST), regardless of grade. Among other S100 protein–positive spindle cell neoplasms, cellular schwannoma can display focal nuclear atypia but it is encapsulated and diffusely positive. Spindle cell melanoma is also diffusely positive, but it is infiltrative, often arranged in sheaves or nests, and more diffusely pleomorphic, with occasional positivity for HMB45 or melan-A. Synovial sarcoma can be focally positive for S100 protein but the presence of other markers (see earlier in this article) and detection of t(X;18) and related fusion genes is diagnostic. Myoepithelioma expresses focal or widespread S100 protein but most examples are also EMA positive, with cytokeratin demonstrable in many cases. Follicular dendritic cell sarcoma, which can also be S100 protein and EMA positive, additionally expresses CD21 and C35, as well as CD23, fascin, clusterin, and desmoplakin, and D2-40 is also positive in many cases. A minority of gastrointestinal stromal tumors are S100 protein positive but they are readily identifiable by their characteristic morphology and expression of CD117, DOG1, h-caldesmon, and CD34, as well as by demonstration of mutations in *KIT* and *PDGFRA* genes.

About one-third of MPNSTs are S100 protein negative,[35] and diagnosis in these cases depends on an association of the tumor with a large nerve or neurofibroma, as well as exclusion of other spindle cell neoplasms. Electron microscopy can also reveal Schwannian differentiation in S100 protein–negative cases,[35] but this technique is now rarely applied. Some MPNSTs express CD34, and other CD34-positive tumors need to be excluded. The principal mimic is solitary fibrous tumor, which can be identified by its circumscription, focal fibrosis, short spindle cells in patternless pattern, pericytomatous vasculature, and concomitant immunoreactivity for bcl-2 and CD99.

PROGNOSIS

Large tumors have a worse prognosis and presence of tumor at surgical resection margin is an adverse prognostic factor. MPNSTs tend to increase in grade with successive recurrences (grade progression), but most are high grade from the outset, and grade is not considered to be of prognostic value in this tumor type.[36] The recurrence rate is about 40%, and about 65% metastasize. The 5-year survival is less than 50%.[37]

△△ *Differential Diagnosis*
    MPNST

- Cellular neurofibroma
- Cellular schwannoma
- Perineurioma
- Adult fibrosarcoma
- Synovial sarcoma
- Spindle cell melanoma
- Spindle cell rhabdomyosarcoma (adult type)
- Follicular dendritic cell sarcoma
- Ectopic thymoma

 Pitfalls
    MPNST

! Diffuse S100 protein positivity in a high-grade spindle cell tumor is more likely to indicate melanoma than MPNST.

! Nuclear palisading can be seen in benign and malignant nerve sheath neoplasms, smooth muscle tumors, and synovial sarcoma.

ADULT-TYPE FIBROSARCOMA

OVERVIEW

Before the availability of modern diagnostic techniques, clinical and pathologic studies of fibrosarcoma included a variety of different neoplasms. Unspecified types of fibrosarcoma in adults have now become increasingly rare.[38] There is no specific immunohistochemical marker of fibroblasts and electron microscopy has fallen into disuse. Therefore, spindle cell sarcomas displaying a fascicular pattern but lacking morphologic or immunohistochemical evidence of a definite lineage are sometimes labeled as fibrosarcoma as a diagnosis of exclusion. They are gradable tumors that recur and have metastatic potential, especially when arising in deep soft tissue of extremities where they are most commonly located. Some subcutaneous fibrosarcomas are genetically similar to fibrosarcoma arising in dermatofibrosarcoma,[39] but lack an obvious associated dermatofibrosarcomatous component. Fibrosarcoma can also arise following therapeutic irradiation, or in a scar resulting from a burn many years earlier.

MACROSCOPIC FEATURES

Deep tumors form a firm, white, circumscribed mass with hemorrhage and necrosis in higher-grade neoplasms. Superficial tumors tend to have more infiltrative margins.

MICROSCOPIC FEATURES

Fibrosarcoma is composed of elongated spindle cells with tapered nuclei and minimal cytoplasm, arranged in sweeping parallel or herringbone-patterned fascicles (**Figs. 8** and **9**). Pleomorphism is variable, but tumors in which this is a prominent feature are conventionally classified as malignant fibrous histiocytoma or pleomorphic undifferentiated sarcoma. Intercellular collagen also varies but most tumors have closely packed cells at least focally.

OTHER DIAGNOSTIC INVESTIGATIONS

Fibrosarcoma is immunoreactive for vimentin (which is wholly nonspecific) and sometimes displays focal positivity for SMA, although to a much lesser extent than in low-grade myofibrosarcoma. Some fibrosarcomas are CD34 positive; of these, some represent malignant solitary fibrous tumors, and several superficial examples show *PDGFRB1-COL1AI* fusion gene transcripts, as in dermatofibrosarcoma (but without a typical dermatofibrosarcomatous component). Other than in the specific fibrosarcoma subtypes, there are no characteristic genetic findings.

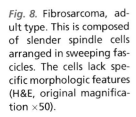

Fig. 8. Fibrosarcoma, adult type. This is composed of slender spindle cells arranged in sweeping fascicles. The cells lack specific morphologic features (H&E, original magnification ×50).

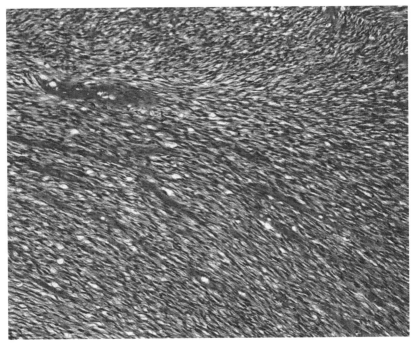

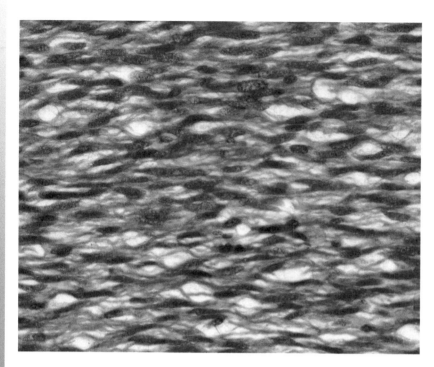

Fig. 9. Fibrosarcoma arising in dermatofibrosarcoma. The cells have elongated tapered nuclei and minimal cytoplasm. There is little nuclear pleomorphism (H&E, original magnification ×150).

INFLAMMATORY MYOFIBROBLASTIC TUMOR

OVERVIEW

Inflammatory myofibroblastic tumor (IMT) is a histologically low-grade neoplasm of myofibroblasts[40] categorized as intermediate (rarely metastasizing) in the World Health Organization (WHO) 2002 classification.[36] IMT differs in several respects from low-grade myofibrosarcoma,[41] and it has been postulated that the former represents a neoplasm of fibroblastic reticulum (myoid) cells.[42] It is most common in children and in females, and the commonest location is the lung. Fever, anemia, leukocytosis, and hypergammaglobulinemia sometimes occur. Extrapulmonary IMT mostly arises within the abdomen or pelvis (retroperitoneum, mesentery, liver, gastrointestinal tract, urinary tract),[43–47] and less frequently in the head and neck (eg, larynx[48]), limbs, or trunk. So-called inflammatory pseudotumor of lymph node appears to be a separate entity.[49] IMT in the urinary tract[46,47] involves the bladder[50,51] and other anatomic sites,[46,47] and some are associated with prior instrumentation. The latter cases (eg, postoperative spindle cell nodule) are said to be more fasciitis-like with fewer plasma cells and lacking hyalinized areas,[47,52] although some investigators do not separate them.[46,53]

GROSS FEATURES

IMT can be solitary or multiple, as firm, white tumors with focal hyalinization or calcification. Mesenteric lesions can infiltrate the intestinal wall. The lesions are infiltrative and can involve

Key Features
INFLAMMATORY MYOFIBROBLASTIC TUMOR

- Can have fascicular, fasciitis-like, and sclerosing patterns

- Composed of elongated myofibroblasts

- Occasional larger "ganglionlike" cells are seen.

- There is a mixed inflammatory infiltrate with numerous plasma cells.

- Sarcomatous transformation is a rare complication.

- About 60% are anaplastic lymphoma kinase (ALK) positive, mainly in childhood visceral lesions.

- Many have ALK gene rearrangements with a variety of fusion partners.

- ALK-negative tumors in adults have a less-favorable outcome.

viscera including the bowel wall. Bladder tumors can be polypoid and also infiltrative.

MICROSCOPIC FEATURES

The typical IMT (**Fig. 10**) comprises bland spindle or stellate cells with ovoid nuclei and small nucleoli forming cellular fascicles, ill-defined storiform whorls often with myxoid change, or dispersed within a hypocellular fibrous stroma. There is a mixed inflammatory infiltrate, with polyclonal plasma cells and lymphocytes (including follicle formation) and sometimes eosinophils or neutrophils. Polygonal "ganglionlike"[54] cells can occur, similar to those in proliferative fasciitis,[55,56] but pleomorphism is unusual.[57] More recently, a variant with epithelioid or more pleomorphic cytomorphology (**Fig. 11**), associated with *ALK-RANBP2* fusion, has been described, which, based on its aggressive behavior, has been termed epithelioid inflammatory myofibroblastic sarcoma.[58] In general, anaplastic lymphoma kinase (ALK)1-negative tumors tend to display more nuclear pleomorphism and atypical mitoses.[54]

OTHER DIAGNOSTIC TESTS

IMT displays focal or widespread immunoreactivity for smooth muscle and muscle-specific actins, and less often for desmin. However, 10 of 11 epithelioid inflammatory myofibroblastic sarcomas expressed desmin and all were CD30 positive.[58] Cytokeratins are occasionally demonstrable in intra-abdominal tumors. ALK (**Fig. 12**) is positive in 50% to 60% of cases, mostly in childhood.[54,59–61] The *ALK* gene located on 2p23 is rearranged with various fusion partners. Of these, tropomyosin 3 (*TPM3-ALK*) or tropomyosin 4 (*TPM4-ALK*) are most common,[62] and result in diffuse cytoplasmic immunostaining for ALK. Fusion of *ALK* with clathrin heavy chain gene, localized to 17q23[63] is associated with a granular staining pattern on immunohistochemistry. *ALK* fusion with *RANBP2* at 2q13, results in nuclear membrane staining in a distinct ringlike pattern (**Fig. 13**), and is associated with epithelioid morphology.[58] Other partner genes include *SEC31L1* at 4q21, and *CARS* at 11p15. In IMT arising in the bladder, there is immunoreactivity for cytokeratins, SMA, and desmin in about 75%, 75%, and 60% of cases respectively, and h-caldesmon is expressed in more than 50%. ALK positivity is found in 46% to 62% of cases, with good correlation between immunohistochemistry and fluorescence in situ hybridization (FISH) for *ALK* gene rearrangements.[51] The treatment of choice is surgical.

DIAGNOSIS AND DIFFERENTIAL DIAGNOSIS

ALK immunohistochemistry is useful but is positive mostly in childhood visceral examples only, and

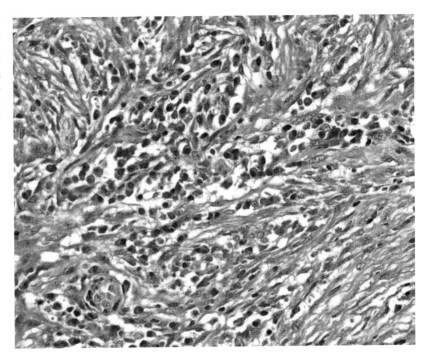

Fig. 10. Inflammatory myofibroblastic tumor. Fascicles of spindled myofibroblastic cells are interspersed with inflammatory cells that comprise predominantly plasma cells (H&E, original magnification ×100).

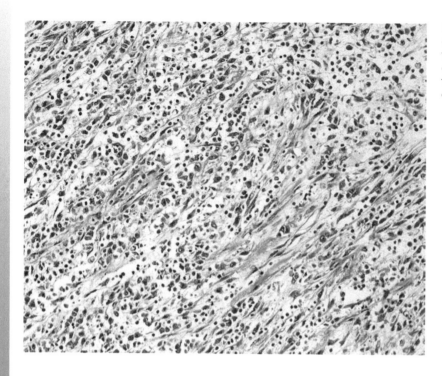

Fig. 11. Inflammatory myofibroblastic sarcoma. This tumor has epithelioid myofibroblasts in an edematous inflamed stroma (H&E, original magnification ×50).

the diagnosis depends on a synthesis of clinical features with morphology; the coexistence of the fascicular, fasciitis-like, and sclerosing patterns is particularly useful. The differential diagnosis is wide and includes benign and malignant myofibroblastic lesions and spindle cell sarcomas. Nodular fasciitis lacks atypia, necrosis, hyaline sclerosis, and a plasma cell or mixed inflammatory infiltrate.

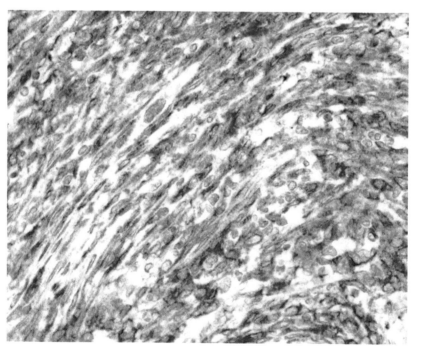

Fig. 12. Inflammatory myofibroblastic tumor. There is diffuse immunoreactivity for ALK in lesional cells. This is most commonly seen in IMT in viscera in childhood, and is prognostically more favorable (immunoperoxidase, original magnification ×100).

Fig. 13. Inflammatory myofibroblastic sarcoma. This tumor displays a distinctive ringlike immunoreactivity for ALK, reflecting the *ALK-RANBP2* gene fusion (immunoperoxidase, original magnification ×200).

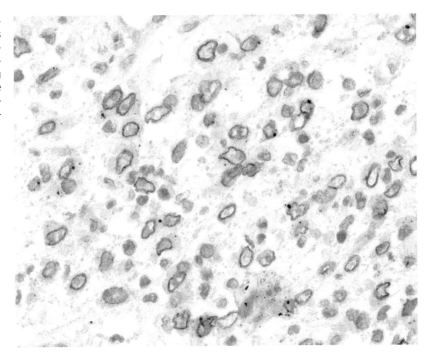

Retroperitoneal fibrosis and other sclerosing and fibroinflammatory lesions are clinically distinct, and have a sparse spindle cell component without pleomorphism; there are often increased numbers of immunoglobulin (Ig)G4 secreting plasma cells and sometimes raised serum IgG4 levels in this group of lesions, unlike in most IMTs.[64–66] However, a subset of IMTs have a raised IgG4/IgG ratio that is within the range for IgG4-related sclerosing disease, so the 2 conditions might have some overlap.[67] Solitary fibrous tumor has variable cellularity, short randomly arranged cells, and CD34 positivity. Fibromatosis has myofibroblasts evenly dispersed in collagen (intra-abdominal fibromatosis can have prominent keloidal collagen bundles), features mast cells rather than

plasma cells, and in many cases shows nuclear positivity for beta catenin. Low-grade myofibrosarcoma is more cellular and fascicular, and lacks the marked inflammatory infiltrate; however, its appearances can overlap with those of IMT. Regular leiomyosarcoma has nontapered cells, and is immunohistochemically positive for desmin and h-caldesmon. Inflammatory leiomyosarcoma also appears more smooth musclelike than myofibroblastic, has a lymphocytic infiltrate, and tends to express desmin diffusely with only with very focal SMA.[68]

Among other spindle cell tumors, follicular dendritic cell sarcoma has cells with a prominent nuclear membrane and speckled chromatin, an intimately admixed lymphocytic infiltrate, and a diagnostic immunophenotype that includes CD21, CD35, CD23, D2-40,[69] and fascin,[70] as well as S100 protein and EMA in some. Gastrointestinal stromal tumor can be identified by immunoreactivity for CD117 and DOG1,[71] as well as for CD34 and h-caldesmon, which are frequently expressed. Dedifferentiated liposarcoma with inflammatory myofibroblastic tumorlike features has been described and can be recognized by MDM2 amplification and ALK negativity, as well as the association in some cases of a well-differentiated liposarcomatous component.[72] Finally, inflammatory fibroid polyps of the bowel, which are benign lesions of focally whorled spindle and stellate cells

△△ ***Differential Diagnosis***
INFLAMMATORY MYOFIBROBLASTIC
TUMOR

- Nodular fasciitis
- Low-grade myofibrosarcoma
- Inflammatory leiomyosarcoma
- Dedifferentiated liposarcoma
- Gastrointestinal stromal tumor

> **Pitfalls**
> **INFLAMMATORY MYOFIBROBLASTIC TUMOR**
>
> ! Fewer cellular areas resemble IgG4-related sclerosing disease and IMT can sometimes have a raised IgG4/IgG ratio.
>
> ! An IMT-like pattern is a rare manifestation of dedifferentiated liposarcoma. It is positive for MDM2 and CDK4 and negative for ALK.
>
> ! ALK is negative in most adult cases and its absence does not rule out the diagnosis.

in an inflamed fibromyxoid stroma (including eosinophils) are CD34 positive. They can arise in the submucosa and mucosa of the stomach, small bowel, colon, and rarely esophagus, and the presence in some of *PGFRA* mutations has been reported.[73]

PROGNOSIS

After excision, 25% to 35% of IMTs recur.[44,57] There are no histologic features predictive of recurrence, although complete surgical removal helps to prevent it.[74] With the exception of nuclear membrane positivity in epithelioid IMT, absence of immunoreactivity for ALK is in general associated with a worse outcome.[54] Metastases are rare in usual IMT,[75,76] but sarcomatous transformation is an occasional event.[77] In one series, 12% of cases progressed to a pleomorphic neoplasm, and atypical tumors had a recurrence rate of 56%, with metastases (all ALK-negative) in 17%.[54]

LOW-GRADE MYOFIBROSARCOMA

OVERVIEW

A rare subset of spindle cell sarcomas shows diffuse myofibroblastic differentiation. These occur in both children and adults (range 9–75, mean 40 years) and more often in males.[78] They usually involve deep soft tissue, and favor head and neck locations, such as tongue, cheek, maxilla, and mandible, as well as the extremities, including the hand. Occasional cases have arisen in the trunk, retroperitoneum, and other parts of skeleton. They are slowly growing masses between 2 and 17 cm in diameter. Although designated as intermediate (rarely metastasizing) in the WHO 2002 classification, more than a third of examples recur, especially if incompletely excised, and metastasis as a low-grade neoplasm or

transformation to a higher-grade sarcoma are well documented.[79] Surgical excision is the usual initial management.

GROSS FEATURES

The tumors are circumscribed or infiltrative and solid, with white cut surface and usually lack necrosis or hemorrhage except in grade 2 tumors.

MICROSCOPIC FEATURES

Low-grade myofibrosarcomas are usually moderately cellular and composed of spindle cells with ovoid nuclei, with a distinct small nucleolus, and often amphophilic cytoplasm. The nuclei are mostly uniform, but focal (or very focal) nuclear enlargement or hyperchromasia is found, as well as mitotic activity. The cells are arranged in parallel fascicles, with minimal stroma, which infiltrate skeletal muscle or subcutaneous fat. Variations include a storiform pattern, focal myxoid change, and a scanty lymphocytic infiltrate, somewhat as in nodular fasciitis (**Figs. 14** and **15**).

OTHER DIAGNOSTIC TECHNIQUES

The cells are positive for SMA (with subplasmalemmal linear accentuation) and occasionally express desmin focally but lack h-caldesmon,[80] smooth muscle myosin, CD34, and S100 protein. Electron microscopy shows abundant rough endoplasmic reticulum, subplasmalemmal stress fibers, and very rarely a fibronexus structure, which is diagnostic of myofibroblastic differentiation.[78] There are no specific translocations, but abnormalities in 12p11 and 12q13-q22 regions, with multiple ring chromosomes, have been found.[81]

DIAGNOSIS AND DIFFERENTIAL DIAGNOSIS

Myofibrosarcoma differs clinically from nodular fasciitis in having a longer history, or one of a previous similar lesion elsewhere, and continuing to grow to a larger size. Unlike in nodular fasciitis, this sarcoma has an infiltrative growth pattern, focal nuclear atypia, and occasionally necrosis. Some examples, however, including metastatic deposits, are remarkably fasciitislike and subtle clues, including mild or focal nuclear pleomorphism, as well as lack of zonation, need to be sought. Fibromatosis is less cellular, lacks nuclear atypia, and has evenly dispersed interstitial collagen with slitlike or gaping thin-walled vessels and mast cells. Many cases, especially when deeply located, are immunoreactive for beta-catenin in nuclei. Fibrosarcomas have longer,

Fig. 14. Low-grade myofibrosarcoma. This tumor is characterized by cellular fascicles of mostly uniform myofibroblastic cells that infiltrate surrounding tissues. There is focal nuclear enlargement or hyperchromasia (H&E, original magnification ×100).

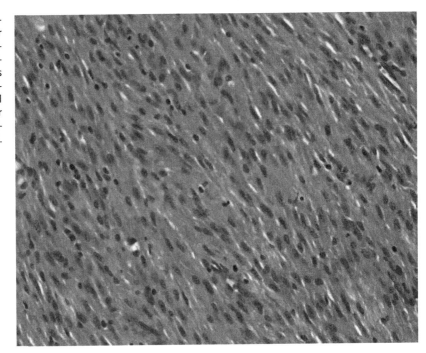

Fig. 15. Low-grade myofibrosarcoma. Immunostaining for smooth muscle actin shows accentuation beneath the cell membrane on either side of the cell ("tram-track" appearance) (immunoperoxidase, original magnification ×400).

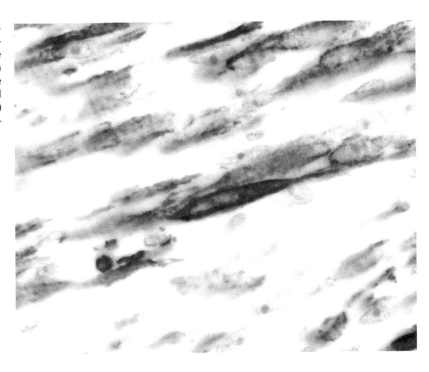

more tapered nuclei with scanty cytoplasm and absence of SMA except very focally. The spindle cells of smooth muscle tumors have blunt-ended nuclei, and more abundant eosinophilic cytoplasm with longitudinal fibrils and, in addition to SMA, they express h-caldesmon and desmin.

LEIOMYOSARCOMA

OVERVIEW

Leiomyosarcomas are malignant tumors showing smooth muscle differentiation that can arise in any anatomic site but their biologic behavior varies according to location. Cutaneous and superficial subcutaneous tumors with histologic features of malignancy are found on extensor surfaces of extremities and in the head and neck region especially in older adults and mostly in men. They are presumed to arise in relation to arrector pili muscle, and present as a firm nodule with or without skin discoloration, and can be painful, ulcerated, or bleeding, but rarely metastasize. Most smooth muscle tumors of deep soft tissue, on the other hand, are frankly malignant, with behavior relating to grade. The retroperitoneum is a common site, especially in older women, with less frequent occurrence in extremities in either sex. Deep leiomyosarcomas often originate in the wall of a large vein, such as inferior vena cava, or femoral or long saphenous vein, and extend into adjacent soft tissue, giving rise to

a tumor mass or causing venous obstruction. Inflammatory leiomyosarcoma occurs in deep soft tissue of trunk or proximal limbs, and can cause systemic symptoms. Epstein-Barr virus–positive smooth muscle tumors can arise in immunosuppressed patients.[82]

GROSS FEATURES

Leiomyosarcoma forms a solid, white tumor that can be circumscribed or infiltrative (especially in retroperitoneum), and can display hemorrhage and necrosis, especially in higher-grade lesions. The associated vein of origin can be seen in some cases.

MICROSCOPIC FEATURES

Cutaneous leiomyosarcomas have a diffuse or nodular growth pattern. The former, of supposed arrector pili origin, are usually well differentiated and contained within the dermis. The latter, which are likely of vascular origin, are more circumscribed but more pleomorphic and mitotically active, and more likely to extend into subcutis. Most leiomyosarcomas (**Fig. 16**) typically display fascicles, intersecting at right angles, of nontapered cells with markedly eosinophilic cytoplasm and blunt-ended nuclei (often unexpectedly pleomorphic with few mitoses). Paranuclear vacuoles are a distinctive feature. Nuclear palisading is also sometimes seen in lower-grade neoplasms and some tumors show marked myxoid change,

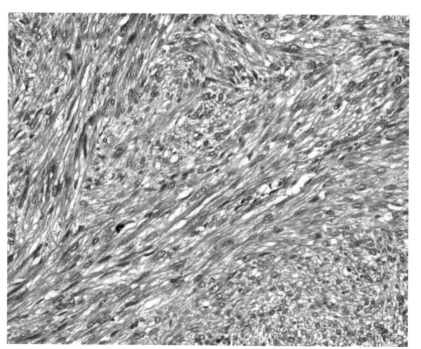

Fig. 16. Leiomyosarcoma. Spindle cells with focal nuclear pleomorphism, mitotic activity, and obvious eosinophilic cytoplasm, are arranged in fascicles that abut each other at right angles (H&E, original magnification ×100).

Key Features
LEIOMYOSARCOMA

- Often associated with wall of vein.
- Epstein-Barr virus–positive examples can arise in immunosuppressed patients.
- Nontapered spindle cells with abundant eosinophilic cytoplasm.
- Blunt-ended nuclei with paranuclear vacuoles.
- Fascicles arranged at right angles.
- Osteoclastic aggregates in some.
- Inflammatory variant shows marked chronic inflammatory infiltrate and psammoma bodies.

Differential Diagnosis
LEIOMYOSARCOMA

- Nodular fasciitis
- Cellular schwannoma
- Leiomyoma
- Inflammatory myofibroblastic tumor
- Low-grade myofibrosarcoma
- Gastrointestinal stromal tumor
- Perivascular epithelioid cell tumor
- Pleomorphic sarcoma (malignant fibrous histiocytoma)

stromal fibrosis, or prominent clusters of osteoclastlike giant cells.[83] Inflammatory leiomyosarcoma is a minimally pleomorphic tumor with a marked lymphocytic infiltrate, xanthoma cells, and foci of calcification, including psammoma bodies.[84] Epithelioid leiomyosarcoma occurs mostly in the female genital tract.[85]

OTHER DIAGNOSTIC TECHNIQUES

Leiomyosarcoma is usually diffusely positive for SMA, calponin, and (to a variable extent) desmin and h-caldesmon. Some examples, especially in women, display nuclear immunoreactivity for estrogen receptor and progesterone receptor. Dot-like (or rarely diffuse cytoplasmic) expression of cytokeratins can additionally be seen in some cases, and there is occasionally CD34 positivity. There are no diagnostic molecular genetic abnormalities. A subset in the female genital tract, including those with epithelioid morphology, expresses HMB45.[86] Inflammatory leiomyosarcoma shows diffuse positivity for desmin but only focal SMA expression and usually none for h-caldesmon.[68,84] A few examples have shown genetic abnormalities with a near-haploid karyotype,[68] but there are no ultrastructural studies and it is not clear that these tumors show smooth muscle differentiation.

DIAGNOSIS AND DIFFERENTIAL DIAGNOSIS

The identification of smooth muscle differentiation is usually straightforward, but diagnosis of malignancy can be challenging. The distinction from leiomyoma is not necessarily critical in dermal smooth muscle tumors because they rarely metastasize, and it has been suggested that such lesions, provided they do not extend into subcutaneous fat, be termed atypical leiomyomas.[87] There is a significant recurrence rate in tumors with a mitotic index of more than 1 mitosis per 10 high-power fields (HPF), any significant pleomorphism with or without mitoses, or necrosis, however. Such lesions should be completely excised with observation in case of recurrence. Although deep leiomyomas are very rare, it can be difficult to assess malignant potential in well-differentiated deep smooth muscle tumors especially in a small biopsy. A diagnosis of leiomyoma can be suggested in the absence of atypia, pleomorphism, or mitoses (while noting if required that the biopsy might not be representative); however, necrosis[88-90] or pleomorphism alone or with any mitoses indicate a diagnosis of leiomyosarcoma.[91] Tumors without pleomorphism or necrosis, but with a mitotic index of 1 to 5 per 50 HPF, can be regarded as neoplasms of uncertain malignant potential.[90] Retroperitoneal leiomyosarcomas generally have greater than 5 mitoses per 10 HPF,[91] retroperitoneal uterine-type leiomyomas can have up to 5 mitoses per 10 HPF,[91,92] but 5 to 10 mitoses per 50 HPF (women) indicates uncertain malignant potential. In retroperitoneal smooth muscle tumors in men, the presence of 1 to 5 mitoses per 50 HPF without pleomorphism or necrosis also indicates smooth muscle tumor of uncertain malignant potential.

Nodular fasciitis is sometimes mistaken for leiomyosarcoma, but the cells in the former are myofibroblastic and express SMA with rare focal desmin positivity and absence of h-caldesmon. Among spindle cell sarcomas, low-grade myofibrosarcoma has more tapered cells with less cytoplasm, and also displays a myofibroblastic immunophenotype. In the abdomen, gastrointestinal stromal tumor (GIST) can be distinguished from leiomyosarcoma (including those with CD34 expression) by the presence of CD117 and DOG1, and by analysis for mutations in *KIT* or *PDGFRA* genes. Dedifferentiated liposarcoma can have fascicular areas and focally express desmin and SMA[93]; however, the diagnosis can be made by finding additional features such as an atypical lipomatous component, meningothelial-like whorls,[94] or heterologous elements, and by showing amplification of MDM2 or CDK by FISH or immunohistochemistry.[95] Perivascular epithelioid cell tumor expresses SMA, h-caldesmon, and sometimes desmin, but has spindle cells with clear or granular cytoplasm and rounded nuclei and coexpresses the melanocytic markers HMB45, melan-A, and MiTF. Some examples are also immunoreactive for TFE3.[96]

PROGNOSIS

In one large series of cutaneous leiomyosarcomas, 27% recurred locally and 7% (4 cases) metastasized.[97] In another, however, leiomyosarcomas confined to the dermis or very superficial subcutis did not metastasize, leading to the suggestion that they be termed atypical intradermal smooth muscle tumors.[87] Similar tumors involving subcutis, however, behave as sarcomas with recurrence in more than 50% and metastasis in more than 30%. Lesions should be removed with clear excision margins. The metastatic rate in deep leiomyosarcomas is 45% with a 5-year survival of 64%.[98] Retroperitoneal leiomyosarcoma has an especially poor outcome with survival rates between 10% and 50%.[99] Tumor grade is an important prognostic factor in smooth muscle tumors.[100,101] Older age, large size, and occurrence of vascular invasion are prognostically adverse, and prior biopsy or incomplete excision are additional risk factors for metastasis[101]; however, even small leiomyosarcomas and those with very low mitotic indices have been known to metastasize.[102] Leiomyosarcomas with less than 50% of myxoid change in the stroma are usually of low-grade malignancy, but in one study, 38% of cases recurred and 15% metastasized.[85]

SPINDLE CELL RHABDOMYOSARCOMA

OVERVIEW

Embryonal rhabdomyosarcoma has variable morphology, which includes spindling of cells, but it is a clinicopathologically distinct entity predominantly occurring in childhood as a rapidly growing tumor in the paratesticular region, bladder, prostate, orbit, middle ear, paranasal sinuses, pharynx, bile duct, and other viscera. More uniformly spindled rhabdomyosarcomas occur in 2 forms. In children and young adults, spindle cell rhabdomyosarcoma is a better differentiated or low-grade tumor, which has been placed in the WHO classification as a variant of embryonal rhabdomyosarcoma, and in the International Prognostic Classification of Pediatric Rhabdomyosarcoma in the superior prognosis category. About 15% of cases metastasize, mainly to lymph nodes,[103] and more than 95% survive for 5 years.[104] Sites of predilection are head and neck and paratesticular regions. In older adults, spindle cell rhabdomyosarcoma also arises in the head and neck area or trunk, but it is a highly aggressive neoplasm that frequently recurs and metastasizes to lungs.[105] Foci of spindled rhabdomyosarcoma can also occur in other sarcoma types, such as malignant peripheral nerve sheath tumor, dedifferentiated liposarcoma, and ectomesenchymoma, and as a divergent component of germ cell tumors, renal cell carcinoma, nephroblastoma, pleuropulmonary blastoma, and medulloblastoma. Sclerosing (pseudovascular) rhabdomyosarcoma is a variant of adult spindle cell rhabdomyosarcoma in deep soft tissue in which the lesional cells are dispersed in hyalinized stroma.[106,107]

GROSS FEATURES

Spindle cell rhabdomyosarcoma manifests as a circumscribed, firm mass with whorled cut surface. Necrosis can be seen in aggressive examples.

MICROSCOPIC FEATURES

The childhood/young adult variant comprises fascicles or whorls of uniform, elongated, tapered

Pitfalls
LEIOMYOSARCOMA

! Usually immunoreactive for SMA, desmin, and h-caldesmon. Tumors expressing SMA only are more likely to be myofibroblastic.

! A subset of uterine leiomyosarcoma can express HMB45.

! A subset can be CD34 positive and in the abdomen need to be distinguished from GIST by demonstration of CD117 and DOG1 positivity, and in some cases by mutational analysis.

Fig. 17. Spindle cell rhabdomyosarcoma. This is a high-grade spindle cell sarcoma without apparent rhabdomyoblastic differentiation (*A*); however, immuno-staining for desmin is strong and diffuse (*B*), and nuclei are immunoreactive for myogenin (*C*). (*A*, H&E, original magnification ×100; *B*, immunoperoxidase, original magnification ×100; *C*, immunoperoxidase, original magnification ×150.)

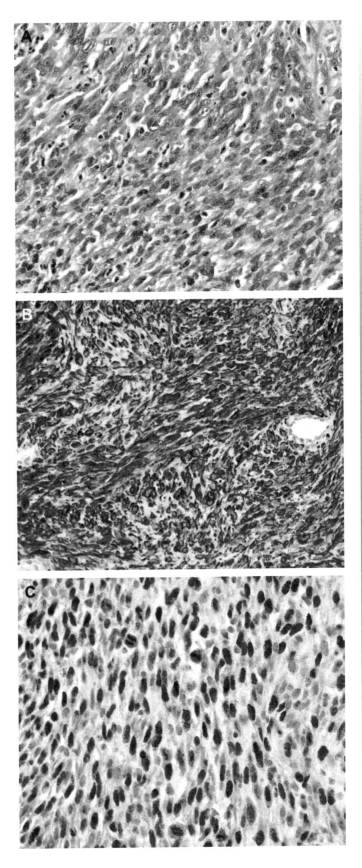

spindle cells with focally blunt-ended nuclei, and highly eosinophilic cytoplasm in which cross-striations can sometimes be identified. Round, large rhabdomyoblasts are also sometimes seen, usually singly. The quantity of intercellular stroma is of no prognostic significance but childhood spindle cell rhabdomyosarcoma are sometimes termed either "collagen-rich," like fibrosarcoma, or "collagen-poor," simulating leiomyosarcoma.

Adult spindle cell rhabdomyosarcoma (Fig. 17) is a highly cellular and fibrosarcomalike spindle cell tumor with pleomorphism, mitotic activity, scanty eosinophilic cytoplasm, variable numbers of rhabdomyoblasts, and focal necrosis.[108] Areas of sclerosing pseudovascular rhabdomyosarcoma[109] can be seen in some cases.

Sclerosing pseudovascular rhabdomyosarcoma comprises "pseudovascular" nests or cords of small round cells or spindle cells with frequent mitoses in a densely hyalinized or chondroid stroma.[107] Rhabdomyoblastic differentiation is rarely identified.

OTHER DIAGNOSTIC TECHNIQUES

Like other types of rhabdomyosarcoma, the spindle cell variant is diffusely or multifocally immunoreactive for desmin, and (in nuclei) for myogenin and MyoD1 (cytoplasmic staining is of no diagnostic significance) (see Fig. 17). Some also express SMA focally, but h-caldesmon is absent. In sclerosing pseudovascular rhabdomyosarcoma, desmin is often focally positive, with a dot-like pattern, and MyoD1 is more often expressed than myogenin.[106]

DIAGNOSIS AND DIFFERENTIAL DIAGNOSIS

The tumor can be differentiated from the juvenile (intermediate) variant of fetal rhabdomyoma by the presence of mitoses, pleomorphism, and necrosis, as well as the clinical picture. The diffuse expression of desmin and myogenin, and absence of h-caldesmon, enables the distinction from leiomyosarcoma, and essentially excludes other spindle cell sarcomas, such as synovial sarcoma. This immunophenotype also allows identification of the rhabdomyosarcomatous component of Triton tumor (MPNST with focal rhabdomyoblastic differentiation), in which the Schwannian component shows focal positivity for S100 protein and lacks skeletal muscle markers.

PROGNOSIS

Spindle cell rhabdomyosarcoma in adolescents has a better outcome than in adults, where it is an aggressive high-grade neoplasm. Favorable prognostic factors for embryonal rhabdomyosarcoma include young age, orbital or paratesticular location, botryoid morphology, spindle cell histology (in childhood but not in adults), and low stage. Some reported cases of sclerosing pseudovascular rhabdomyosarcoma have behaved aggressively, but there are few cases with long-term follow-up.[106]

ENDOTHELIAL NEOPLASMS

Angiosarcoma can assume spindle cell morphology and resemble other spindle cell sarcomas. This can be a particular diagnostic problem in cutaneous lesions. Morphologic features supportive of the diagnosis include features of areas of vasoformation, foci of epithelioid angiosarcoma, hemorrhagic stroma, and a prominently marked hemorrhage. CD31 is the most sensitive (and specific) marker and shows diffuse membranous positivity. CD34 and FLI1 (in nuclei) are sometimes positive and HHV8 is absent. Kaposi sarcoma (KS) in advanced stages can manifest as a cellular spindle cell sarcoma, composed of curved fascicles of tapered narrow spindle cells with mild pleomorphism and mitotic activity, disposed in curved fascicles. There is often interstitial red cell extravasation, and hyaline globules are characteristic. Nuclear immunostaining for HHV8 is a specific and diagnostic feature of KS. Endothelial markers, including CD31, CD34, FLI-1, and podoplanin (D2-40), are also positive.

REFERENCES

1. Lejars M, Rubens-Duval M. Les sarcomes primitifs des synoviales articulaires. Rev Chir 1910;41: 751–83.
2. Fisher C. Synovial sarcoma. Ann Diagn Pathol 1998;2(6):401–21.
3. Michal M, Fanburg-Smith JC, Lasota J, et al. Minute synovial sarcomas of the hands and feet: a clinicopathologic study of 21 tumors less than 1 cm. Am J Surg Pathol 2006;30(6):721–6.
4. van de Rijn M, Barr FG, Xiong QB, et al. Radiation-associated synovial sarcoma. Hum Pathol 1997; 28(11):1325–8.
5. Egger JF, Coindre JM, Benhattar J, et al. Radiation-associated synovial sarcoma: clinicopathologic and molecular analysis of two cases. Mod Pathol 2002;15(9):998–1004.
6. Deraedt K, Debiec-Rychter M, Sciot R. Radiation-associated synovial sarcoma of the lung following radiotherapy for pulmonary metastasis of Wilms' tumour. Histopathology 2006;48(4):473–5.
7. van de Rijn M, Barr FG, Xiong QB, et al. Poorly differentiated synovial sarcoma: an analysis of

clinical, pathologic, and molecular genetic features. Am J Surg Pathol 1999;23(1):106–12.

8. Jagdis A, Rubin BP, Tubbs RR, et al. Prospective evaluation of TLE1 as a diagnostic immunohistochemical marker in synovial sarcoma. Am J Surg Pathol 2009;33(12):1743–51.

9. Terry J, Saito T, Subramanian S, et al. TLE1 as a diagnostic immunohistochemical marker for synovial sarcoma emerging from gene expression profiling studies. Am J Surg Pathol 2007;31(2): 240–6.

10. Matsuyama A, Hisaoka M, Iwasaki M, et al. TLE1 expression in malignant mesothelioma. Virchows Arch 2010;457(5):577–83.

11. Pilotti S, Mezzelani A, Azzarelli A, et al. bcl-2 expression in synovial sarcoma. J Pathol 1998; 184(3):337–9.

12. Fisher C, Schofield J. S100 protein positive synovial sarcoma. Histopathology 1991;19:375–7.

13. Dei Tos AP, Wadden C, Calonje E, et al. Immunohistochemical demonstration of glycoprotein p30/32mic2 (CD99) in synovial sarcoma. A potential cause of diagnostic confusion. Appl Immunohistochem 1995;3:168–73.

14. Miettinen M, Cupo W. Neural cell adhesion molecule distribution in soft tissue tumors. Hum Pathol 1993;24(1):62–6.

15. Kohashi K, Oda Y, Yamamoto H, et al. Reduced expression of SMARCB1/INI1 protein in synovial sarcoma. Mod Pathol 2010;23(7):981–90.

16. He R, Patel RM, Alkan S, et al. Immunostaining for SYT protein discriminates synovial sarcoma from other soft tissue tumors: analysis of 146 cases. Mod Pathol 2007;20(5):522–8.

17. Crew AJ, Clark J, Fisher C, et al. Fusion of SYT to two genes, SSX1 and SSX2, encoding proteins with homology to the Kruppel-associated box in human synovial sarcoma. EMBO J 1995;14(10): 2333–40.

18. Agus V, Tamborini E, Mezzelani A, et al. Re: A novel fusion gene, SYT-SSX4, in synovial sarcoma. J Natl Cancer Inst 2001;93(17):1347–9.

19. Terry J, Nielsen T. Expression of CD133 in synovial sarcoma. Appl Immunohistochem Mol Morphol 2010;18(2):159–65.

20. Mancuso T, Mezzelani A, Riva C, et al. Analysis of SYT-SSX fusion transcripts and bcl-2 expression and phosphorylation status in synovial sarcoma. Lab Invest 2000;80(6):805–13.

21. Antonescu CR, Kawai A, Leung DH, et al. Strong association of SYT-SSX fusion type and morphologic epithelial differentiation in synovial sarcoma. Diagn Mol Pathol 2000;9(1):1–8.

22. Nakayama R, Mitani S, Nakagawa T, et al. Gene expression profiling of synovial sarcoma: distinct signature of poorly differentiated type. Am J Surg Pathol 2010;34(11):1599–607.

23. van de Rijn M, Barr FG, Collins MH, et al. Absence of SYT-SSX fusion products in soft tissue tumors other than synovial sarcoma. Am J Clin Pathol 1999;112(1):43–9.

24. Tamborini E, Agus V, Perrone F, et al. Lack of SYT-SSX fusion transcripts in malignant peripheral nerve sheath tumors on RT-PCR analysis of 34 archival cases. Lab Invest 2002;82(5):609–18.

25. Steigen SE, Schaeffer DF, West RB, et al. Expression of insulin-like growth factor 2 in mesenchymal neoplasms. Mod Pathol 2009;22(7):914–21.

26. Fernebro J, Francis P, Eden P, et al. Gene expression profiles relate to SS18/SSX fusion type in synovial sarcoma. Int J Cancer 2006;118(5):1165–72.

27. Schmitt T, Kasper B. New medical treatment options and strategies to assess clinical outcome in soft-tissue sarcoma. Expert Rev Anticancer Ther 2009;9(8):1159–67.

28. Toretsky JA, Gorlick R. IGF-1R targeted treatment of sarcoma. Lancet Oncol 2010;11(2):105–6.

29. Ladanyi M, Antonescu CR, Leung DH, et al. Impact of SYT-SSX fusion type on the clinical behavior of synovial sarcoma: a multi-institutional retrospective study of 243 patients. Cancer Res 2002;62(1): 135–40.

30. Spillane AJ, A'Hern R, Judson IR, et al. Synovial sarcoma: a clinicopathologic, staging, and prognostic assessment. J Clin Oncol 2000;18(22): 3794–803.

31. Ferner RE. Neurofibromatosis 1. Eur J Hum Genet 2007;15(2):131–8.

32. Bottillo I, Ahlquist T, Brekke H, et al. Germline and somatic NF1 mutations in sporadic and NF1-associated malignant peripheral nerve sheath tumours. J Pathol 2009;217(5):693–701.

33. Sabah M, Cummins R, Leader M, et al. Loss of p16 (INK4A) expression is associated with allelic imbalance/loss of heterozygosity of chromosome 9p21 in microdissected malignant peripheral nerve sheath tumors. Appl Immunohistochem Mol Morphol 2006;14(1):97–102.

34. Hirose T, Scheithauer BW, Sano T. Perineurial malignant peripheral nerve sheath tumor (MPNST). A clinicopathologic, immunohistochemical, and ultrastructural study of seven cases. Am J Surg Pathol 1998;22:1368–78.

35. Fisher C, Carter RL, Ramachandra S, et al. Peripheral nerve sheath differentiation in malignant soft tissue tumours: an ultrastructural and immunohistochemical study. Histopathology 1992;20(2):115–25.

36. Fletcher C, Unni K, Mertens F, editors. World Health Organization Classification of Tumours. Pathology and genetics of tumours of soft tissue and bone. Lyon (France): IARC Press; 2002.

37. Wanebo JE, Malik JM, VandenBerg SR, et al. Malignant peripheral nerve sheath tumors. A clinicopathologic study of 28 cases. Cancer 1993;71(4):1247–53.

38. Bahrami A, Folpe AL. Adult-type fibrosarcoma: a reevaluation of 163 putative cases diagnosed at a single institution over a 48-year period. Am J Surg Pathol 2010;34(10):1504–13.

39. Sheng WQ, Hashimoto H, Okamoto S, et al. Expression of COL1A1-PDGFB fusion transcripts in superficial adult fibrosarcoma suggests a close relationship to dermatofibrosarcoma protuberans. J Pathol 2001;194(1):88–94.

40. Coffin CM, Humphrey PA, Dehner LP. Extrapulmonary inflammatory myofibroblastic tumor: a clinical and pathological survey. Semin Diagn Pathol 1998;15(2):85–101.

41. Qiu X, Montgomery E, Sun B. Inflammatory myofibroblastic tumor and low-grade myofibroblastic sarcoma: a comparative study of clinicopathologic features and further observations on the immunohistochemical profile of myofibroblasts. Hum Pathol 2008;39(6):846–56.

42. Nonaka D, Birbe R, Rosai J. So-called inflammatory myofibroblastic tumour: a proliferative lesion of fibroblastic reticulum cells? Histopathology 2005; 46(6):604–13.

43. Coden DJ, Hornblass A. Orbital hemangiopericytoma. JAMA 1990;264(14):1861.

44. Coffin CM, Watterson J, Priest JR, et al. Extrapulmonary inflammatory myofibroblastic tumor (inflammatory pseudotumor). A clinicopathologic and immunohistochemical study of 84 cases. Am J Surg Pathol 1995;19(8):859–72.

45. Coffin CM, Dehner LP, Meis-Kindblom JM. Inflammatory myofibroblastic tumor, inflammatory fibrosarcoma, and related lesions: an historical review with differential diagnostic considerations. Semin Diagn Pathol 1998;15(2):102–10.

46. Montgomery EA, Shuster DD, Burkart AL, et al. Inflammatory myofibroblastic tumors of the urinary tract: a clinicopathologic study of 46 cases, including a malignant example inflammatory fibrosarcoma and a subset associated with high-grade urothelial carcinoma. Am J Surg Pathol 2006;30(12):1502–12.

47. Hirsch MS, Dal Cin P, Fletcher CD. ALK expression in pseudosarcomatous myofibroblastic proliferations of the genitourinary tract. Histopathology 2006;48(5):569–78.

48. Wenig BM, Devaney K, Bisceglia M. Inflammatory myofibroblastic tumor of the larynx. A clinicopathologic study of eight cases simulating a malignant spindle cell neoplasm. Cancer 1995;76(11): 2217–29.

49. Moran CA, Suster S, Abbondanzo SL. Inflammatory pseudotumor of lymph nodes: a study of 25 cases with emphasis on morphological heterogeneity. Hum Pathol 1997;28(3):332–8.

50. Harik LR, Merino C, Coindre JM, et al. Pseudosarcomatous myofibroblastic proliferations of the bladder: a clinicopathologic study of 42 cases. Am J Surg Pathol 2006;30(7):787–94.

51. Sukov WR, Cheville JC, Carlson AW, et al. Utility of ALK-1 protein expression and ALK rearrangements in distinguishing inflammatory myofibroblastic tumor from malignant spindle cell lesions of the urinary bladder. Mod Pathol 2007;20(5):592–603.

52. Gleason BC, Hornick JL. Inflammatory myofibroblastic tumours: where are we now? J Clin Pathol 2008;61(4):428–37.

53. Freeman A, Geddes N, Munson P, et al. Anaplastic lymphoma kinase (ALK 1) staining and molecular analysis in inflammatory myofibroblastic tumours of the bladder: a preliminary clinicopathological study of nine cases and review of the literature. Mod Pathol 2004;17(7):765–71.

54. Coffin CM, Hornick JL, Fletcher CD. Inflammatory myofibroblastic tumor: comparison of clinicopathologic, histologic, and immunohistochemical features including ALK expression in atypical and aggressive cases. Am J Surg Pathol 2007;31(4): 509–20.

55. Mirra M, Falconieri G, Zanconati F, et al. Inflammatory fibrosarcoma: another imitator of Hodgkin's disease? Pathol Res Pract 1996;192(5):474–8 [discussion: 479–82].

56. Meis-Kindblom JM, Kjellstrom C, Kindblom LG. Inflammatory fibrosarcoma: update, reappraisal, and perspective on its place in the spectrum of inflammatory myofibroblastic tumors. Semin Diagn Pathol 1998;15(2):133–43.

57. Meis JM, Enzinger FM. Inflammatory fibrosarcoma of the mesentery and retroperitoneum. A tumor closely simulating inflammatory pseudotumor. Am J Surg Pathol 1991;15(12):1146–56.

58. Marino-Enriquez A, Wang WL, Roy A, et al. Epithelioid inflammatory myofibroblastic sarcoma: an aggressive intra-abdominal variant of inflammatory myofibroblastic tumor with nuclear membrane or perinuclear ALK. Am J Surg Pathol 2011;35(1): 135–44.

59. Chan JK, Cheuk W, Shimizu M. Anaplastic lymphoma kinase expression in inflammatory pseudotumors. Am J Surg Pathol 2001;25(6):761–8.

60. Cessna MH, Zhou H, Sanger WG, et al. Expression of ALK1 and p80 in inflammatory myofibroblastic tumor and its mesenchymal mimics: a study of 135 cases. Mod Pathol 2002;15(9):931–8.

61. Cook JR, Dehner LP, Collins MH, et al. Anaplastic lymphoma kinase (ALK) expression in the inflammatory myofibroblastic tumor: a comparative immunohistochemical study. Am J Surg Pathol 2001;25(11):1364–71.

62. Lawrence B, Perez-Atayde A, Hibbard MK, et al. TPM3-ALK and TPM4-ALK oncogenes in inflammatory myofibroblastic tumors. Am J Pathol 2000; 157(2):377–84.

63. Bridge JA, Kanamori M, Ma Z, et al. Fusion of the ALK gene to the clathrin heavy chain gene, CLTC, in inflammatory myofibroblastic tumor. Am J Pathol 2001;159(2):411–5.

64. Miyajima N, Koike H, Kawaguchi M, et al. Idiopathic retroperitoneal fibrosis associated with IgG4-positive-plasmacyte infiltrations and idiopathic chronic pancreatitis. Int J Urol 2006;13(11):1442–4.

65. Taniguchi T, Kobayashi H, Fukui S, et al. A case of multifocal fibrosclerosis involving posterior mediastinal fibrosis, retroperitoneal fibrosis, and a left seminal vesicle with elevated serum IgG4. Hum Pathol 2006;37(9):1237–9 [author reply: 1239].

66. Yamamoto H, Yamaguchi H, Aishima S, et al. Inflammatory myofibroblastic tumor versus IgG4-related sclerosing disease and inflammatory pseudotumor: a comparative clinicopathologic study. Am J Surg Pathol 2009;33(9):1330–40.

67. Saab ST, Hornick JL, Fletcher CD, et al. IgG4 plasma cells in inflammatory myofibroblastic tumor: inflammatory marker or pathogenic link? Mod Pathol 2011;24(4):606–12.

68. Chang A, Schuetze SM, Conrad EU 3rd, et al. So-called "inflammatory leiomyosarcoma": a series of 3 cases providing additional insights into a rare entity. Int J Surg Pathol 2005;13(2):185–95.

69. Yu H, Gibson JA, Pinkus GS, et al. Podoplanin (D2-40) is a novel marker for follicular dendritic cell tumors. Am J Clin Pathol 2007;128(5):776–82.

70. Grogg KL, Macon WR, Kurtin PJ, et al. A survey of clusterin and fascin expression in sarcomas and spindle cell neoplasms: strong clusterin immunostaining is highly specific for follicular dendritic cell tumor. Mod Pathol 2005;18(2):260–6.

71. Espinosa I, Lee CH, Kim MK, et al. A novel monoclonal antibody against DOG1 is a sensitive and specific marker for gastrointestinal stromal tumors. Am J Surg Pathol 2008;32(2):210–8.

72. Lucas DR, Shukla A, Thomas DG, et al. Dedifferentiated liposarcoma with inflammatory myofibroblastic tumor-like features. Am J Surg Pathol 2010;34(6):844–51.

73. Schildhaus HU, Cavlar T, Binot E, et al. Inflammatory fibroid polyps harbour mutations in the platelet-derived growth factor receptor alpha (PDGFRA) gene. J Pathol 2008;216(2):176–82.

74. Kovach SJ, Fischer AC, Katzman PJ, et al. Inflammatory myofibroblastic tumors. J Surg Oncol 2006;94(5):385–91.

75. Morotti RA, Legman MD, Kerkar N, et al. Pediatric inflammatory myofibroblastic tumor with late metastasis to the lung: case report and review of the literature. Pediatr Dev Pathol 2005;8(2):224–9.

76. Petridis AK, Hempelmann RG, Hugo HH, et al. Metastatic low-grade inflammatory myofibroblastic tumor (IMT) in the central nervous system of a 29-year-old male patient. Clin Neuropathol 2004;23(4):158–66.

77. Hussong JW, Brown M, Perkins SL, et al. Comparison of DNA ploidy, histologic, and immunohistochemical findings with clinical outcome in inflammatory myofibroblastic tumors. Mod Pathol 1999;12(3):279–86.

78. Fisher C. Myofibroblastic malignancies. Adv Anat Pathol 2004;11(4):190–201.

79. Eyden B, Banerjee SS, Shenjere P, et al. The myofibroblast and its tumours. J Clin Pathol 2009;62(3):236–49.

80. Perez-Montiel MD, Plaza JA, Dominguez-Malagon H, et al. Differential expression of smooth muscle myosin, smooth muscle actin, h-caldesmon, and calponin in the diagnosis of myofibroblastic and smooth muscle lesions of skin and soft tissue. Am J Dermatopathol 2006;28(2):105–11.

81. Lestou VS, O'Connell JX, Ludkovski O, et al. Coamplification of 12p11 and 12q13 approximately q22 in multiple ring chromosomes in a spindle cell sarcoma resolved by novel multicolor fluorescence in situ hybridization analysis. Cancer Genet Cytogenet 2002;139(1):44–7.

82. Deyrup AT, Lee VK, Hill CE, et al. Epstein-Barr virus-associated smooth muscle tumors are distinctive mesenchymal tumors reflecting multiple infection events: a clinicopathologic and molecular analysis of 29 tumors from 19 patients. Am J Surg Pathol 2006;30(1):75–82.

83. Mentzel T, Calonje E, Fletcher CD. Leiomyosarcoma with prominent osteoclast-like giant cells. Analysis of eight cases closely mimicking the so-called giant cell variant of malignant fibrous histiocytoma. Am J Surg Pathol 1994;18(3):258–65.

84. Merchant W, Calonje E, Fletcher CD. Inflammatory leiomyosarcoma: a morphological subgroup within the heterogeneous family of so-called inflammatory malignant fibrous histiocytoma. Histopathology 1995;27(6):525–32.

85. Rubin BP, Fletcher CD. Myxoid leiomyosarcoma of soft tissue, an underrecognized variant. Am J Surg Pathol 2000;24(7):927–36.

86. Vang R, Kempson RL. Perivascular epithelioid cell tumor ('PEComa') of the uterus: a subset of HMB-45-positive epithelioid mesenchymal neoplasms with an uncertain relationship to pure smooth muscle tumors. Am J Surg Pathol 2002;26(1):1–13.

87. Kraft S, Fletcher CD. Atypical intradermal smooth muscle neoplasms: clinicopathologic analysis of 84 cases and a reappraisal of cutaneous "leiomyosarcoma". Am J Surg Pathol 2011;35(4):599–607.

88. Fletcher CD, Kilpatrick SE, Mentzel T. The difficulty in predicting behavior of smooth-muscle tumors in deep soft tissue. Am J Surg Pathol 1995;19(1):116–7.

89. Miettinen M, Fetsch JF. Evaluation of biological potential of smooth muscle tumours. Histopathology 2006;48(1):97–105.

90. Weiss SW. Smooth muscle tumors of soft tissue. Adv Anat Pathol 2002;9(6):351–9.

91. Paal E, Miettinen M. Retroperitoneal leiomyomas: a clinicopathologic and immunohistochemical study of 56 cases with a comparison to retroperitoneal leiomyosarcomas. Am J Surg Pathol 2001; 25(11):1355–63.

92. Billings SD, Folpe AL, Weiss SW. Do leiomyomas of deep soft tissue exist? An analysis of highly differentiated smooth muscle tumors of deep soft tissue supporting two distinct subtypes. Am J Surg Pathol 2001;25(9):1134–42.

93. Hasegawa T, Seki K, Hasegawa F, et al. Dedifferentiated liposarcoma of retroperitoneum and mesentery: varied growth patterns and histological grades—a clinicopathologic study of 32 cases. Hum Pathol 2000;31:717–27.

94. Thway K, Robertson D, Thway Y, et al. Dedifferentiated liposarcoma with meningothelial-like whorls, metaplastic bone formation, and CDK4, MDM2, and p16 expression: a morphologic and immunohistochemical study. Am J Surg Pathol 2011; 35(3):356–63.

95. Binh MB, Sastre-Garau X, Guillou L, et al. MDM2 and CDK4 immunostainings are useful adjuncts in diagnosing well-differentiated and dedifferentiated liposarcoma subtypes: a comparative analysis of 559 soft tissue neoplasms with genetic data. Am J Surg Pathol 2005;29(10):1340–7.

96. Folpe AL, Kwiatkowski DJ. Perivascular epithelioid cell neoplasms: pathology and pathogenesis. Hum Pathol 2010;41(1):1–15.

97. Massi D, Franchi A, Alos L, et al. Cutaneous leiomyosarcoma: clinico-pathologic analysis of 76 cases. Lab Invest 2008;88:98A.

98. Gustafson P, Willen H, Baldetorp B, et al. Soft tissue leiomyosarcoma. A population-based epidemiologic and prognostic study of 48 patients, including cellular DNA content. Cancer 1992;70(1):114–9.

99. Stoeckle E, Coindre JM, Bonvalot S, et al. Prognostic factors in retroperitoneal sarcoma: a multivariate analysis of a series of 165 patients of the French Cancer Center Federation Sarcoma Group. Cancer 2001;92(2):359–68.

100. Fisher C, Goldblum JR, Epstein JI, et al. Leiomyosarcoma of the paratesticular region: a clinicopathologic study. Am J Surg Pathol 2001; 25(9):1143–9.

101. Farshid G, Pradhan M, Goldblum J, et al. Leiomyosarcoma of somatic soft tissues: a tumor of vascular origin with multivariate analysis of outcome in 42 cases. Am J Surg Pathol 2002;26(1):14–24.

102. Berlin O, Stener B, Kindblom LG, et al. Leiomyosarcomas of venous origin in the extremities. A correlated clinical, roentgenologic, and morphologic study with diagnostic and surgical implications. Cancer 1984;54:2147–59.

103. Leuschner I, Newton WA Jr, Schmidt D, et al. Spindle cell variants of embryonal rhabdomyosarcoma in the paratesticular region. A report of the Intergroup Rhabdomyosarcoma Study. Am J Surg Pathol 1993;17(3):221–30.

104. Parham DM, Ellison DA. Rhabdomyosarcomas in adults and children: an update. Arch Pathol Lab Med 2006;130(10):1454–65.

105. Nascimento AF, Fletcher CD. Spindle cell rhabdomyosarcoma in adults. Am J Surg Pathol 2005; 29(8):1106–13.

106. Folpe AL, McKenney JK, Bridge JA, et al. Sclerosing rhabdomyosarcoma in adults: report of four cases of a hyalinizing, matrix-rich variant of rhabdomyosarcoma that may be confused with osteosarcoma, chondrosarcoma, or angiosarcoma. Am J Surg Pathol 2002;26(9):1175–83.

107. Kuhnen C, Herter P, Leuschner I, et al. Sclerosing pseudovascular rhabdomyosarcoma-immunohistochemical, ultrastructural, and genetic findings indicating a distinct subtype of rhabdomyosarcoma. Virchows Arch 2006;449(5):572–8.

108. Stock N, Chibon F, Binh MB, et al. Adult-type rhabdomyosarcoma: analysis of 57 cases with clinicopathologic description, identification of 3 morphologic patterns and prognosis. Am J Surg Pathol 2009;33(12):1850–9.

109. Mentzel T, Kuhnen C. Spindle cell rhabdomyosarcoma in adults: clinicopathological and immunohistochemical analysis of seven new cases. Virchows Arch 2006;449(5):554–60.

MYOFIBROMA, MYOPERICYTOMA, MYOEPITHELIOMA, AND MYOFIBROBLASTOMA OF SKIN AND SOFT TISSUE

Robert E. LeBlanc, MD[a], Janis Taube, MD, MSc[b],*

KEYWORDS

- Myofibroma • Myopericytoma • Myoepithelioma • Myofibroblastoma

ABSTRACT

The authors address a group of loosely associated, characteristically benign soft tissue neoplasms that exhibit partial myoid differentiation. The entities share similarities in morphology and in nomenclature that have historically created confusion. The authors attempt to clarify the distinct architectural patterns and the corresponding immunophenotypic and ulrastructural features that distinguish myofibroma, myopericytoma, myoepithelioma, and myofibroblastoma.

entity is distinguished from other neoplasms with dual myofibroblastic and fibroblastic differentiation, including a subset of solitary fibrous tumors and pleomorphic myofibrosarcoma; and it is distinguished from purely reactive myofibroblastic proliferations, including nodular fasciitis, proliferative fasciitis, and ischemic fasciitis.

MYOFIBROMA AND MYOFIBROMATOSIS

OVERVIEW

Myofibromas were first described in 1951 as *congenital fibrosarcoma* by Williams and Schrum[1] but were later reclassified as *congenital generalized fibromatosis* by Stout,[2] who distinguished a good prognostic variant characterized by skin and soft tissue tumors from a poor prognostic variant involving the viscera.[2] Chung and Enzinger[3] were the first to determine that the neoplasms were myofibroblastic in origin and, thus, renamed them *infantile myofibromatosis*. The currently accepted nomenclature is *myofibroma* for solitary lesions and *myofibromatosis* for multiple lesions. This

Myofibromas occur at a variety of ages, although they are most common in childhood and are the most frequent fibrous tumors of infancy.[4] Male children and adults are more frequently affected than females; however, multicentricity is more commonly observed in females. Most lesions are sporadic, although rare autosomal dominant familial myofibromatosis has been described.[5] The neoplasms usually arise in the head, neck, trunk, and proximal extremities but can involve skeletal muscle, bone, and the maxillofacial region where they may be misconstrued as malignant given their propensity to trap adjacent muscle, nerve, and salivary tissue.[6–8] The category myofibromatosis has subsumed the entity previously called *infantile hemangiopericytoma*, and is associated with high mortality when neoplasms involve the heart, lungs, gastrointestinal tract, and central nervous system.[5] There are rare reports of myofibromas involving the eyelid, conjunctiva, and orbit,[9–13] and there is a report of a myofibroma involving the cranial vault.[14]

[a] Department of Pathology, The Johns Hopkins Hospital, 600 North Wolfe Street, Baltimore, MD 21287, USA
[b] Departments of Dermatology and Pathology, The Johns Hopkins Hospital, 600 North Wolfe Street, Baltimore, MD 21287, USA
* Corresponding author.
E-mail address: Jtaube1@jhmi.edu

Surgical Pathology 4 (2011) 745–759
doi:10.1016/j.path.2011.08.003
1875-9181/11/$ – see front matter © 2011 Elsevier Inc. All rights reserved.

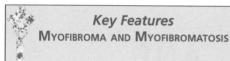

Key Features
MYOFIBROMA AND MYOFIBROMATOSIS

1. Benign solitary or multiple myofibroblastic neoplasms that occur predominantly in childhood and infancy, carrying an excellent prognosis in most cases that do not involve viscera

2. Biphasic zonation pattern with light-staining fascicles to whorls of myofibroblastic cells and dark-staining cellular areas of polygonal cells in association with hemangiopericytomatous vascular spaces; Hyalinized areas with low cellularity and central necrosis are common

3. Smooth muscle actin (SMA) positive, desmin and cytokeratin negative

4. Treated with conservative local excision and infrequently recur

GROSS FEATURES

Myofibromas are generally circumscribed, purple macules to nodules that can grow to be as large as 3 cm and may mimic a vascular neoplasm. On a cut surface, however, they have a fibrous, white-brown rubbery appearance.

MICROSCOPIC FEATURES

Myofibromas have a biphasic zonation pattern comprised of variably light and dark staining areas. The light staining areas tend to be present along the periphery of the neoplasm and consist of irregular to whorled fascicles of pale, eosinophilic myofibroblastic cells with abundant cytoplasm, elongated to tapered nuclei, and vesicular chromatin. The darker staining zones have dense cellularity and are comprised of polygonal cells with amphophilic cytoplasm, indistinct cell borders, subtle nuclear hyperchromasia, and pleomorphism (**Fig. 1**). There are often associated hemangiopericytomalike vessels. Mitotic activity is variable and does not predict behavior.[15] Myxoid change, hyalinization, and foci of calcification are common, (**Fig. 2**) and there may be prominent central necrosis within tumor nodules. The presence of subendothelial intravascular growth should not be misconstrued as vascular invasion.[15]

IMMUNOPHENOTYPE

The neoplastic cells stain with smooth muscle actin (SMA), vimentin, and muscle-specific actin monoclonal antibody HHF35. They are negative for desmin, S100, and cytokeratins.[15]

ULTRASTRUCTURAL FEATURES

The neoplastic cells contain abundant rough endoplasmic reticulum reminiscent of fibroblasts

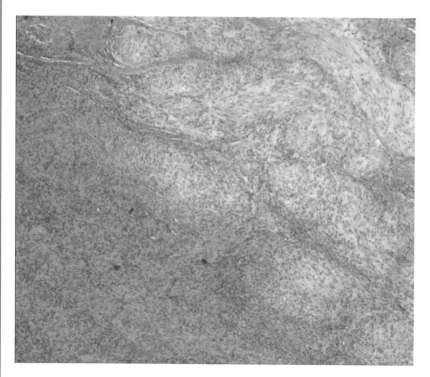

Fig. 1. Myofibroma. Biphasic morphology of hypercellular and hypocellular zones, which seem dark and light, respectively (hematoxylin-eosin [H&E], original magnification ×40).

Fig. 2. Myofibroma. Whorled fascicles with intervening hyalinized stroma in the peripheral, lighter staining zones (H&E, original magnification ×100).

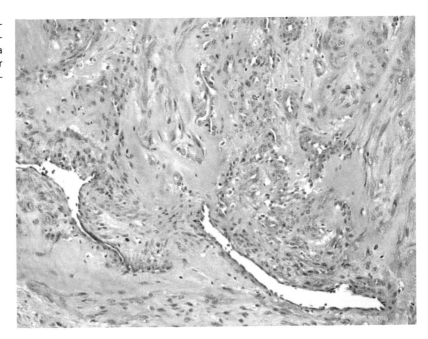

and peripheral contractile filaments suggestive of smooth muscle differentiation; however, they lack a lamina and feature a cell-to-matrix junction termed the *fibronexus* that is characteristic of myofibroblasts.[15–17]

MOLECULAR FEATURES

Cytogenetic analyses of myofibromas have revealed nonspecific chromosome 8 abnormalities.[15] It is important to note that myofibromas do not exhibit the ETV6-NTRK3 translocation that defines infantile fibrosarcoma and cellular mesoblastic nephroma.[15,18]

DIFFERENTIAL DIAGNOSIS

The differential diagnosis of myofibroma depends on whether the lighter or darker zones in an individual neoplasm predominate. The less cellular, lighter-staining zones may mimic a reactive myofibroblastic proliferation, such as nodular fasciitis, infantile fibromatosis, or inflammatory myofibroblastic tumor. Nodular fasciitis may be distinguished by its infiltrative growth, accompanying inflammation, and clinical presentation. Infantile fibromatosis usually involves muscle and lacks the hemangiopericytomatous vascular pattern that is typically seen with myofibromas. Inflammatory myofibroblastic tumors have prominent inflammation with abundant plasma cells and also lack the hemangiopericytomatous vascular pattern. The lighter areas around the periphery may also

resemble neurofibroma, which can be differentiated by S100 staining, if necessary.

Partial sampling of the more cellular zones of a myofibroma may raise the differential diagnosis of a myopericytoma, which may also feature hemangiopericytomatous morphology and stain positive with SMA and negative with desmin; however, they lack the biphasic zonation and show a concentric perivascular arrangement of plump, spindled cells. The more cellular areas may also resemble a sarcoma, such as malignant solitary fibrous tumor, which is Bcl-2 positive and tends to be actin negative. Recognition of the biphasic morphology and immunostains, if necessary, may be used to help distinguish myofibroma from more aggressive neoplasms.

Pitfalls
MYOFIBROMA AND MYOFIBROMATOSIS

! Myofibromas arising in the maxillofacial region can be misconstrued as malignant given their propensity to trap adjacent muscle, nerve, and salivary tissue.

! Mitotic activity and mild pleomorphism in myofibromas are variable and do not predict aggressive behavior.

! Subendothelial intravascular growth can occur with myofibromas and should not be misconstrued as vascular invasion.

PROGNOSIS

Myofibromas are treated by conservative local excision and infrequently recur. Lesions may regress, undergoing spontaneous apoptosis. Multicentric disease is associated with greater morbidity and mortality, which approaches 75% when there is involvement of the viscera.[15,19]

MYOPERICYTOMA

OVERVIEW

Myopericytomas encompass a family of characteristically benign, pericytic neoplasms of the dermis and superficial subcutis that represent one end of the spectrum of entities once grouped together as hemangiopericytomas. In 1942, Stout and Murray[20] coined the term *hemangiopericytoma* to describe a tumor of the extremities comprised of plump, polygonal to bluntly fusiform cells arranged around prominent thin-walled, branching blood vessels. However, the hemangiopericytomatous vascular pattern was unable to predict clinical behavior; it was gradually accepted that the initial morphologic classification encompassed a heterogeneous group of both benign and malignant neoplasms, which do not fall under the rubrics of solitary fibrous tumors, myofibromas, synovial sarcomas, mesenchymal chondrosarcomas, infantile fibrosarcomas, and endometrial stromal sarcomas, among others.[21] Hemangiopericytomatous neoplasms with pericytic differentiation have more recently been classified as *myopericytoma* and *glomangiopericytoma*.

Myopericytomas are slow growing and generally painless, solitary, benign soft tissue neoplasms that arise from perivascular modified smooth muscle cells. They demonstrate a range of morphologies overlapping those of glomus tumors and myofibromas. Myopericytomas occur over a wide age range; however, they are most common in adult men and frequently arise on the lower extremities.[22] Occasionally they are found on the head and neck or on the trunk, and there are reports of visceral involvement, including the lungs,[23] parotid gland,[24] oral cavity,[25] and gastrointestinal tract.[26] A distinct subset of intravascular myopericytomas has been described with occasional desmin positivity[27,28]; rare malignant myopericytomas have been reported, including one subgroup associated with Epstein-Barr virus and immunosuppression.[29] Multicentric myopericytomas are rare.[22]

GROSS FEATURES

Myopericytomas are poorly circumscribed, fibrous tumors of the skin, subcutaneous tissue, and

Key Features
MYOPERICYTOMA

1. Benign, usually solitary myopericytic neoplasm with a predilection to involve the lower extremities of adults

2. Hemangiopericytomatous pattern with concentric, perivascular arrangement of plump, spindled to glomoid cells with SMA and caldesmon positivity

3. Morphologic overlap with glomus tumors and myofibromas

4. Rarely recur following excision

superficial soft tissue, which range in size from 1 to 3 cm.

MICROSCOPIC FEATURES

Myopericytomas are demarcated, nonencapsulated neoplasms that can adopt different patterns; however, the most characteristic feature is the concentric, perivascular arrangement of plump to spindled, eosinophilic cells with bland, round-to-ovoid nuclei (**Fig. 3**). A myofibromalike pattern consists of sheets and fascicles of plump, eosinophilic spindle cells. The pericytomatous pattern is comprised of spindled cells with elongated nuclei that form concentric layers in the walls of small vessels and extend around adjacent blood vessels at the periphery of the tumor, mimicking true vascular invasion. The glomangiomatous pattern consists of rounded, eosinophilic glomoid cells that may be large and multinucleated. Pleomorphism, necrosis, and infiltration are rare, and mitotic figures usually do not exceed 2 per 10 high-powered fields.

ULTRASTRUCTURAL FEATURES

Myopericytes are modified smooth muscle cells identified by prominent cytoplasmic filaments with dense bodies and continuous external lamina. They lack a fibronexus.

IMMUNOPHENOTYPE

Myopericytomas are SMA and h-caldesmon positive.[22] They are typically desmin negative, but occasional weak expression may be seen. They are also characteristically negative for S100.[30]

MOLECULAR FEATURES

There are descriptions of t(7;12) (p21–22;q13–15) myopericytomas resulting in ACTB-GLI fusion and activation of the GLI oncogene, which is an

Fig. 3. Myopericytoma. Bland, spindled tumor cells with ample eosinophilic cytoplasm surrounding hemangiopericytomalike-vessels (H&E, original magnification ×100).

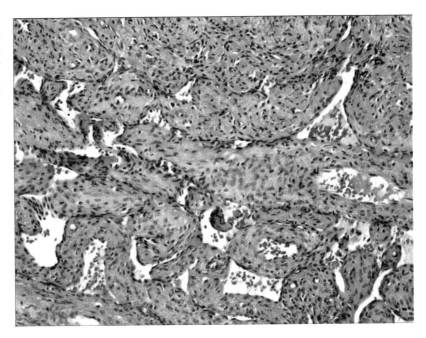

integral component of the sonic hedgehog signaling pathway.[31]

DIFFERENTIAL DIAGNOSIS

Myopericytomas need to be differentiated from other entities in the adult hemangiopericytoma spectrum. Two closely related neoplasms that exhibit overlapping differentiation and morphology are glomus tumor/glomangioma and glomangiopericytoma, the latter of which was formerly called sinonasal-type hemangiopericytoma. Myopericytomas differ from glomus tumors in their location and their characteristic concentric perivascular

Fig. 4. Glomus tumor. Regular cords of uniform tumor cells with characteristically round nuclei, which immediately abut vessels. Foci demonstrate a prominent basement membrane (H&E, original magnification ×200).

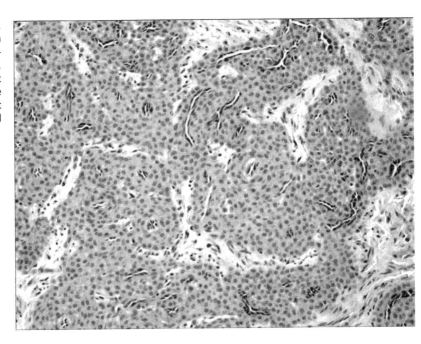

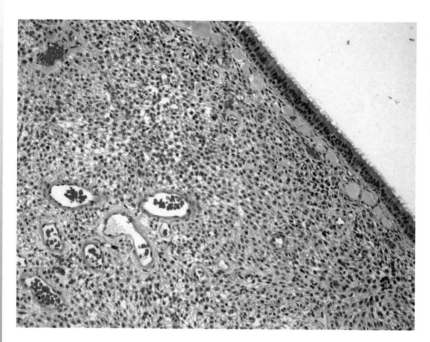

Fig. 5. Glomangiopericytoma. Sheets of monomorphous cells with prominent vasculature surrounded by hyalinized material. Interspersed inflammatory and red blood cells are a readily identified (H&E, original magnification ×100).

growth. Cases that show glomuslike cytology and architecture typically have some areas of elongated spindled cells more characteristic of a myopericytoma, aiding in the distinction (**Fig. 4**). Glomangiopericytomas may be differentiated from myopericytomas based on location, hyalinization around the staghorn vasculature, and tumor cells that form a syncytium with indistinct cell borders. Inflammatory cells are abundant in the stroma, which can seem myxoid and exhibit variable hemorrhage and fibrosis (**Fig. 5**).[32,33]

Myopericytomas differ from the more frequently observed solitary fibrous tumor, which is a circumscribed, lobulated neoplasm comprised of a patternless arrangement of monomorphous, small basophilic, ovoid to spindled cells with ill-defined cytoplasmic borders. Solitary fibrous tumors are Bcl-2 and CD99 positive. They can be differentiated from myofibromas by their lack of biphasic morphology. Angiomyomas may also share a similar concentric arrangement of myoid cells around vessels but also display a mature muscle phenotype replete with SMA and desmin positivity.

Pitfalls
MYOPERICYTOMA

! Subendothelial intravascular growth can occur with myopericytomas and should not be misconstrued as vascular invasion.

PROGNOSIS

Myopericytomas are characteristically benign neoplasms. Some regress spontaneously following biopsy and only rarely recur following excision.[34] Malignant myopericytoma is exceedingly rare and associated with a high mitotic rate, hypercellularity, pleomorphism, and necrosis.[35]

MYOEPITHELIOMA OF SOFT TISSUE

OVERVIEW

Myoepithelioma of soft tissue is a myoepithelial cell-derived neoplasm closely related to myoepithelial-predominant benign mixed tumors (chondroid syringoma) but lacking ductal differentiation. It occurs in the dermis, subcutis, or deep soft tissue and is similar in behavior and appearance to that of the analogous salivary gland neoplasm. Myoepitheliomas of soft tissue most commonly occur in older adults; however, they may occur over a wide age range with no gender predilection.[36] The usually painless neoplasms are found mainly on the limb girdles, extremities, and head and neck of patients, growing to approximately 5 cm, although there are reports of neoplasms growing to as large as 20 cm in diameter.[37]

GROSS FEATURES

Myoepitheliomas usually measure 0.5 to 2.5 cm and arise in the subcutis and less frequently involve the dermis.[38–40] They are typically

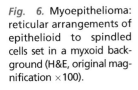

Key Features
MYOEPITHELIOMA OF SOFT TISSUE

1. Benign, pseudoencapsulated neoplasm of myoepithelial cells closely related to parachordoma that recurs following excision in approximately 20% of cases

2. May exhibit 2 distinct patterns, including fascicles to sheets of spindle cells with syncytial cytoplasm and no stroma and reticular arrangements of epithelioid, plasmacytoid, and spindled cells in a myxoid or hyalinized stroma

3. Stains with epithelial markers and show variable SMA and S100 staining

4. Myxoid chondrosarcoma may be distinguished by a lack of cytokeratin and actin staining and by identification of the t(9;22)(q22;q12) translocation

circumscribed with a yellow-white cut surface and focal myxoid or gelatinous change. Necrosis is generally not a predominant feature.

MICROSCOPIC FEATURES

Myoepitheliomas of soft tissue are roughly circumscribed, pseudoencapsulated neoplasms of the dermis and subcutaneous tissues. They may seem microscopically infiltrative.[37] There are 2 distinct patterns. The first, most prevalent architecture consists of reticular growth with cords of epithelioid, ovoid, and spindled cells in a myxoid or hyalinized stroma (Fig. 6). The second pattern is comprised of sheets of plump spindle cells with abundant eosinophilic, syncytial cytoplasm and little stroma (Fig. 7). Focal osteochondroid or adipocytic differentiation has been reported.

Malignant myoepithelioma is also referred to as myoepithelial carcinoma and exhibits nuclear atypia with prominent nucleoli, high mitotic activity, and necrosis.[37,40]

IMMUNOPHENOTYPE

Myoepitheliomas are positive for cytokeratins and epithelial membrane antigen. Approximately half are positive for SMA and there is variable reactivity with desmin and h-caldesmon. They may also exhibit positivity with S100, calponin, and glial fibrillary acidic protein.[41] Some lack INI1 staining.

ULTRASTRUCTURAL FEATURES

By electron microscopy, myoepithelioma shows incomplete epithelial differentiation with microvillous surface projections, primitive cell junctions, and fragmented basal lamina.[42]

MOLECULAR FEATURES

There are reports of a myoepithelioma harboring a balanced translocation t(1;22)(q23;q12) resulting in the fusion of EWSR1 and PBX[43] and of

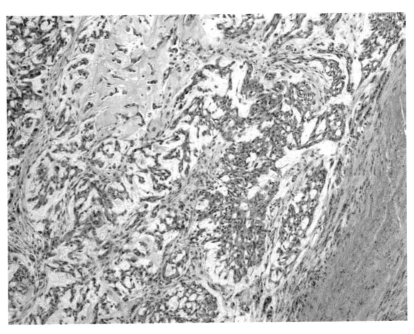

Fig. 6. Myoepithelioma: reticular arrangements of epithelioid to spindled cells set in a myxoid background (H&E, original magnification ×100).

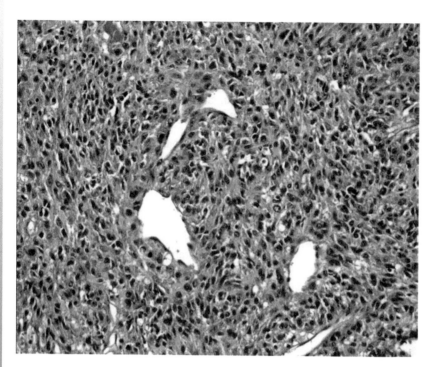

Fig. 7. Myoepithelioma: sheetlike arrangement of epithelioid to spindled cells arranged around hemangiopericytomalike vessels (H&E, original magnification ×200).

a myoepithelial carcinoma involving a translocation t(19;22)(q13;q12) resulting in EWSR1-ZNF444 fusion.[44]

DIFFERENTIAL DIAGNOSIS

The differential diagnosis is broad because myoepithelial cells may adopt spindled, epithelioid, and plasmacytoid morphologies in a myxoid or hyalinized stroma. Neoplasms that show obvious ductal differentiation are better classified as mixed tumors.

Parachordomas are comprised of a small nest of S100-positive and often cytokeratin-positive cells with epithelial differentiation and pale eosinophilic cytoplasm set in a myxoid background. They contain small, cellular islands with focal cytoplasmic vacuolization, reminiscent of the physaliferous cells of chordoma, which help distinguish this entity from myoepitheliomas. Additionally, parachordomas are often calponin negative. Extraskeletal myxoid chondrosarcomas are also comprised of small nests of cells set in a mucoid matrix. Although there is variable S100

reactivity, this malignancy is rarely positive for cytokeratins or actin. Most extraskeletal myxoid chondrosarcomas contain a t(9;22)(q22;q12) resulting in a EWSR1-NR4A3 fusion.[45]

Schwannomas stain positive with S100 and may resemble the spindled variant of myoepithelioma. In addition to nuclear psuedopallisading, which is not a feature of myoepithelioma, schwannomas are cytokeratin and calponin negative. Leiomyomas, which may exhibit a background of myxoid degenerative change, do not stain with cytokeratin or S100.

Synovial sarcoma is a characteristically deep soft tissue tumor of young adults in contrast to the more superficial myoepithelioma. They are distinguishable by hyalinization and calcification that do not occur in the latter entity and by an abrupt transition from spindled to epithelial cells in biphasic tumors. Synovial sarcomas are also S100 and cytokeratin positive; however, they are actin negative.[38]

Lastly, myoepithelioma of soft tissue may also be mimicked by ectopic hamartomatous thymomas, which are slow-growing, supraclavicular or

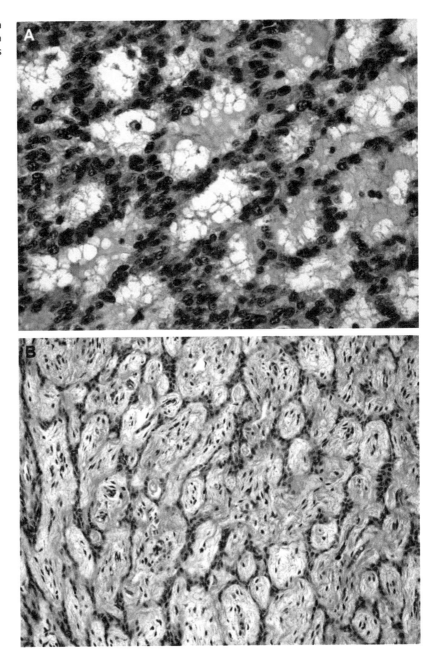

Fig. 8. Myoepithelioma (*A*) comparison with ectopic hamartomatous thymoma (*B*).

presternal tumors that, despite nomenclature, are presumed to be mixed tumors arising from the branchial anlage. They almost always arise in adult men.[46] These lobulated tumors are comprised of fascicles of spindle cells that can have solid, cystic, glandular, or tubular epithelial differentiation (**Fig. 8**). Negative staining with S100 may be used to help distinguish them from myoepitheliomas of soft tissue.[46]

PROGNOSIS

Complete excision of myoepitheliomas of soft tissue is standard therapy; however, approximately 1 of 5 of patients experience local recurrence. Frequent recurrence and rare metastases in isolated cases have been described.[36] Approximately 40% of neoplasms meeting the criteria for myoepithelial carcinoma recur and 30% metastasize.[37,40]

Pitfalls
MYOEPITHELIOMA OF
SOFT TISSUE

! May seem microscopically infiltrative despite benign behavior

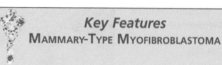

Key Features
MAMMARY-TYPE MYOFIBROBLASTOMA

1. Benign, slow growing neoplasm predominantly occurring in older men with a bulging, rubbery appearance similar to fibroadenoma

2. Bands of hyalinized collagen with intervening, irregular fascicles of bland spindle cells in a myxoid background with frequent mast cells

3. CD34 and desmin positivity; neoplasms rarely stain with SMA or cytokeratin markers

MAMMARY-TYPE MYOFIBROBLASTOMA

OVERVIEW

Mammary-type myofibroblastoma is a rare, slow-growing, and painless subcutaneous neoplasm comprised of modified smooth muscle cells seen predominantly in older men in whom it may resemble gynecomastia or arise in the setting of gynecomastia. Sizes up to 4 cm in diameter have been reported in the breast and up to 6 cm in other locations, including inguinal soft tissue, abdominal wall, and buttock.[47] Bilateral myofibroblastomas are rarely observed.

GROSS FEATURES

Mammary-type myofibroblastoma is a circumscribed to multilobular, bulging rubbery mass with a pale, gray-pink cut surface resembling fibroadenoma.

MICROSCOPIC FEATURES

Mammary-type myofibroblastomas are well-delineated, circumscribed nodules with pushing borders and bands of wiry, hyalinized collagen intermixed with irregular, cellular fascicles of bland spindle cells (**Fig. 9**). Fat trapping is observed; however, the lesion does not invade breast tissue. Myxoid change is common and focal hyalinization of blood vessels and hemangiopericytomatous change may also occur. The neoplastic spindle cells have eosinophilic cytoplasm with bland, tapered nuclei featuring a few small nucleoli and occasional nuclear grooves. Minor nuclear pleomorphism and mitotic figures are common. Atypia and necrosis are infrequent and focal chondroid differentiation is rare. Mast cells are sometimes prominent in the stroma.

ULTRASTRUCTURAL FEATURES

Electron microscopy reveals moderate amounts of rough endoplasmic reticulum, peripheral bundles of myofilaments with focal densities, intermediate filaments, attachment plaques alternating with plasmalemmal caveolae, and fragments of external lamina.[48,49] Myofibroblastomas lack the characteristic fibronexus junction of myofibroblastic differentiation. The features suggest incomplete smooth muscle differentiation with myofibroblastic features.

IMMUNOPHENOTYPE

Mammary-type myofibroblastomas uniformly express CD34. Bcl2 and desmin are typically positive and h-caldesmon is often negative. Only a minority of myofibroblastomas is SMA positive. Estrogen and progesterone receptor positivity has been reported. S100 and epithelial markers, including cytokeratins, are negative.[50]

MOLECULAR FEATURES

Mammary-type myofibroblastoma is associated with 13q- and 16q-, and there is a report of losses at the RB/13q14 and FKHR/13q14 loci reminiscent of changes observed in spindle cell lipoma and in cellular angiofibroma.[51–53]

DIFFERENTIAL DIAGNOSIS

Mammary-type myofibroblastoma should be distinguished from fibromatosis, which is not circumscribed or delineated, and consists of more diffuse fibrosis without the thick collagen bands characteristic of myofibroblastoma. Solitary fibrous tumors and myofibroblastomas can each feature a hemangiopericytomatous pattern and express CD34 and Bcl2; however, the former does not feature bands of wiry hyalinized collagen or typically express any smooth muscle markers. Leiomyosarcomas infrequently express CD34 and are comprised of perpendicularly arranged fascicles with blunt-ended nuclei and paranuclear vacuoles. Myoepitheliomas of soft tissue expresses S100 and keratin and often form nests of cells in a myxoid background. Metaplastic carcinoma may seem

Fig. 9. Mammary-type myofibroblastoma. Low-power (*A*) and high-power (*B*) views of wiry, hyalinized collagen intermixed with irregular, cellular fascicles of bland spindle cells.

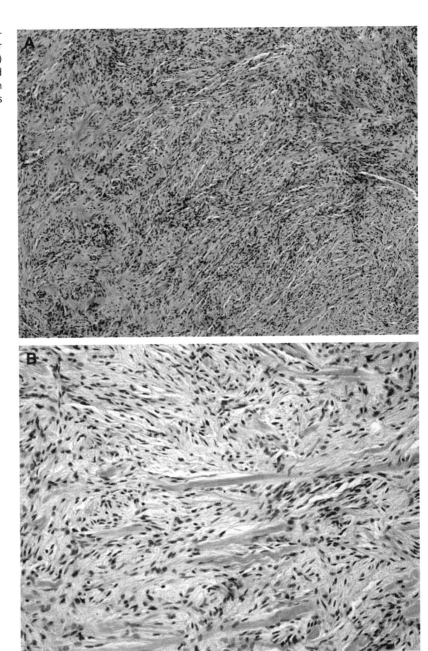

similar to mammary-type myofibroblastoma when particularly well differentiated; however, myofibromas usually do not express cytokeratins and they do not infiltrate breast tissue.

PROGNOSIS

Mammary-type myofibroblastoma is a benign neoplasm. Excision is considered curative.[49]

INTRANODAL PALISADED MYOFIBROBLASTOMA

OVERVIEW

Intranodal palisaded myofibroblastoma is a distinct spindle cell neoplasm of lymph nodes described in 1989 that has previously been described as intranodal hemorrhagic spindle cell tumor with amianthoid fibers, palisaded myofibroblastoma,

Key Features
INTRANODAL PALISADED MYOFIBROBLASTOMA

1. Benign solid neoplasm with a predilection for inguinal nodes of older men

2. Sheets of uniform, pale spindle cells with vague palisading around hyalinized foci with blood vessels

3. Brightly eosinophilic, stellate, thick amianthoid collagen fibers and marked hemosiderin deposition

4. SMA and calponin positivity, negative CD34

and solitary spindle cell tumor with myoid differentiation of the lymph node. This neoplasm exhibits modified smooth muscle and myofibroblastic differentiation and most frequently involves the inguinal lymph nodes of middle-aged men. There are reports of submandibular lymph node involvement[54] and of multicentric disease in an infant.[55]

GROSS FEATURES

Intranodal palisaded myoepitheliomas are solid tumors occurring in distended lymph nodes with focally hemorrhagic cut surfaces.

MICROSCOPIC FEATURES

Intranodal palisaded myofibroblastoma is comprised of highly vascular fascicles to sheets of uniform pale, eosinophilic spindle cells with elongated nuclei and minimal mitotic activity. Involved lymph nodes are often completely effaced, leaving a thin, compressed rim of nodal parenchyma at the perimeter of the neoplasm.[56] There is characteristic, vague palisading of neoplastic fascicles around hyalinized foci that occasionally contain blood vessels. Hemorrhage and hemosiderin deposition may be prominent (**Figs. 10** and **11**). There is a scattered, stellate arrangement of abnormally thickened, brightly eosinophilic amianthoid collagen fibers around blood vessels with occasional calcification.[57] Small, clustered intracellular eosinophilic globules comprised of actin are occasionally identified.[56] There is a solitary report of metaplastic bone formation within an intranodal palisaded myofibroblastoma.[58]

ULTRASTRUCTURAL FEATURES

Intranodal palisaded myofibroblastomas contain moderate amounts of rough endoplasmic reticulum, abundant actin-sized filaments in cell processes, external lamina, and absence of fibronectin fibrils and fibronexus, favoring myoid differentiation over myofibroblastic differentiation.[59,60]

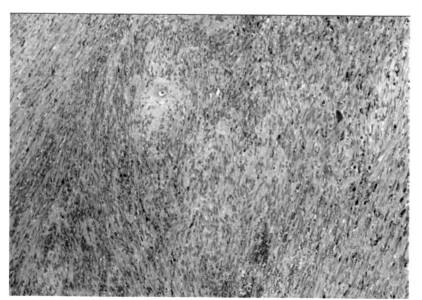

Fig. 10. Intranodal palisaded myofibroblastoma. Vague palisading around a hyalinized area with a central blood vessel. Note the red blood cells and marked hemosiderin deposition (hematoxylin-eosin, original magnification ×40).

Fig. 11. Intranodal palisaded myofibroblastoma (hematoxylin-eosin, original magnification ×40).

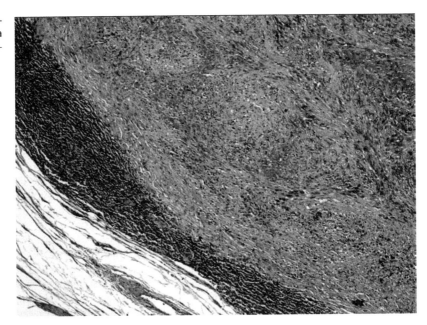

IMMUNOPHENOTYPE

Intranodal palisaded myofibroblastomas are CD34 negative. They stain positive with SMA and calponin, and some overexpress cyclin D1. The neoplasms are negative for desmin, h-caldesmon, S100, and CD31.[56]

DIFFERENTIAL DIAGNOSIS

Intranodal palisaded myofibroblastomas can mimic an intranodal schwannoma, which is S100. Intranodal palisaded myofibroblastoma may also be misconstrued as a metastatic sarcoma or as nodal involvement of Kaposi sarcoma, which in contrast is CD34 positive.

Pitfalls
INTRANODAL PALISADED MYOFIBROBLASTOMA

! They may be misdiagnosed as metastatic sarcoma, but can be distinguished by bland cytology, lack of mitotic activity, and by immunohistochemistry.

! They may be mistaken for schwannoma; however, there are only rare reports of schwannoma arising in a lymph node.

PROGNOSIS

Intranodal palisaded myofibroblastomas are benign and occasionally recur following excision. There have been no reports of metastasis.[58,59]

REFERENCES

1. Williams JO, Schrum D. Congenital fibrosarcoma; report of a case in a newborn infant. AMA Arch Pathol 1951;51(5):548–52.
2. Stout AP. Juvenile fibromatosis. Cancer 1954;7:953.
3. Chung EB, Enzinger FM. Infantile myofibromatosis. Cancer 1981;48(8):1807–18.
4. Daimaru Y, Hashimoto H, Enjoji M. Myofibromatosis in adults (adult counterpart of infantile myofibromatosis). Am J Surg Pathol 1989;13(10):859–65.
5. Mentzel T, Calonje E, Nascimento AG, et al. Infantile hemangiopericytoma versus infantile myofibromatosis: study of a series suggesting a continuous spectrum of infantile myofibroblastic lesions. Am J Surg Pathol 1994;18:922–30.
6. Montgomery E, Speight PM, Fisher C. Myofibromas presenting in the oral cavity: a series of 9 cases. Oral Surg Oral Med Oral Pathol Oral Radiol Endod 2000;89(3):343–8.
7. Foss RD, Ellis GL. Myofibromas and myofibromatosis of the oral region: a clinicopathologic analysis of 79 cases. Oral Surg Oral Med Oral Pathol Oral Radiol Endod 2000;89(1):57–65.

8. Oliver RJ, Coulthard P, Carre C, et al. Solitary adult myofibroma of the mandible simulating an odontogenic cyst. Oral Oncol 2003;39(6):626–9.

9. Asadi Amoli F, Sina AH, Kasai A, et al. A well-known lesion in an unusual location: infantile myofibroma of the eyelid: a case report and review of literature. Acta Med Iran 2010;48(6):412–6.

10. Lascaratos G, Gupta M, Bridges L, et al. Myofibroma of the conjunctiva invading the cornea in infancy. J Pediatr Ophthalmol Strabismus 2010;47:e1–3.

11. Mynatt CJ, Feldman KA, Thompson LD. Orbital infantile myofibroma: a case report and clinicopathologic review of 24 cases from the literature. Head Neck Pathol 2011. [Epub ahead of print].

12. Yazici B, Bilge AD, Yazici Z, et al. Congenital cranioorbital myofibroma. Ophthal Plast Reconstr Surg 2011;27(4):e108–111.

13. Larsen AC, Prause JU, Petersen BL, et al. Solitary infantile myofibroma of the orbit. Acta Ophthalmol 2010. [Epub ahead of print].

14. Merciadri P, Pavanello M, Nozza P, et al. Solitary infantile myofibromatosis of the cranial vault: case report. Childs Nerv Syst 2011;27(4):643–7.

15. Hicks J, Mierau G. The spectrum of pediatric fibroblastic and myofibroblastic tumors. Ultrastruct Pathol 2004;28(5–6):265–81.

16. Eyden B. Electron microscopy in the study of myofibroblastic lesions. Semin Diagn Pathol 2003;20(1):13–24.

17. Eyden B, Banerjee SS, Shenjere P, et al. The myofibroblast and its tumours. J Clin Pathol 2009;62(3):236–49.

18. Sandberg AA, Bridge JA. Updates on the cytogenetics and molecular genetics of bone and soft tissue tumor: congenital (infantile) fibrosarcoma and mesoblastic nephroma. Cancer Genet Cytogenet 2002;132:1–13.

19. Wiswell TE, Davis J, Cunningham BE, et al. Infantile myofibromatosis: the most common fibrous tumor of infancy. J Pediatr Surg 1988;23(4):315–8.

20. Stout AP, Murray MR. Hemangiopericytoma: a vascular tumor featuring Zimmermann's pericytes. Ann Surg 1942;116(1):26–33.

21. Nappi O, Ritter JH, Pettinato G, et al. Hemangiopericytoma: histopathological pattern or clinicopathologic entity? Semin Diagn Pathol 1995;12(3):221–32.

22. Mentzel T, Dei Tos AP, Sapi Z, et al. Myopericytoma of skin and soft tissues: clinicopathologic and immunohistochemical study of 54 cases. Am J Surg Pathol 2006;30(1):104–13.

23. Jian-Hua CA, Jin-Ping XU, Yong-Cheng LI, et al. Pulmonary myopericytoma: a case report and review of the literatures. Chin Med J 2009;122:755–7.

24. Chu ZG, Yu JQ, Yang ZG, et al. Myopericytoma involving the parotid gland as depicted on multidetector CT. Korean J Radiol 2009;10:398–401.

25. Datta V, Rawal YB, Mincer HH, et al. Myopericytoma of the oral cavity. Head Neck 2007;29:605–8.

26. Ramdial PK, Sing Y, Deonarain J, et al. Periampullary Epstein-Barr virus-associated myopericytoma. Hum Pathol 2011. [Epub ahead of print].

27. Ko JY, Choi WJ, Kang HS, et al. Intravascular myopericytoma: an interesting case of a long-standing large, painful subcutaneous tumor. Pathol Int 2011;61(3):161–4.

28. Park HJ, Lee DR, Park MY, et al. A case of intravascular myopericytoma. J Clin Pathol 2010;63(9):847–8.

29. Lau PP, Wong OK, Lui PC, et al. Myopericytoma in patients with AIDS. A new class of Epstein-Barr virus–associated tumor. Am J Surg Pathol 2009;33:1666–72.

30. Fisher C. Myofibrosarcoma. Virchows Arch 2004;445(3):215–23.

31. Dahlén A, Fletcher CD, Mertens F, et al. Activation of the GLI oncogene through fusion with the beta-actin gene (ACTB) in a group of distinctive pericytic neoplasms: pericytoma with t(7;12). Am J Pathol 2004;164(5):1645–53.

32. Dandekar M, McHugh JB. Sinonasal glomangiopericytoma: case report with emphasis on the differential diagnosis. Arch Pathol Lab Med 2010;134(10):1444–9.

33. Thompson LD. Sinonasal tract glomangiopericytoma (hemangiopericytoma). Ear Nose Throat J 2004;83(12):807.

34. Granter SR, Badizadegan K, Fletcher CD. Myofibromatosis in adults, glomangiopericytoma, and myopericytoma: a spectrum of tumors showing perivascular myoid differentiation. Am J Surg Pathol 1998;22(5):513–25.

35. McMenamin ME, Fletcher CD. Malignant myopericytoma: expanding the spectrum of tumours with myopericytic differentiation. Histopathology 2002;41(5):450–60.

36. Kilpatrick SE, Limon J. Mixed tumour/myoepithelioma/parachordoma. In: Fletcher CD, Unni K, Mertens F, editors. WHO classification of tumours. Pathology and genetics. Tumours of soft tissue and bone. Lyon (France): IARC Press; 2002. p. 198–9.

37. Hornick JL, Fletcher CD. Myoepithelial tumors of soft tissue: a clinicopathologic and immunohistochemical study of 101 cases with evaluation of prognostic parameters. Am J Surg Pathol 2003;27(9):1183–96.

38. Michal M, Miettinen M. Myoepitheliomas of the skin and soft tissues. Report of 12 cases. Virchows Arch 1999;434(5):393–400.

39. Kutzner H, Mentzel T, Kaddu S, et al. Cutaneous myoepithelioma: an under-recognized cutaneous neoplasm composed of myoepithelial cells. Am J Surg Pathol 2001;25(3):348–55.

40. Hornick JL, Fletcher CD. Cutaneous myoepithelioma: a clinicopathologic and immunohistochemical study of 14 cases. Hum Pathol 2004;35(1):14–24.

41. Mentzel T. Myoepithelial neoplasms of skin and soft tissues. Pathologe 2005;26(5):322–30.

42. Kuhnen C, Herter P, Kasprzynski A, et al. Myoepithelioma of soft tissue – case report with clinicopathologic, ultrastructural, and cytogenetic findings. Pathologe 2005;26(5):331–7 [in German].

43. Brandal P, Panagopoulos I, Bjerkehagen B, et al. Detection of a t(1;22)(q23;q12) translocation leading to an EWSR1-PBX1 fusion gene in a myoepithelioma. Genes Chromosomes Cancer 2008;47(7):558–64.

44. Brandal P, Panagopoulos I, Bjerkehagen B, et al. t(19;22)(q13;q12) Translocation leading to the novel fusion gene EWSR1-ZNF444 in soft tissue myoepithelial carcinoma. Genes Chromosomes Cancer 2009;48(12):1051–6.

45. Noguchi H, Mitsuhashi T, Seki K, et al. Fluorescence in situ hybridization analysis of extraskeletal myxoid chondrosarcomas using EWSR1 and NR4A3 probes. Hum Pathol 2010;41(3):336–42.

46. Fetsch JF, Laskin WB, Michal M, et al. Ectopic hamartomatous thymoma: a clinicopathologic and immunohistochemical analysis of 21 cases with data supporting reclassification as a branchial anlage mixed tumor. Am J Surg Pathol 2004;28(10):1360–70.

47. McMenamin ME, Fletcher CD. Mammary-type myofibroblastoma of soft tissue: a tumor closely related to spindle cell lipoma. Am J Surg Pathol 2001;25(8):1022–9.

48. Eyden BP, Shanks JH, Ioachim E, et al. Myofibroblastoma of breast: evidence favoring smooth-muscle rather than myofibroblastic differentiation. Ultrastruct Pathol 1999;23(4):249–57.

49. Wargotz ES, Weiss SW, Norris HJ. Myofibroblastoma of the breast. Sixteen cases of a distinctive benign mesenchymal tumor. Am J Surg Pathol 1987;11(7):493–502.

50. Magro G, Gurrera A, Bisceglia M. H-caldesmon expression in myofibroblastoma of the breast: evidence supporting the distinction from leiomyoma. Histopathology 2003;42(3):233–8.

51. Maggiani F, Debiec-Rychter M, Verbeeck G, et al. Extramammary myofibroblastoma is genetically related to spindle cell lipoma. Virchows Arch 2006;449(2):244–7.

52. Mandahl N, Mertens F, Willén H. A new cytogenetic subgroup in lipomas: loss of chromosome 16 material in spindle cell and pleomorphic lipomas. J Cancer Res Clin Oncol 1994;120(12):707–11.

53. Maggiani F, Debiec-Rychter M, Vanbockrijck M, et al. Cellular angiofibroma: another mesenchymal tumour with 13q14 involvement, suggesting a link with spindle cell lipoma and (extra)-mammary myofibroblastoma. Histopathology 2007;51(3):410–2.

54. Alguacil-Garcia A. Intranodal myofibroblastoma in a submandibular lymph node. A case report. Am J Clin Pathol 1992;97(1):69–72.

55. Rahimi S, Onetti Muda A, Faraggiana T. Multicentric intranodal myofibroblastoma in an infant. Histopathology 1995;27(5):477–8.

56. Weiss SW, Gnepp DR, Bratthauer GL. Palisaded myofibroblastoma. A benign mesenchymal tumor of lymph node. Am J Surg Pathol 1989;13(5):341–6.

57. Suster S, Rosai J. Intranodal hemorrhagic spindle-cell tumor with "amianthoid" fibers. Report of six cases of a distinctive mesenchymal neoplasm of the inguinal region that simulates Kaposi's sarcoma. Am J Surg Pathol 1989;13(5):347–57.

58. Creager AJ, Garwacki CP. Recurrent intranodal palisaded myofibroblastoma with metaplastic bone formation. Arch Pathol Lab Med 1999;123(5):433–6.

59. Lee JY, Abell E, Shevechik GJ. Solitary spindle cell tumor with myoid differentiation of the lymph node. Arch Pathol Lab Med 1989;113(5):547–50.

60. Eyden B, Chorneyko KA. Intranodal myofibroblastoma: study of a case suggesting smooth-muscle differentiation. J Submicrosc Cytol Pathol 2001;33(1–2):157–63.

PERIPHERAL NERVE SHEATH TUMORS

Ashley M. Cimino-Mathews, MD

KEYWORDS

• Nerve sheath tumors • Neoplasms • Schwann cells • Peripheral nerve

ABSTRACT

This article presents an overview of the diagnostic categories of benign and malignant nerve sheath tumors, including neuroma, neurofibroma, nerve sheath myxoma, perineurioma, schwannoma, and malignant peripheral nerve sheath tumor. The discussion emphasizes histologic patterns; ancillary studies, such as immunohistochemistry; and differential diagnoses. The information is of value to practicing pathologists in both community and academic settings.

OVERVIEW OF PERIPHERAL NERVE SHEATH TUMORS

Peripheral nerve sheath tumors consist of a heterogeneous group of neoplasms derived from one or more of the cell types that accompany peripheral nerve fibers. The predominant cell types include Schwann cells and perineurial cells, which are described in this article, as well as nerve sheath dendritic cells and fibroblasts. Schwann cells are neural crest-derived spindle cells that form the innermost layer of the endoneurium and are intimately associated with the nerve fibers.[1] Schwann cell nuclei are wavy, spindled, and characteristically pointed at both ends. Schwann cells are diffusely and strongly immunoreactive for the S-100 protein[2] as well as Leu7 and laminin while negative for epithelial membrane antigen (EMA), desmin, and muscle-specific actin. Schwann cells are typically negative for cytokeratin expression; however, schwannomas with focal cytokeratin immunoreactivity have been described.[3] Perineurial cells are slender spindled cells with similarity to arachnoid mater cells, and they form an external layer outside of the endoneurium.[4] Perineurial cells are immunoreactive for claudin-1,[5] EMA (focally),[6] and glucose transporter 1 (GLUT1)[6] but are negative for the S-100 protein.

Benign nerve sheath tumors include neuromas, neurofibromas, nerve sheath myxomas, perineuriomas, and schwannomas. Benign nerve sheath tumors arise in the differential of bland spindle cell lesions of the superficial and deep soft tissues, which includes leiomyoma, fibromatosis, solitary fibrous tumor and low-grade fibromyxoid sarcoma. Benign nerve sheath tumors, however, may also display diverse cytomorphologic features, such as epithelioid morphology, hypercellularity, myxoid matrix, and degenerative atypia. Malignant peripheral nerve sheath tumors (MPNSTs) are the malignant and aggressive counterparts to the benign neoplasms. MPNSTs arise in the differential of intermediate to high-grade soft tissue neoplasms, which includes synovial sarcoma, fibrosarcoma, leiomyosarcoma, sarcomatoid carcinoma, and melanoma. A more detailed discussion of each of these individual non-nerve sheath entities can be found in the accompanying articles elsewhere in this issue.

NEUROMA

Neuroma is a benign, disordered proliferation of nerves that include all the cellular components of the nerve sheath in otherwise normal relationships to each other. Each component can be highlighted by the appropriate immunohistochemical stain (eg, neurofilament for axons, the S-100 protein for Schwann cells, and EMA for perineurial cells).

Traumatic neuroma presents as a painful or tender nodule arising adjacent to a nerve after trauma or surgery. Microscopically, it consists of a non-neoplastic, nonencapsulated, disorganized

Department of Pathology, The Johns Hopkins Hospital, Weinberg 2242, 401 North Broadway, Baltimore, MD 21231-2410, USA
E-mail address: acimino@jhmi.edu

Surgical Pathology 4 (2011) 761–782
doi:10.1016/j.path.2011.08.004
1875-9181/11/$ – see front matter © 2011 Elsevier Inc. All rights reserved.

Key Features
PERIPHERAL NERVE SHEATH TUMORS

1. May be associated with syndromes, such as neurofibromatosis type 1 or 2, multiple endocrine neoplasia (MEN), type II, and Carney complex

2. Composed of varying proportions of perineurial cells, Schwann cells, and nerve axons

3. Benign tumors include neuroma, neurofibroma, nerve sheath myxoma, perineurioma, and schwannoma

4. Benign tumors typically composed of bland spindle cells characterized by wavy nuclei with pointed ends

5. Benign tumors may display degenerative atypia, epithelioid morphology, myxoid stroma, or hyper-cellular regions

6. Neurofibromas characteristically contain dense collagen fibers and prominent mast cells

7. Schwannomas commonly display regions of alternating cellularity (Antoni A and Antoni B areas), Verocay bodies, fibrous capsules, and peripheral lymphoid cuffs

8. Schwannomas are diffusely and strongly immunoreactive for the S-100 protein

9. MPNSTs typically have sweeping fascicles of atypical spindle cells with wavy nuclei, tumor cell condensation around large vessels, frequent mitoses, and necrosis

10. MPNSTs are usually only focally immunoreactive for the S-100 protein

mass of nerve bundles embedded in scar tissue (**Fig. 1**). Mucosal neuroma presents as a small nodule located beneath the mucosal epithelial surfaces of the eyelids, intestines, and oral cavity. Clinically, mucosal neuroma is associated with MEN, type IIb, which is characterized by thyroid medullary carcinoma, pheochromocytoma, and parathyroid hyperplasia. Microscopically, it consists of nonencapsulated, disorganized bundles of nerve fibers with distinct perineurium (**Fig. 2**). Palisaded

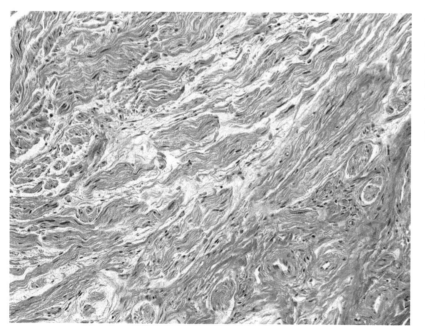

Fig. 1. Traumatic neuroma. Disorganized nerve bundles containing all normal cell types of the peripheral nerve are embedded in scar tissue and represent a non-neoplastic response to injury to a nerve (hematoxylin-eosin [H&E], original magnification ×64).

Fig. 2. Mucosal neuroma. Small bundles of nerve fibers containing all normal cell types of the peripheral nerve, with prominent perineurium, are arranged haphazardly within connective tissue (H&E, original magnification ×64).

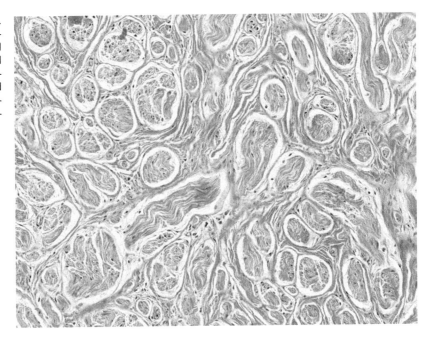

encapsulated neuroma (solitary circumscribed neuroma) presents as a small, solitary painless nodule arising on the face of middle-aged individuals. Microscopically, it consists of a well-circumscribed, dermal proliferation of nerve bundles with closely intermixed axons and palisading Schwann cells surrounded by a thin capsule of perineurial cells (**Fig. 3**).

The differential diagnosis for neuroma includes neurofibroma and schwannoma. Neuroma, however,

Fig. 3. Palisaded encapsulated neuroma. A well-circumscribed dermal nodule of tightly packed Schwann cells and axons is surrounded by a thin layer of perineurial cells (H&E, original magnification ×20).

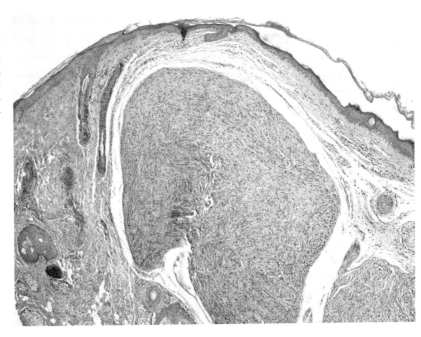

lacks the characteristic collagenous stroma and mast cells of neurofibroma and lacks the biphasic appearance of schwannoma. Clinical outcomes for neuroma are excellent.

NEUROFIBROMA

Neurofibroma is a neoplastic but benign proliferation of the peripheral nerve that contains all the cellular components of the peripheral nerve sheath as well as the axon. Single neurofibromas may be nonsyndromic, but multiple neurofibromas suggest neurofibromatosis (NF) type 1 (von Recklinghausen disease), which is an autosomal dominant defect in the neurofibromin gene located on chromosome 17q11.[7] Patients with NF1 develop multiple neurofibromas (solitary or plexiform) along with an array of associated lesions, including café-au-lait skin pigmentation, pigmented iris hamartomas (Lisch nodules), unilateral acoustic neuromas, and an increased incidence of MPNST and other soft tissue tumors.[8]

Grossly, the growth pattern of a neurofibroma may be localized, diffuse, or plexiform. A typical localized neurofibroma is a solitary, well-circumscribed nodule that is associated with an adjacent peripheral nerve. Microscopically, a typical neurofibroma consists of bland, spindled Schwann cells, and fibroblasts (**Fig. 4**) dispersed in loose collagen fibers that may condense to form a shredded carrot–like appearance. The stroma can be variably myxoid and has prominent mast cells (**Fig. 5**). Neurofibroma may have scattered atypia, including nuclear hyperchromasia and enlargement, but necrosis and brisk mitotic activity are absent.

A diffuse neurofibroma lacks a capsule and is characterized by an infiltrative growth pattern of spindled Schwann cells that entrap adipose tissue, skeletal muscle, or adnexal structures (**Figs. 6** and **7**). The presence of round, laminated eosinophilic structures, called Wagner-Meissner bodies, is a characteristic feature. Plexiform neurofibroma has a complex, multilobulated, and tortuous growth pattern consisting of expanded nerves that are contiguous with the normal nerve (**Fig. 8**). Plexiform neurofibromas only occur in NF1. Pigmented neurofibroma contains focal pigmented melanocytes (**Fig. 9**), which are immunoreactive for melanocytic markers, such as HMB45 and Melan-A.[9] Additional rare subtypes of neurofibroma include dendritic cell[10] and epithelioid variants.[11]

The differential diagnosis of a neurofibroma includes neuroma and schwannoma as well as bland non-nerve sheath spindle cell lesions. In contrast to a schwannoma, a neurofibroma lacks nuclear palisading and Verocay bodies, alternating Antoni A and Antoni B areas, and prominent

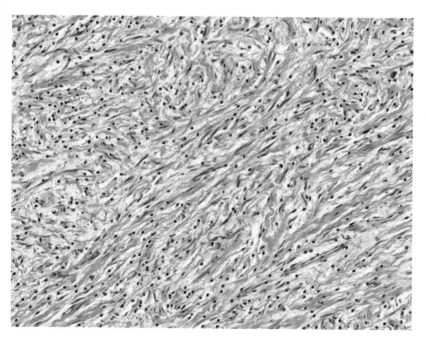

Fig. 4. Localized neurofibroma. Short spindle cells with wavy nuclei and tapered ends are arranged in a collagenous stroma with prominent mast cells (H&E, original magnification ×64).

Fig. 5. Myxoid neurofibroma. The stroma is highly myxoid and scantly cellular, containing small, bland spindle cells with tapered nuclei and scattered mast cells (H&E, original magnification ×100).

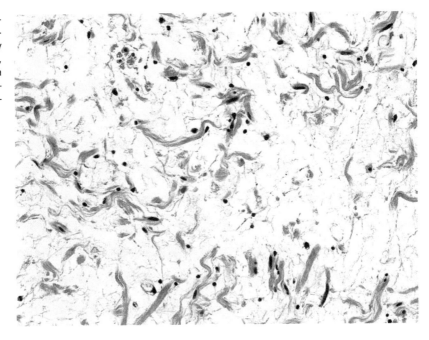

Fig. 6. Diffuse neurofibroma. Bands of short spindled Schwann cells with wavy nuclei entrap skeletal muscle and adipose tissue (H&E, original magnification ×64).

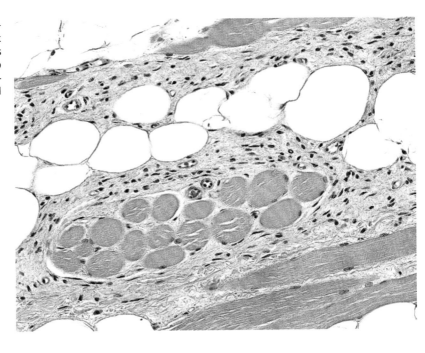

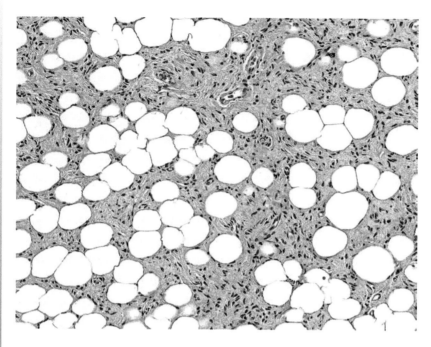

Fig. 7. Diffuse neurofibroma. Sheets of short spindle Schwann cells with wavy nuclei and fine collagen infiltrate through adipose tissue with a poorly defined border (H&E, original magnification ×64).

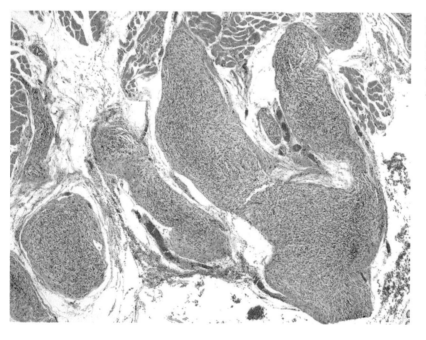

Fig. 8. Plexiform neurofibroma. Multiple nodules of expanded nerve bundles involve the subcutaneous tissue and skeletal muscle (H&E, original magnification ×20).

Fig. 9. Pigmented neurofibroma. Epithelioid melanocytes containing granular melanin pigment are interspersed between delicate collagen fibers and spindle cells with short wavy nuclei (H&E, original magnification ×100).

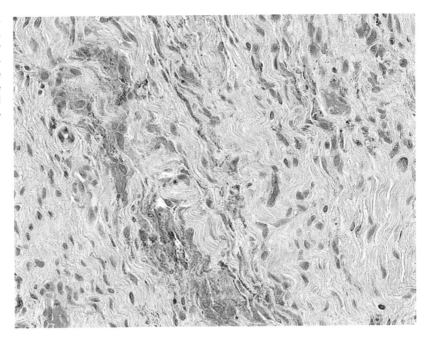

hyalinized vessels. Furthermore, in contrast to a schwannoma in which the spindle cells are diffusely immunoreactive for the S-100 protein, the spindle cells of a conventional neurofibroma are only focally positive. The risk of malignant transformation of a neurofibroma in patients with NF1 is approximately 4.6%.[8]

MYXOMA

Nerve sheath myxoma is a rare benign neural lesion involving the extremities of adults, affecting men and women equally with a peak incidence in the fourth decade.[12] Grossly, nerve sheath myxoma is a superficial, myxoid, and multilobulated lesion

Fig. 10. Nerve sheath myxoma. The superficial nodule is slightly lobulated, well-circumscribed with a smooth border, and contains spindled cells in a highly myxoid stroma (H&E, original magnification ×40).

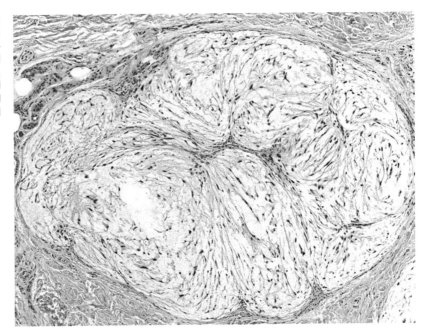

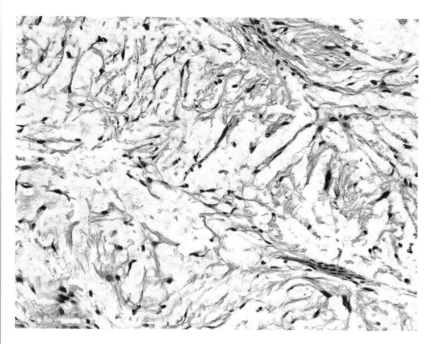

Fig. 11. Nerve sheath myxoma. Stellate and spindle cells with short, wavy, and hyperchromatic nuclei are dispersed in a myxoid stroma with fine vasculature (H&E, original magnification ×100).

with smooth borders. Microscopically, it is characterized by stellate, spindle, or epithelioid cells dispersed in a highly myxoid stroma (**Figs. 10** and **11**). These cells are strongly immunoreactive for the S-100 protein (**Fig. 12**), confirming their schwannian origin, as well as glial fibrillary acidic protein (GFAP), neuron-specific enolase (NSE), and CD57. EMA-positive perineurial cells may be seen at the periphery of the lesion. Nerve sheath myxoma frequently recurs if incompletely excised.

Nerve sheath myxoma was previously grouped with the entity neurothekeoma, which is similarly myxoid, superficial, and benign; however, the two lesions are now understood to be distinct

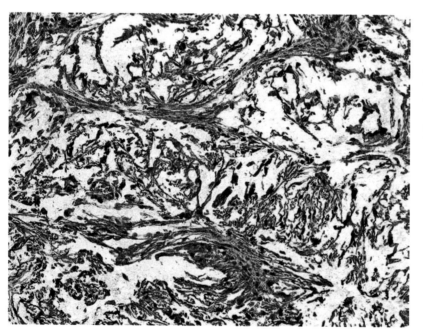

Fig. 12. Nerve sheath myxoma. Stellate, spindle, and epithelial cells are diffusely immunoreactive for the S-100 protein, confirming the nerve sheath origin of this neoplasm (S-100 protein immunostain, original magnification ×100).

and have nonoverlapping clinical and pathologic features. Briefly, neurothekeoma preferentially affects female patients over a wide age range (pediatric to adult), is commonly found on the head and upper extremity, rarely recurs, and consists of epithelioid cells that are not immunoreactive for the S-100 protein.[13,14] The differential diagnosis of nerve sheath myxoma and neurothekeoma includes other nerve sheath tumors with myxoid stroma as well as other superficial myxoid lesions, such as cutaneous myxoma (superficial angiomyxoma), superficial acral fibromyxoma, and spindle cell lipoma.

PERINEURIOMA

Perineurioma is a rare benign neoplasm comprised of perineurial cells, most often occurring in the extremities or trunks of adults.[15–17] Like NF2, perineurioma is associated with abnormalities of chromosome 22.[18,19] Grossly, perineurioma is typically well-circumscribed and not associated with a nerve. Microscopically, a conventional perineurioma is composed of bland, elongated spindle cells arranged in parallel rows (Fig. 13) with variably whorled or storiform patterns (Fig. 14) and little to no atypia or mitotic activity. The spindled perineurial cells are immunoreactive for EMA (often focal) (Fig. 15), GLUT1 (Fig. 16), and claudin-1 and are negative for the S-100 protein. Intraneural perineurioma is a benign neoplasm in which the perineurial cells grow within and expand a nerve, characterized by a classic concentric onion-bulb appearance to the layers of perineurial cells (Fig. 17).[20] Additional perineurioma variants include the intestinal,[21] reticular,[22,23] and sclerosing subtypes.[24]

The differential diagnosis of perineurioma includes the other benign nerve sheath tumors, meningioma, and low-grade fibromyxoid sarcoma. Unlike neurofibroma, perineurioma is typically composed of one cell type; however, hybrid lesions, such as mixed perineurioma/schwannoma[25] and mixed perineurioma/neurofibroma,[26,27] have been described. Like perineurioma, meningioma has a whorled architecture and displays EMA and claudin-1 positivity; however, the clinical location of the lesion (ie, head and neck region) may be helpful. Like perineurioma, low-grade fibromyxoid sarcoma is composed of bland, monotonous spindle cells that are immunoreactive for EMA and claudin-1; however, it is characterized by a diagnostic translocation t(7;16) (q34; p11), forming the fusion product FUS-CREB3L2 or FUS-CREB3L1.[28] Recurrence or malignant transformation of perineurioma is rare.[29]

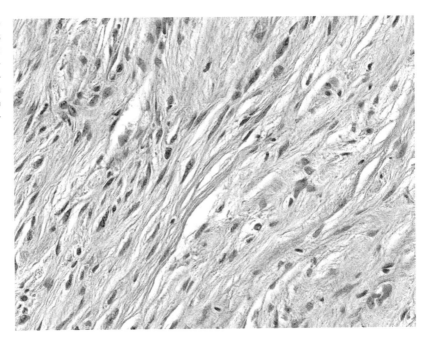

Fig. 13. Perineurioma. Elongated spindle cells with thin nuclei with tapering ends and terminal cytoplasmic processes are arranged in a delicate fibrous stroma (H&E, original magnification ×160).

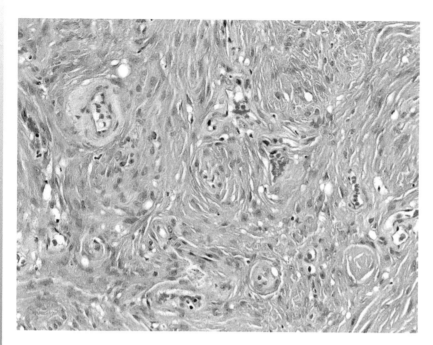

Fig. 14. Perineurioma. Spindled to epithelioid cells with delicate, open chromatin are arranged in a storiform pattern with meningothelial-like perivascular whorls (H&E, original magnification ×160).

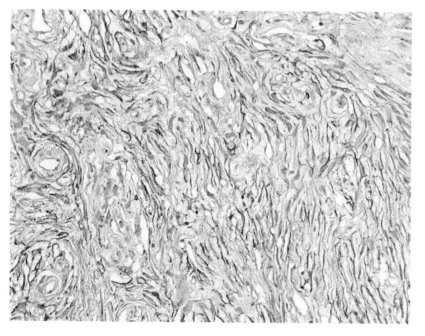

Fig. 15. Perineurioma. An immunostain for EMA highlights the thin, tapered cytoplasmic processes of perineurial cells (EMA immunostain, original magnification ×100).

Fig. 16. Perineurioma. An immunostain for GLUT1 is immunoreactive in the cytoplasm of perineurial cells (GLUT1 immunostain, original magnification ×100).

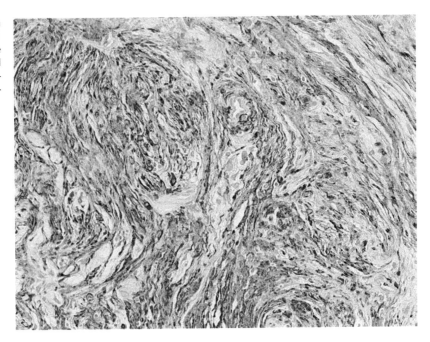

Fig. 17. Intraneural perineurioma. Concentric rings of short, spindled perineurial cells surround axons within a nerve, creating an onion bulb–like appearance (H&E, original magnification ×100).

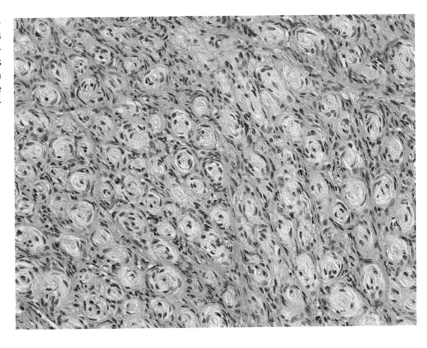

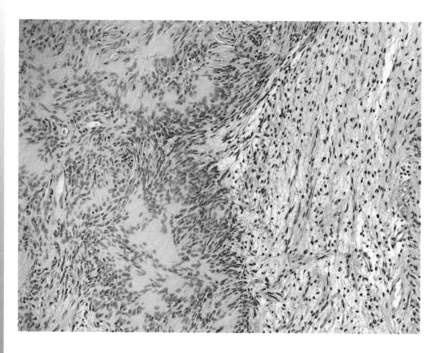

Fig. 18. Schwannoma. The typical biphasic pattern consists of alternating cellular Antoni A areas with palisading wavy Schwann cell nuclei (Verocay bodies) (*left*) adjacent to myxoid and less cellular Antoni B areas (*right*) (H&E, original magnification ×64).

SCHWANNOMA

Schwannoma is a benign neoplastic proliferation of Schwann cells with a wide anatomic distribution, including superficial and deep soft tissues as well as the gastrointestinal tract. Schwannomas of the cerebellopontine angle (acoustic neuromas) are associated with NF2, which is an autosomal dominant disorder with a defect in the merlin gene located on chromosome 22q12.[8] Patients with NF2 develop bilateral acoustic neuromas and an array of associated lesions, including glial hamartomas, meningiomas, and ependymomas.[7,8]

Grossly, the growth pattern of schwannoma is most often solitary, well-circumscribed, and encapsulated but rarely can be plexiform. A nerve

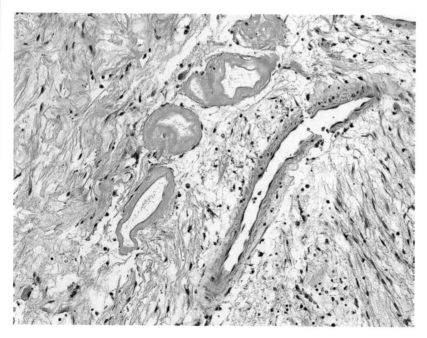

Fig. 19. Schwannoma. Prominent gaping vessels with hyalinized walls are a characteristic feature, here seen in a hypocellular, Antoni B areas (H&E, original magnification ×64).

Fig. 20. Myxoid schwannoma. The stroma may be focally or extensively myxoid and contain scattered spindled and stellate cells with wavy, tapered nuclei and focal hyperchromasia (H&E, original magnification ×100).

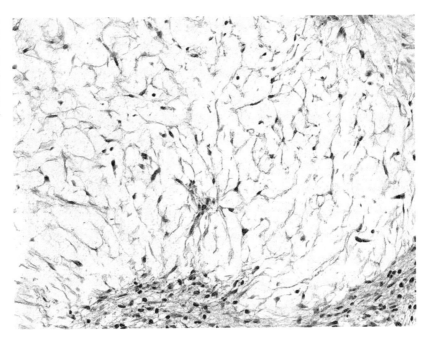

of origin may be seen attached to the tumor. Microscopically, a conventional schwannoma is a biphasic tumor comprised of bland spindle cells with wavy nuclei arranged in alternating cellular areas (Antoni A) with nuclear palisading (Verocay bodies) and less cellular, myxoid, or hyalinized areas (Antoni B) (**Fig. 18**). Schwannoma also characteristically features a fibrous capsule, a peripheral lymphoid cuff, and prominent hyalinized vessels containing luminal thrombi (**Fig. 19**). The stroma of a schwannoma is occasionally myxoid (**Fig. 20**). Ancient schwannoma displays widespread degenerative change, including cystic degeneration, hemorrhage, and marked nuclear

Fig. 21. Cellular schwannoma. Bland-appearing spindle cells with wavy nuclei and tapered ends are tightly arranged in sweeping fascicles with no Verocay bodies or Antoni B areas (H&E, original magnification ×100).

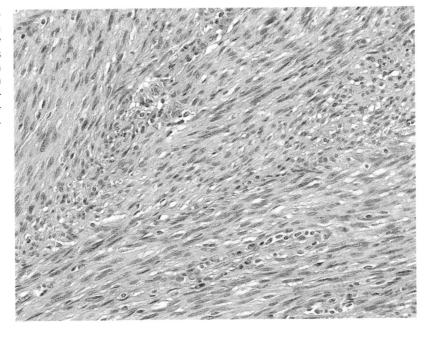

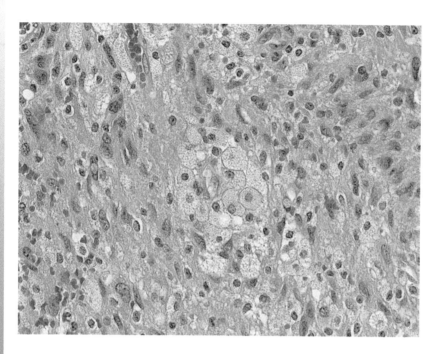

Fig. 22. Cellular schwannoma. Aggregates of foamy macrophages are frequently seen dispersed among spindled to epithelioid cells (H&E, original magnification ×160).

atypia, such as nuclear enlargement and hyperchromasia. Mitotic activity and necrosis, however, are rare.

Cellular schwannoma consists of primarily densely cellular Antoni A areas (**Fig. 21**) without the presence of Verocay bodies or Antoni B areas.[30,31] Cellular schwannoma often displays scattered aggregates of foamy macrophages (**Fig. 22**), increased mitotic activity, and focal atypia. Epithelioid schwannoma is a rare, well-circumscribed lesion characterized by plump rounded Schwann cells arranged in cords or nests (**Fig. 23**).[11,32] Epithelioid schwannoma, like all other schwannoma variants, is strongly and

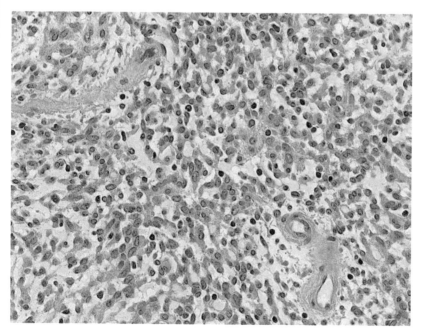

Fig. 23. Epithelioid schwannoma. Plump cells with uniform, rounded nuclei and minimal atypia are arranged in a slightly myxoid stroma (H&E, original magnification ×160).

Fig. 24. Epithelioid schwannoma. The round Schwann cells are diffusely and strongly immunoreactive for the S-100 protein in the nucleus and cytoplasm (S-100 protein immunostain, original magnification ×160).

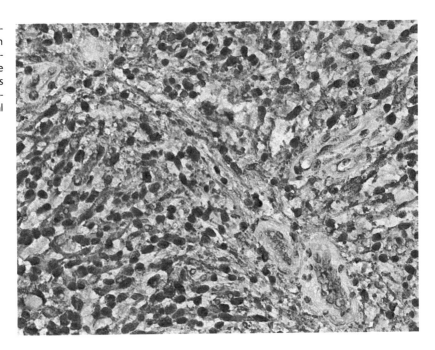

diffusely immunoreactive for the S-100 protein in the nuclei and cytoplasm (**Fig. 24**). Melanotic (pigmented) schwannoma displays hyperchromatic nuclei with evidence of both schwannian and melanocytic differentiation, including granular melanin within the tumor cells (**Fig. 25**). Melanotic schwannoma is associated with the Carney complex of cardiac and cutaneous myxomas, endocrine hyperactivity, and hyperpigmentation.[33]

Ganglioneuroma is a differentiated neoplasm typically arising in the mediastinum or retroperitoneum that consists of mature ganglion cells embedded within schwannian stroma (**Fig. 26**). It is the fully differentiated form of neuroblastoma

Fig. 25. Melanotic (pigmented) schwannoma. Epithelioid and spindled cells display hyperchromatic, enlarged nuclei and coarsely granular cytoplasmic melanin pigment (H&E, original magnification ×100).

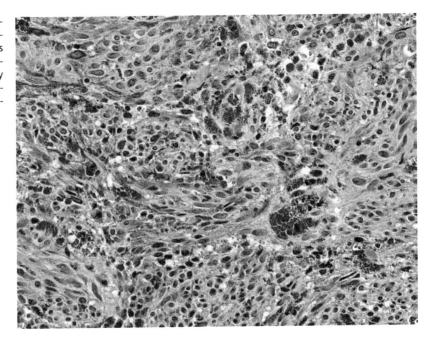

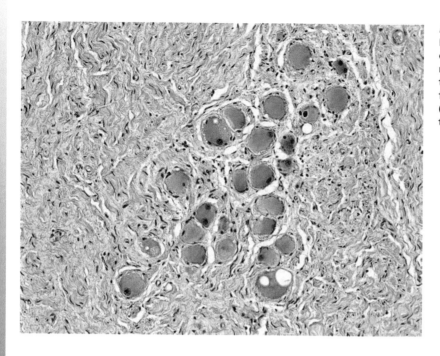

Fig. 26. Ganglioneuroma. Mature ganglion cells are embedded in a schwannian stroma and represent the fully differentiated form of neuroblastoma (H&E, original magnification ×64).

and lacks immature elements. Multiple ganglioneuromas are seen in NF1 and MEN, type II. Additional schwannoma variants include neuroblastoma-like schwannoma (neurilemmoma)[34] and plexiform schwannoma.[35–37]

The differential diagnosis of a cellular schwannoma includes other benign nerve sheath tumors as well as non-neural, bland-appearing spindle cell lesions, such as fibromatosis, leiomyoma, and low-grade fibromyxoid sarcoma. In addition to the distinctive cytomorphologic features (described previously), the immunophenotype of the lesion can aid in the diagnosis.[2] For instance, schwannoma is diffusely and strongly immunoreactive

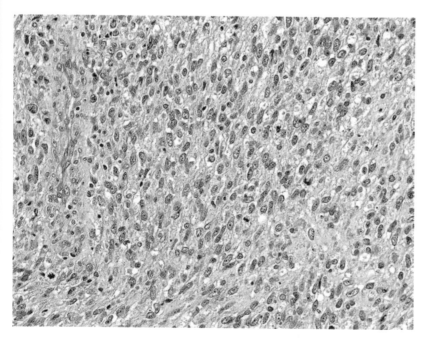

Fig. 27. MPNST. Pleomorphic spindle cells are arranged in a vaguely fascicular pattern and display nuclear enlargement with frequent mitotic figures (H&E, original magnification ×100).

for the S-100 protein; fibromatosis is positive for actin and nuclear β-catenin; leiomyoma is positive for actin and desmin; and low-grade fibromyxoid sarcoma is positive for EMA and claudin-1. In addition, schwannoma with degenerative atypia is also diffusely immunoreactive for the S-100 protein; this aids in distinguishing it from MPNST, which typically only has focal reactivity for the S-100 protein.

MALIGNANT PERIPHERAL NERVE SHEATH TUMOR

MPNST is an intermediate to high-grade, malignant counterpart to the benign nerve sheath tumors (described previously) and may show incomplete differentiation toward one type of the nerve sheath cells.[29,38] MPNST most commonly arises from major nerves of the deep soft tissue in adult patients; however, it may also occur in the pediatric population. It arises either de novo or in association with NF.

Grossly, MPNST is a large infiltrative tumor that is associated with a major nerve. Conventional MPNST is a cellular neoplasm comprised of pleomorphic spindle cells with atypical features, including nuclear enlargement and hyperchromasia (**Fig. 27**), commonly arranged in sweeping fascicles. The nuclei are wavy and characteristically pointed at one end and blunt at the other (**Fig. 28**), with occasional triangular forms. The mitotic activity is brisk with atypical mitotic figures. MPNST frequently displays geographic necrosis with peripheral nuclear palisading, similar to what is seen in glioblastoma. MPNST often contains

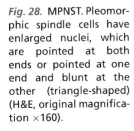

Differential Diagnosis
PERIPHERAL NERVE SHEATH TUMORS

Benign peripheral nerve sheath tumors

Leiomyoma

Fibromatosis

Solitary fibrous tumor

Inflammatory myofibroblastic tumor

Low-grade fibromyxoid sarcoma

MPNSTs

Synovial sarcoma

Fibrosarcoma

Leiomyosarcoma

Clear cell sarcoma

Sarcomatoid carcinoma

Melanoma

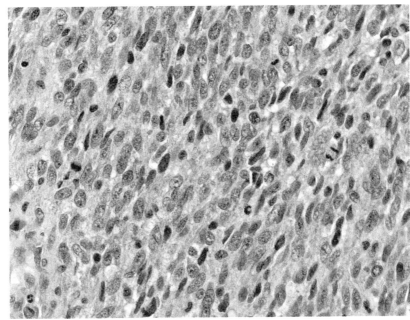

Fig. 28. MPNST. Pleomorphic spindle cells have enlarged nuclei, which are pointed at both ends or pointed at one end and blunt at the other (triangle-shaped) (H&E, original magnification ×160).

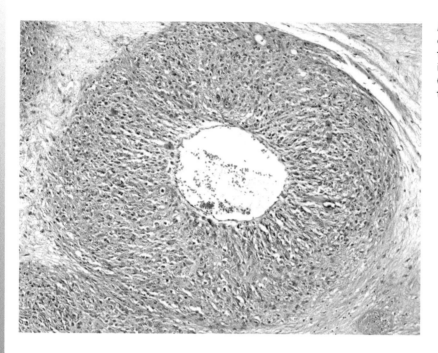

Fig. 29. MPNST. Neoplastic cells condense beneath the prominent vessels and infiltrate the vessel walls (H&E, original magnification ×40).

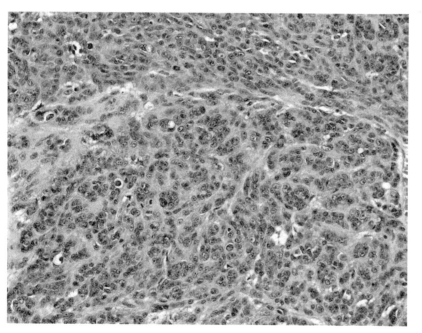

Fig. 30. Epithelioid MPNST. Neoplastic cells are round with prominent nucleoli, eosinophilic cytoplasm, and frequent mitotic figures (H&E, original magnification ×64).

Fig. 31. Epithelioid MPNST. Large cells with round nuclei, prominent nucleoli, and eosinophilic cytoplasm are arranged in islands and nests (H&E, original magnification ×64).

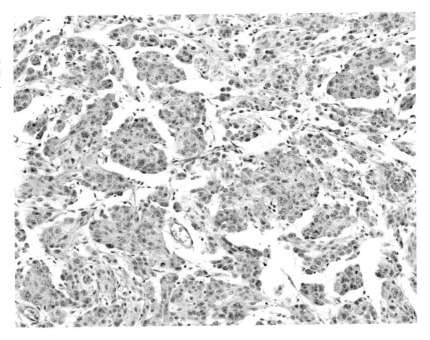

Fig. 32. MPNST with divergent differentiation. Heterologous elements including cartilage and bone are seen within fascicular malignant spindle cells (H&E, original magnification ×64).

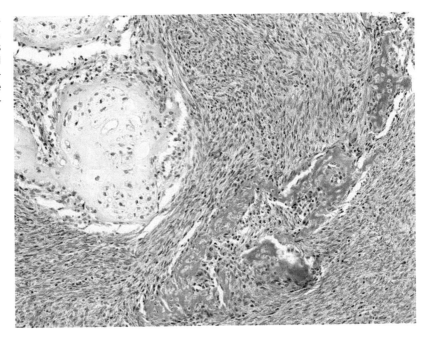

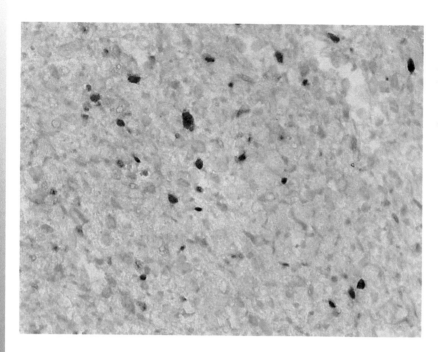

Fig. 33. Malignant triton tumor. Nuclear labeling for myogenin highlights focal skeletal muscle differentiation within an MPNST (myogenin immunostain, original magnification ×160).

prominent hyalinized vessels with cellular condensation adjacent to the vessels and infiltration of the malignant cells into the vessel walls (**Fig. 29**). Epithelioid MPNST is a rare variant comprised of rounded epithelial cells with prominent nucleoli

Pitfalls
PERIPHERAL NERVE SHEATH TUMORS

! Benign nerve sheath tumors can display degenerative atypia, including nuclear enlargement and hyperchromasia, often accompanied by cystic degeneration and hemorrhage, which should not be mistaken for malignancy. Note that benign schwannomas with degenerative atypia are diffusely and strongly immunoreactive for the S-100 protein, whereas true MPNSTs are usually only focally positive.

! Benign and malignant nerve sheath tumors can display extensive epithelioid morphology and should not be confused with carcinomas or melanoma.

! Nerve sheath tumors, such as neurofibroma and schwannoma, may contain melanin pigment and should not be confused with melanoma.

! Schwannomas may display focal immunoreactivity for cytokeratins and should not be confused with epithelial neoplasms.

(**Fig. 30**) that may form discrete islands and nests (**Fig. 31**).[39–41] Variant MPNST with divergent differentiation displays heterologous elements, such as bone and cartilage (**Fig. 32**). Malignant triton tumor is an MPNST containing focal skeletal muscle differentiation as highlighted by immunohistochemial stains for myogenin or desmin (**Fig. 33**).

The differential diagnosis of conventional MPNST includes intermediate to high-grade malignant sarcomas of soft tissue, such as undifferentiated pleomorphic sarcoma (malignant fibrous histiocytoma), pleomorphic liposarcoma, leiomyosarcoma, fibrosarcoma, and synovial sarcoma. The differential diagnosis for epithelioid MPNST also includes sarcomatoid carcinoma and melanoma. An immunohistochemical panel, including the S-100 protein, HMB45, Melan-A, cytokeratins, smooth muscle actin, desmin, calponin, INI1, CD34, β-catenin, and ALK can aid in the diagnosis.[2] Spindled MPNST is only focally immunoreactive for the S-100 protein, whereas epithelioid MPNST is diffusely positive. MPNST has a poor prognosis, with frequent local recurrence and distant hematogenous metastasis and a 5-year survival of 44%.[38]

REFERENCES

1. Jessen KR, Mirsky R. The origin and development of glial cells in peripheral nerves. Nat Rev Neurosci 2005;6(9):671–82.
2. Fisher C. Immunohistochemistry in diagnosis of soft tissue tumours. Histopathology 2011;58(7):1001–12.

3. Fanburg-Smith JC, Majidi M, Miettinen M. Keratin expression in schwannoma; a study of 115 retroperitoneal and 22 peripheral schwannomas. Mod Pathol 2006;19(1):115–21.

4. Pina-Oviedo S, Ortiz-Hidalgo C. The normal and neoplastic perineurium: a review. Adv Anat Pathol 2008;15(3):147–64.

5. Folpe AL, Billings SD, McKenney JK, et al. Expression of claudin-1, a recently described tight junction-associated protein, distinguishes soft tissue perineurioma from potential mimics. Am J Surg Pathol 2002; 26(12):1620–6.

6. Hirose T, Tani T, Shimada T, et al. Immunohistochemical demonstration of EMA/Glut1-positive perineurial cells and CD34-positive fibroblastic cells in peripheral nerve sheath tumors. Mod Pathol 2003;16(4): 293–8.

7. McClatchey AI. Neurofibromatosis. Annu Rev Pathol 2007;2:191–216.

8. Ferner RE. Neurofibromatosis 1 and neurofibromatosis 2: a twenty first century perspective. Lancet Neurol 2007;6(4):340–51.

9. Fetsch JF, Michal M, Miettinen M. Pigmented (melanotic) neurofibroma: a clinicopathologic and immunohistochemical analysis of 19 lesions from 17 patients. Am J Surg Pathol 2000;24(3):331–43.

10. Michal M, Fanburg-Smith JC, Mentzel T, et al. Dendritic cell neurofibroma with pseudorosettes: a report of 18 cases of a distinct and hitherto unrecognized neurofibroma variant. Am J Surg Pathol 2001;25(5):587–94.

11. Laskin WB, Fetsch JF, Lasota J, et al. Benign epithelioid peripheral nerve sheath tumors of the soft tissues: clinicopathologic spectrum of 33 cases. Am J Surg Pathol 2005;29(1):39–51.

12. Fetsch JF, Laskin WB, Miettinen M. Nerve sheath myxoma: a clinicopathologic and immunohistochemical analysis of 57 morphologically distinctive, S-100 protein- and GFAP-positive, myxoid peripheral nerve sheath tumors with a predilection for the extremities and a high local recurrence rate. Am J Surg Pathol 2005;29(12):1615–24.

13. Fetsch JF, Laskin WB, Hallman JR, et al. Neurothekeoma: an analysis of 178 tumors with detailed immunohistochemical data and long-term patient follow-up information. Am J Surg Pathol 2007;31(7):1103–14.

14. Hornick JL, Fletcher CD. Cellular neurothekeoma: detailed characterization in a series of 133 cases. Am J Surg Pathol 2007;31(3):329–40.

15. Hornick JL, Fletcher CD. Soft tissue perineurioma: clinicopathologic analysis of 81 cases including those with atypical histologic features. Am J Surg Pathol 2005;29(7):845–58.

16. Macarenco RS, Ellinger F, Oliveira AM. Perineurioma: a distinctive and underrecognized peripheral nerve sheath neoplasm. Arch Pathol Lab Med 2007; 131(4):625–36.

17. Rankine AJ, Filion PR, Platten MA, et al. Perineurioma: a clinicopathological study of eight cases. Pathology 2004;36(4):309–15.

18. Lasota J, Fetsch JF, Wozniak A, et al. The neurofibromatosis type 2 gene is mutated in perineurial cell tumors: a molecular genetic study of eight cases. Am J Pathol 2001;158(4):1223–9.

19. Brock JE, Perez-Atayde AR, Kozakewich HP, et al. Cytogenetic aberrations in perineurioma: variation with subtype. Am J Surg Pathol 2005;29(9):1164–9.

20. Boyanton BL Jr, Jones JK, Shenaq SM, et al. Intraneural perineurioma: a systematic review with illustrative cases. Arch Pathol Lab Med 2007;131(9): 1382–92.

21. Hornick JL, Fletcher CD. Intestinal perineuriomas: clinicopathologic definition of a new anatomic subset in a series of 10 cases. Am J Surg Pathol 2005;29(7):859–65.

22. Graadt van Roggen JF, McMenamin ME, Belchis DA, et al. Reticular perineurioma: a distinctive variant of soft tissue perineurioma. Am J Surg Pathol 2001;25(4):485–93.

23. Mentzel T, Kutzner H. Reticular and plexiform perineurioma: clinicopathological and immunohistochemical analysis of two cases and review of perineurial neoplasms of skin and soft tissues. Virchows Arch 2005;447(4):677–82.

24. Fetsch JF, Miettinen M. Sclerosing perineurioma: a clinicopathologic study of 19 cases of a distinctive soft tissue lesion with a predilection for the fingers and palms of young adults. Am J Surg Pathol 1997;21(12):1433–42.

25. Hornick JL, Bundock EA, Fletcher CD. Hybrid schwannoma/perineurioma: clinicopathologic analysis of 42 distinctive benign nerve sheath tumors. Am J Surg Pathol 2009;33(10):1554–61.

26. Kazakov DV, Pitha J, Sima R, et al. Hybrid peripheral nerve sheath tumors: schwannoma-perineurioma and neurofibroma-perineurioma. A report of three cases in extradigital locations. Ann Diagn Pathol 2005;9(1):16–23.

27. Shelekhova KV, Danilova AB, Michal M, et al. Hybrid neurofibroma-perineurioma: an additional example of an extradigital tumor. Ann Diagn Pathol 2008; 12(3):233–4.

28. Thway K, Fisher C, Debiec-Rychter M, et al. Claudin-1 is expressed in perineurioma-like low-grade fibromyxoid sarcoma. Hum Pathol 2009;40(11):1586–90.

29. Hirose T, Scheithauer BW, Sano T. Perineurial malignant peripheral nerve sheath tumor (MPNST): a clinicopathologic, immunohistochemical, and ultrastructural study of seven cases. Am J Surg Pathol 1998;22(11): 1368–78.

30. Lodding P, Kindblom LG, Angervall L, et al. Cellular schwannoma. A clinicopathologic study of 29 cases. Virchows Arch A Pathol Anat Histopathol 1990; 416(3):237–48.

31. White W, Shiu MH, Rosenblum MK, et al. Cellular schwannoma. A clinicopathologic study of 57 patients and 58 tumors. Cancer 1990;66(6):1266–75.

32. Kindblom LG, Meis-Kindblom JM, Havel G, et al. Benign epithelioid schwannoma. Am J Surg Pathol 1998;22(6):762–70.

33. Carney JA. The carney complex (myxomas, spotty pigmentation, endocrine overactivity, and schwannomas). Dermatol Clin 1995;13(1):19–26.

34. Goldblum JR, Beals TF, Weiss SW. Neuroblastoma-like neurilemoma. Am J Surg Pathol 1994;18(3):266–73.

35. Hirose T, Scheithauer BW, Sano T. Giant plexiform schwannoma: a report of two cases with soft tissue and visceral involvement. Mod Pathol 1997;10(11):1075–81.

36. Agaram NP, Prakash S, Antonescu CR. Deep-seated plexiform schwannoma: a pathologic study of 16 cases and comparative analysis with the superficial variety. Am J Surg Pathol 2005;29(8):1042–8.

37. Berg JC, Scheithauer BW, Spinner RJ, et al. Plexiform schwannoma: a clinicopathologic overview with emphasis on the head and neck region. Hum Pathol 2008;39(5):633–40.

38. Wanebo JE, Malik JM, VandenBerg SR, et al. Malignant peripheral nerve sheath tumors. A clinicopathologic study of 28 cases. Cancer 1993;71(4):1247–53.

39. Lodding P, Kindblom LG, Angervall L. Epithelioid malignant schwannoma. A study of 14 cases. Virchows Arch A Pathol Anat Histopathol 1986;409(4):433–51.

40. Laskin WB, Weiss SW, Bratthauer GL. Epithelioid variant of malignant peripheral nerve sheath tumor (malignant epithelioid schwannoma). Am J Surg Pathol 1991;15(12):1136–45.

41. McMenamin ME, Fletcher CD. Expanding the spectrum of malignant change in schwannomas: epithelioid malignant change, epithelioid malignant peripheral nerve sheath tumor, and epithelioid angiosarcoma: a study of 17 cases. Am J Surg Pathol 2001;25(1):13–25.

CLEAR CELL TUMORS OF SOFT TISSUE

Aaron Auerbach, MD, MPH[a], David S. Cassarino, MD, PhD[b],*

KEYWORDS
- Clear cell sarcoma • Malignant melanoma of soft parts • Perivascular epithelioid cell tumor
- Angiomyolipoma • Clear cell myomelanocytic tumor • Lymphangioleiomyomatosis
- Tuberous sclerosis

ABSTRACT

Clear cell lesions of soft tissue include varying morphologic patterns and a range of clinical behaviors and prognoses. Benign lesions include perivascular epithelioid cell tumors, clear cell fibrous papule, and distinctive dermal clear cell mesenchymal tumor; malignant tumors include clear cell sarcoma, liposarcoma, and rare malignant perivascular epithelioid cell tumors. Clear cell variants of other benign and malignant soft tissue tumors include fibrous histiocytoma, atypical fibroxanthoma, myoepithelioma, leiomyoma and leiomyosarcoma, and rhabdomyosarcoma. Metastatic clear cell tumors, including renal cell carcinoma and adrenal cortical carcinoma, should be considered in the differential diagnosis and excluded through clinical history, imaging studies, and immunohistochemical stains.

OVERVIEW OF CLEAR CELL TUMORS OF SOFT TISSUE

Clear cell tumors of soft tissue comprise a heterogenous group of neoplasms with varying morphologic patterns and a wide range of clinical behaviors and prognoses.[1] Benign tumors include most cases of perivascular epithelioid cell tumors (PEComas), clear cell fibrous papule, and distinctive dermal clear cell mesenchymal tumor, and malignant tumors include clear cell sarcoma (malignant melanoma of soft parts), liposarcoma (see article by Singhi and Montgomery elsewhere in this issue), and rare malignant PEComas.[1–3] In addition, clear cell variants of dermatofibroma/

fibrous histiocytoma, atypical fibroxanthoma, pleomorphic sarcoma (malignant fibrous histiocytoma), leiomyoma and leiomyosarcoma, rhabdomyosarcoma, and myoepithelioma have also been described.[4,5] Metastatic clear cell tumors involving the soft tissue, such as renal cell carcinoma (RCC), hepatocellular carcinoma (HCC), and adrenal cortical carcinoma, should also be considered in the differential diagnosis and be excluded through complete clinical history, examination, and imaging studies as well as appropriate immunohistochemical stains.

PEComa

PEComa is the common abbreviation for a heterogeneous group of rare neoplasms with an apparent perivascular epithelioid cell differentiation. PEComas are mesenchymal neoplasms in which the perivascular epithelioid cells have a unique phenotype, in that they are immunoreactive for both melanocytic and smooth muscle markers.[3,6–11] There is a well-known association between PEComas and tuberous sclerosis.[3,6,7] Similar to pleomorphic hyalinizing angiectatic tumor of soft parts, epithelioid sarcoma, and alveolar soft part sarcoma, PEComas are typically classified as tumors of uncertain differentiation, because they do not have a known normal histologic counterpart.[3,7]

In 1992, Bonetti, and colleagues[6] first described PEComas (although they did not use that term specifically) as tumor cells with epithelioid histology, clear cytoplasm, and a perivascular location. As the phenotype and natural history of

[a] Department of Pathology, Joint Pathology Center, 606 Stephen Sitter Avenue, Silver Spring, MD 20910, USA
[b] Department of Pathology, Sunset Medical Center, Southern California Permanente Medical Group, 4867 Sunset Boulevard, 2nd floor, Los Angeles, CA 90027, USA
* Corresponding author.
E-mail address: dsc9w@yahoo.com

Surgical Pathology 4 (2011) 783–798
doi:10.1016/j.path.2011.08.005
1875-9181/11/$ – see front matter © 2011 Published by Elsevier Inc.

surgpath.theclinics.com

Key Features
PECOMAS

1. PEComas are a heterogeneous group of rare neoplasms with perivascular epithelioid cell differentiation, including AML, CCST, CCMMT, and LAM.

2. They often are associated with tuberous sclerosis syndrome (AML, CCST, and LAM types).

3. They often have clear cytoplasm, a perivascular location, and spindled (myoid) cells and/or fat.

4. By immunohistochemistry, the cells express melanocytic markers (Melan-A/MART-1, HMB-45, tyrosinase, MITF, but usually not S100) and myoid markers (desmin, SMA, calponin).

5. Most cases are benign, but criteria for aggressive clinical behavior include size, infiltrative growth pattern, marked hypercellularity, nuclear grade, numerous mitotic figures (>1/50 high-power fields [hpf]), atypical mitotic figures, and necrosis.

PEComas became better understood, other tumors, particularly in the liver and the lung, were discovered to show similarities to PEComas.[7,8] Many of these lesions are now reclassified as PEComa or are included in the family of tumors called PEComas. Currently, PEComas consist of a category of tumors that include angiomyolipoma (AML), clear cell sugar tumor (CCST) of lung, clear cell myomelanocytic tumor (CCMMT) of falciform ligament/ligamentum teres, and lymphangioleiomyomatosis (LAM) as well as a few other rare tumors.[3,6–10] Even though these lesions fall within the family of tumors known as PEComas, it is still common to use their established names (ie, AML, CCST, CCMMT, and LAM), because they correlate with the clinical-anatomic characteristics associated with these lesions.

GROSS AND MICROSCOPIC FEATURES

The gross appearance of PEComas is variable, given the tumor type and location. Most cases appear firm and tan-yellow grossly and can measure up to 5 cm in diameter. The tumor cells in PEComas are epithelioid to spindled in shape and are often arranged around blood vessels and penetrate the smooth muscle of small blood vessels. They have clear to granular eosinophilic cytoplasm; small, round, and centrally located nuclei; and

usually small, indistinct nucleoli (Fig. 1). Some cases have a myoid component with more dense, eosinophilic-staining cytoplasm; these cases usually have more spindle-shaped nuclei (Fig. 2). The tumor cells can be found tightly surrounding blood vessels or may be seen radiating away from the blood vessels. PEComas often have a prominent vasculature with small arching thin-walled blood vessels that divide the tumor into distinct sections. Fatty change can be present, usually in angiomyolipomas. Only rarely is melanin pigmentation identified. Some PEComas show more pronounced nuclear atypia, although these are often only focally present or in scattered cells. Sclerosing PEComas are variants that show extensive dense sclerotic hypocellular collagenous stromal hyalinization and have been described in the uterus, retroperitoneum, and pelvis.[9] Sclerosing PEComas often lack the prominent vascular pattern expected in most PEComas. By ultrastructural analysis, PEComas contain microfilament bundles with electron-dense condensation, increased numbers of mitochondria, and membrane-bound dense granules.[10]

IMMUNOHISTOCHEMICAL FEATURES

PEComas have a unique phenotype, because they are immunoreactive for both melanocytic and muscle markers.[3,9–11] Both the myoid component and the fat component of these tumors typically express these immunomarkers. The epithelioid cells in PEComas, however, are often more strongly positive for melanocytic markers compared with myoid markers.[9–11] Alternatively, the spindle cells stain stronger for myoid markers than melanocytic markers.[9–11] The melanocytic markers include HMB-45 (Fig. 3), MART-1/Melan-A, tyrosinase, and microphthalmia transcription factor (MITF), but S100 is often negative. These immunostains demonstrate cytoplasmic positivity, except for MITF, which is a nuclear stain.[11] Positive in up to 90% of cases, HMB-45 and MART-1/Melan-A are the most sensitive melanocytic markers.[11] Muscle markers that are expressed in PEComas include smooth muscle actin, myosin, calponin, desmin (often weak and focal) and h-caldesmon (only a subset of cases). Desmin is more often expressed in both sclerosing and cutaneous PEComas.[8,9] Although neither a melanocytic nor a myoid marker, CD117 has been found immunoreactive in rare PEComas.[3,9] There can also be aberrant CD1a staining in some tumors, but this may only be endogenous biotin staining and not true immunopositivity.[12,13] Epithelial membrane antigen (EMA) and transcription factor E3 (TFE3) expression have been reported in some cases, the significance of which is undetermined.[14]

Fig. 1. PEComa at high magnification shows epithelioid cells with nuclear hyperchromasia and abundant clear cytoplasm proliferating around vessels.

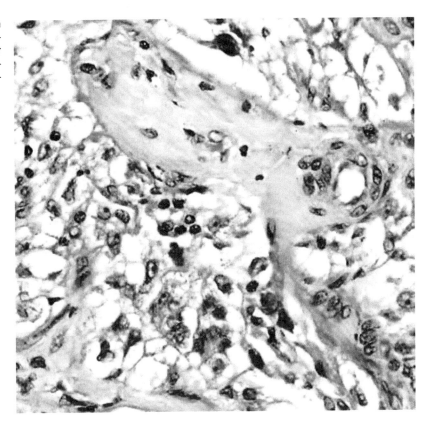

Fig. 2. Another area of the same tumor shows a proliferation of spindle-shaped, myoid-like cells and scattered cells with greater atypia.

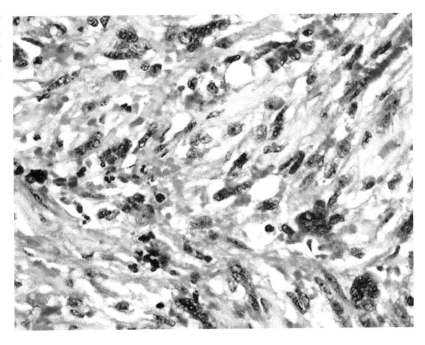

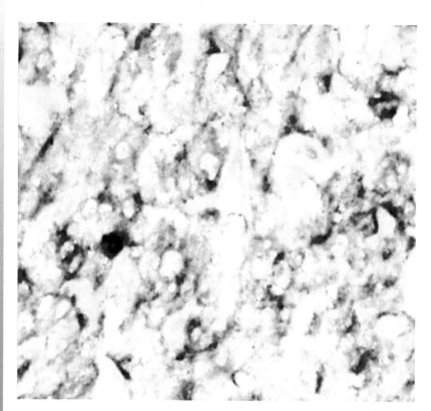

Fig. 3. HMB-45 immunohistochemistry shows strong cytoplasmic expression in PEComa; myoid markers are also immunoreactive (not shown).

EPIDEMIOLOGY OF PEComas

PEComas are rare, but the most common types are AML, CCST, and LAM. They typically occur in adults in their fiftieth and sixtieth decades. In younger patients, PEComas often are associated with tuberous sclerosis.[3,7–9] PEComas are more common in women, with a female-to-male ratio of approximately 5:1.[3,7] Although soft tissue, lungs, kidney, and liver are the most common anatomic locations involved with these tumors, PEComas have recently been described in other sites, such as the gynecologic tract,[9,14,15] bladder,[16] skin,[8,17] and bone.[18] Although CCMMT of falciform ligament/ligamentum teres is included in the PEComa family, it has different epidemiologic characteristics.[3,14,19] CCMT occurs in younger patients than other PEComas and more often in men.[19] Unlike other PEComas, which usually are epithelioid, CCMMT is almost exclusively a spindle cell lesion. These tumors involve, or are next to, the falciform ligament or ligamentum teres in most cases.[19]

TREATMENT AND PROGNOSIS

Most PEComas are benign lesions that are usually treated with full surgical excision. Rarely, there are examples of malignant PEComas with aggressive clinical behavior, including metastasis.[3,14] Recently, criteria have been proposed to classify these tumors as benign, of uncertain malignancy, or malignant.[14] Criteria for malignancy include size, an infiltrative growth pattern, marked hypercellularity, nuclear grade, numerous mitotic figures (>1/50 hpf), atypical mitotic figures, and necrosis.[14] The presence of more than one of these criteria is highly predictive of aggressive clinical course. PEComas that show malignant clinical behavior are usually not AML, LAM, or CCST types.[14] The literature shows that cases of PEComas with only epithelioid cells and no spindle cells exhibit a higher malignant potential.[20]

ANGIOMYOLIPOMA

AML is the most common type of PEComa.[3,10,20] Renal AML is found in more than 40% of patients with tuberous sclerosis, but only approximately 20% of patients with AML also have tuberous sclerosis. AML is most commonly found in the kidney and second-most often in the liver but has also been reported in most other anatomic sites.[3,8,10] Typically, AML shows thick-walled blood vessels, spindled and epithelioid smooth muscle cells, and fat or lipid-like PECs resembling fat (**Fig. 4**).

Fig. 4. An example of an AML with large, eosinophilic-staining myoid-like cells on the left and lipomatous clear cells on the right.

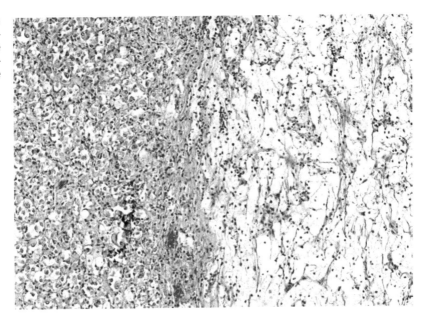

Some blood vessel walls contain perivascular epithelial cells, but others only contain smooth muscle. Tumors with mostly myoid cells may be mistaken for a smooth muscle tumor, such as a leiomyoma, and those with mostly lipid-like PECs can be mistaken for an adipocytic tumor, such as a liposarcoma. Epithelioid cells are dominant in less than 10% of AMLs, most often in hepatic AMLs.[10,20] Although most AMLs are benign, epithelioid AMLs are more likely to be malignant.[20] AMLs in the kidney can involve local lymph nodes, but some case are thought due to a multifocal growth pattern and not true metastasis.[20,21] Cystic AML is another recently described AML variant, which is a solid-cystic lesion with epithelial cysts lined by keratin-positive cuboidal to hobnailed cells with a subepithelial cambium-like layer of HMB-45+, Melan-A+, CD10+ stromal cells.[22]

LYMPHANGIOMYOMATOSIS

LAM is a rare progressive pulmonary disease, which usually presents in young women and rarely can be extrapulmonary.[23,24] Patients usually show a slow progression to respiratory failure due to destruction of lung parenchyma by cyst formation.[23–25] LAM consists of myoid-appearing, spindled to epithelioid-shaped PECs (Fig. 5), which are HMB-45+ and desmin+ and are arranged around thin-walled vascular channels surrounding bronchi, septae, and pleura. Rare cases show prominent clear cell change mimicking CCST but still have an LAM distribution pattern. Multifocal

micronodular penumocyte hyperplasia is also usually present in the lungs.[25] In patients with tuberous sclerosis, LAM is found in less than 3% of cases. Approximately half of the people with LAM also have AML in their kidneys. Unfortunately, patients with LAM have a poor prognosis and are often treated with lung transplantation but show a less than 10-year median survival.[25]

CLEAR CELL SUGAR TUMOR

Initially described by Liebow and Castleman in 1963, CCST is a rare benign, usually primary pulmonary, tumor which is composed of round to spindle-shaped, HMB-45+ epithelioid cells.[26,27] The cells show clear to eosinophilic-staining cytoplasm, and well-delineated prominent cellular borders, which surround blood vessels (Fig. 6). Like other PEComas, there is a well-developed thin-walled vasculature, and the vessels can be hyalinized or dilated. The tumor cells often form a nested or alveolar architecture. There are occasional spindled cells, and the tumor cells often contain glycogen and melanosomes. Extrapulmonary CCST is notable in that it shows increased nuclear atypia and more mitotic figures.[3,26] Some cases of CCST are associated with tuberous sclerosis or LAM, although most occur sporadically.[3,26,27]

PECOMAS AND TUBEROUS SCLEROSIS

PEComas seem related to the genetic alterations of tuberous sclerosis complex (TSC), a genetic disease due to losses of TSC1 on chromosome

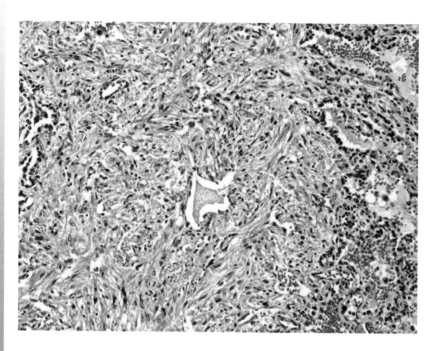

Fig. 5. LAM demonstrating spindled to epithelioid-shaped myoid cells arranged around thin walled vascular channel, similar to angio-myolipoma. Cystic areas were seen elsewhere in the morphologic sections.

9q34 and TSC2 on chromosome 16p13.3, which seem to have a role in the regulation of the Rheb/mTOR/p70S6K pathway.[3,10,26] These genes are involved with catecholamine metabolism and melanin formation, and most of these cases have an autosomal dominant transmission pattern. These patients also present with mental retardation, seizures, subependymal giant cell tumors, cardiac rhabdomyomas, cutaneous angiofibromas, and pulmonary multifocal micronodular hyperplasia. AML, CCST, and LAM are associated with tuberous sclerosis, but the other types of PEComas have not been associated with tuberous sclerosis.[3,8,10,26]

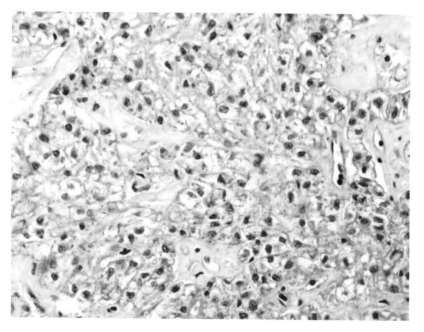

Fig. 6. CCST of the lung showing clear cells with vesicular nuclei and prominent cytoplasmic borders surrounding blood vessels.

Differential Diagnosis
PECOMA

PEComa	Versus Differential Entity	Distinguishing Features that Differ from Major Entity
	Clear Cell Sarcoma	Less prominent vascularity than PEComas Tumor nests and fascicles surrounded by prominent fibrous bands
	Melanoma	Both tumors express melanocytic markers, such as HMB-45, MART-1, and tyrosinase, but S100 is much more likely + in melanoma Melanoma also does not express myoid markers, such as smooth muscle actin and desmin
	Renal Cell Carcinoma	Very prominent small vessels surround the tumor cells Express cytokeratins and EMA, RCC antigen; negative for melanocytic markers
	Smooth Muscle Tumors	Smooth muscle tumors do not contain mature fat and also lack the prominent blood vessels, which are common in PEComas Also, negative for melanocytic markers

DIFFERENTIAL DIAGNOSIS

The differential diagnosis includes other tumors with clear cell morphology, including spindle cell and epithelioid tumors, smooth muscle neoplasms with clear cell features, and tumors expressing melanocytic antigens.[1,3,7–9,14,26] The differential also includes carcinomas, which often show clear cells, including RCC, but these tumors usually do not have the adipose component seen in some PEComas. RCC shows a proliferation of predominantly clear epithelial cells with a prominent vascular pattern, which can mimic PEComa, but RCC often also shows more dilated vessels and areas of hemorrhage (Fig. 7), which are lacking in PEComa. In addition, some cases may present with predominantly spindled cells. RCC also differs from PEComa by showing keratin and

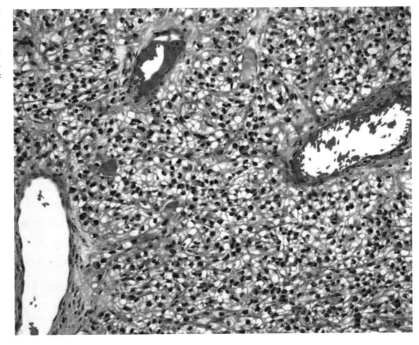

Fig. 7. RCC shows a proliferation of tumor cells with ample clear cytoplasm, small hyperchromatic nuclei, and prominent thin-walled vasculature with areas of hemorrhage.

RCC antibody immunoexpression.[28] HCCs can show a trabecular growth pattern and can produce bile, features that are not seen in other tumors (**Fig. 8**). HCC also has a different phenotype from PEComa, because HCC expresses cytokeratins, HepPar1, Arginase, and glypican 3 as well as showing canalicular staining for CD10 and polyclonal carcinoembryonic antigen (CEA).[29]

Because PEComas express myoid markers, smooth muscle tumors need to be separated from them. Histologically, smooth muscle tumors are composed of fascicles of spindle cells with blunt ends (cigar-shaped nuclei) and eosinophilic cytoplasm.[30] With rare exceptions, smooth muscle tumors do not contain mature fat, unlike many PEComas. Smooth muscle tumors also lack the prominent blood vessels that are common to PEComas. Although smooth muscle tumors express myoid markers, such as desmin and smooth muscle actin, they are negative for melanocytic markers, such as HMB-45, MART-1/Melan-A, and tyrosinase.[30] In addition, it is now known that some smooth muscle tumors in immunocompromised patients are positive for Epstein-Barr virus, a finding not identified in PEComas.[30]

Given the fatty component that can be seen in PEComas, such as angiomyolipoma, they can also be mistaken for well-differentiated liposarcomas. Liposarcoma often contains atypical nuclei, thickened fibrous septae, and lipoblasts within fat. Ultimately, PEComas and liposarcoma should show different phenotypes, with PEComas

Pitfalls
PEComas

! Some PEComas have a predominant epithelioid morphology (ie, epithelioid angiomyolipoma) and could mistaken for an epithelial tumor, including a carcinoma.

! PEComas with the typical clear cell pattern can appear similar to other clear cell tumors, such as liposarcoma and RCC and HCC. The specific phenotype, however, expressing myoid and melanocytic markers, differentiates PEComa from these other tumors.

! If an incomplete immunohistochemical panel is used and PEComa is only tested for either myoid markers or melanocytic markers, then it may be misdiagnosed as a smooth muscle tumor or melanoma, respectively.

highlighted by melanocytic and myoid markers and liposarcomas often marking with MDM2 and CDK4.[4] Rarely, melanoma can present with clear cytoplasm and be confused with PEComa. The melanin pigment, which can be seen in melanoma, is only rarely identified in PEComas.[8] Both melanoma and PEComa express melanocytic markers, such as HMB-45 and tyrosinase, but melanoma does not express myoid markers, such as desmin.

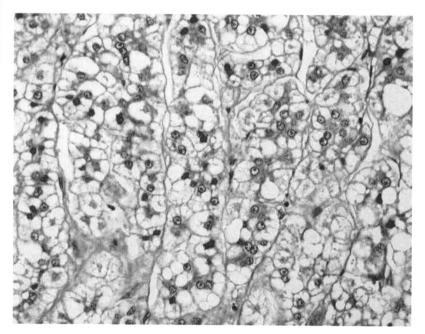

Fig. 8. HCC, clear cell variant, demonstrating a trabecular architecture and abundant clear cytoplasm. The hepatocytes are HepPar1 and arginase positive (not shown).

CLEAR CELL SARCOMA

Clear cell sarcoma (also referred to as *malignant melanoma of soft parts* due to its evidence of melanocytic differentiation) is an uncommon tumor of the soft tissue of the extremities, which usually occurs in young adult patients and is more common in women.[2,31–36] It typically presents as a painless, slowly growing, deep-seated soft tissue mass almost always attached to a tendon or aponeurosis.[2,31] Rare primary gastrointestinal variants of clear cell sarcoma with a distinctive cytogenetic alteration have also been described.[33,34]

GROSS AND MICROSCOPIC FEATURES

Grossly, most tumors appear gray-white and measure between 2 cm and 6 cm in greatest dimensions. The tumors are lobulated or multilobulated and can show focal necrosis in some cases. Only rarely does the tumor appear pigmented grossly. Histologic examination of clear cell sarcoma shows a large, nodular, subcutaneous, or, rarely, dermal, unencapsulated proliferation (**Fig. 9**) of enlarged oval to spindle-shaped cells with pale eosinophilic to clear-staining cytoplasm and vesicular chromatin with prominent nucleoli (**Fig. 10**). The cells are usually arranged in numerous nests, packets, and fascicles surrounded by collageneous tissue bands. Occasional

> **Key Features**
> ### CLEAR CELL SARCOMAS
>
> 1. Rare sarcoma with melanocytic differentiation and distinctive genetic translocation: t(12;22)(q13;q12), corresponds to EWS-ATF1 fusion
>
> 2. Usually presents in young adults on the extremities (foot is most common site). Rare gastrointestinal subtype with distinct translocation (EWS-CREB1)
>
> 3. Deep subcutaneous tumor composed of nests/packets of cells, which often have abundant clear cytoplasm, vesicular nuclei, and prominent nucleoli
>
> 4. By immunohistochemistry, the cells express melanocytic markers (S100, Melan-A/MART-1, HMB-45, tyrosinase, and MITF) and are negative for epithelial and myoid markers

multinucleated cells are often present (see **Fig. 10**). Mitotic figures are identified but are not usually numerous (<2 to 3 per 10 hpf) or atypical appearing. Necrosis is also lacking in most cases. The tumors are often well circumscribed but may show focally infiltrative features as the periphery. Perineural and angiolymphatic invasion are almost

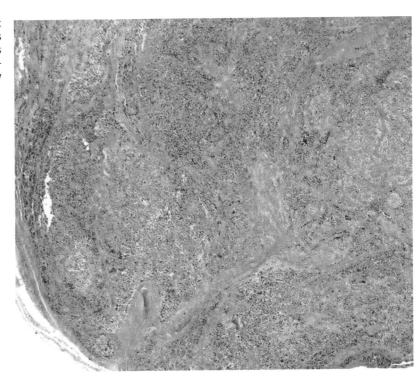

Fig. 9. Clear cell sarcoma at low magnification shows a proliferation of lobules and smaller packets of pale-staining cells surrounded by stromal fibrosis.

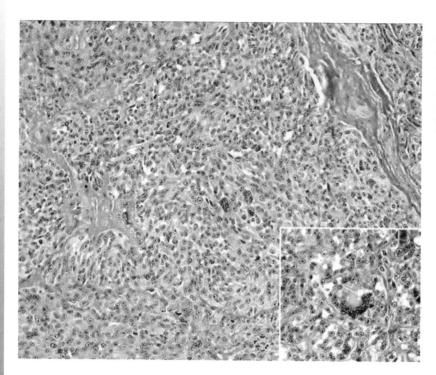

Fig. 10. Higher magnification of clear cell sarcoma shows a proliferation of atypical monotonous cells with enlarged nuclei, vesicular chromatin, and prominent nucleoli. The inset shows a large, wreath-like tumor giant cell.

never seen. The cytoplasmic clearing is due to glycogen, which can be confirmed by periodic acid–Schiff stain, with diastase sensitivity (**Fig. 11**). Melanin pigment can only rarely be identified on hematoxylin-eosin stains, but is much more frequently found with melanin stains (up to 50% of cases) (**Fig. 12**).[2,32,36]

IMMUNOHISTOCHEMICAL AND MOLECULAR FEATURES

Immunohistochemistry shows staining for multiple melanocytic markers, including S100 (**Fig. 13**) in almost all cases and HMB-45 and Melan-A/MART-1 in approximately 80% of cases (although they are usually negative in the gastrointestinal type).[31,32,36] MITF is also positive in the tumor cell nuclei in most cases.[37] A minority of cases may show positivity for synaptophysin, neuron-specific enolase, CD56, CD57, and cytokeratins, but the tumor cells are negative for high molecular weight cytokeratins, EMA, actin, and desmin.[31,32,36]

Cytogenetics, fluorescence in situ hybridization, and polymerase chain reaction studies show a characteristic translocation, t(12;22)(q13;12), in almost all cases of clear cell sarcoma.[32–36] This is a specific translocation involving the EWS and ATF1 genes (or EWS and CREB1 genes in the gastrointestinal cases), which is not seen in other soft tissue tumors. The EWS-CREB1 translocation is also seen in angiomatoid fibrous histiocytoma,

but this tumor has different morphologic and immunohistochemical findings and is easily distinguished from clear cell sarcoma.

EPIDEMIOLOGY

Clear cell sarcoma is a rare soft tissue tumor, which usually occurs in young adult patients, although there is a wide age range (13–90 years old; median age, 27–39 years old). Although it was previously thought to occur more commonly in women, a recent study has suggested a male predominance.[2,31,32] The majority of cases present in the soft tissues, but it has also been documented to occur in visceral sites, especially the gastrointestinal tract.[33,34] Rarely, involvement of other sites, such as the kidney[38] has also been reported.

TREATMENT AND PROGNOSIS

Although these tumors are slow growing, they are considered a high-grade sarcoma, because they have a high recurrence rate and metastatic potential, with metastases typically involving lymph nodes and lung.[2,31,32] There is an average 5-year survival rate of approximately 50% to 60%,[31,32] but the 10-year survival rate is only 25%.[31,32] Treatment typically includes wide local excision and consideration for sentinel lymph node biopsy, because this is a soft tissue sarcoma which often involves the lymph nodes.[3,31,39] Amputation may be necessary for tumors on the distal extremities[31,39]; however,

Fig. 11. Periodic acid–Schiff stain (without diastase digestion) shows prominent cytoplasmic glycogen staining in clear cell sarcoma.

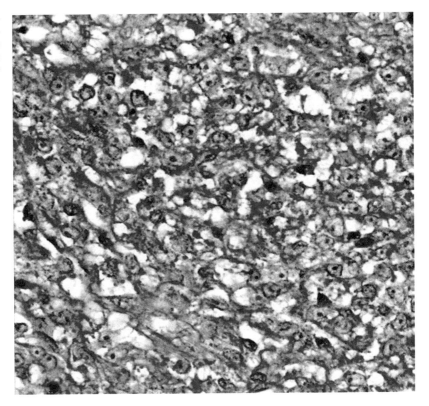

Fig. 12. A minority of clear cell sarcomas shows prominent cytoplasmic pigmentation in a subset of the tumor cells.

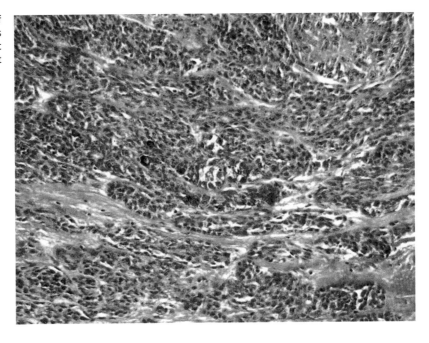

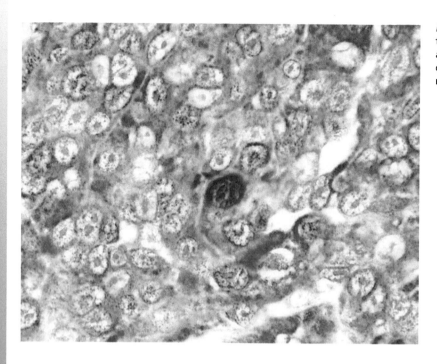

Fig. 13. S100 immunohistochemistry shows strong and diffuse nuclear and cytoplasmic staining in many cases.

once metastatic, the cure rates are dismal.[31,39] Treatment options include chemotherapy and radiation, but the overall response rates are low.[31,39,40]

DIFFERENTIAL DIAGNOSIS

Immunohistochemistry cannot distinguish melanoma from clear cell sarcoma; therefore, the clinical features (ie, patient age and site of the tumor), molecular/cytogenetic studies, and histologic findings are necessary for separating these tumors.[1,3,31–36] Melanoma almost always is a compound tumor, with an in situ component in the overlying epidermis, although it may be minimal in nodular type melanomas (Fig. 14), whereas clear cell sarcoma is a deep subcutaneous (with rare

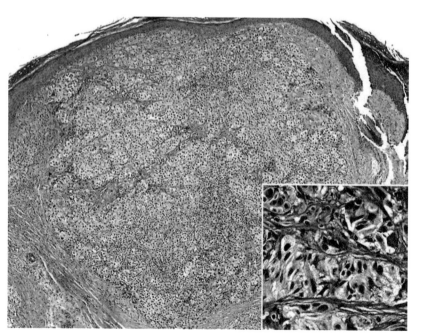

Fig. 14. Nodular type melanoma is usually a large, superficial dermal-based tumor with a predominant dermal component, and a smaller (or minimal) junctional component. This example shows a population of markedly atypical tumor cells with nuclear hyperchromasia and abundant pale to clear-staining cytoplasm (inset).

dermal invasion) tumor without epidermal involvement.[3,31] Metastatic melanoma and the rare primary dermal melanoma can be more difficult to distinguish from clear cell sarcoma due to their deep situation in the dermis and/or subcutis[41,42]; however, these tumors typically show high-grade cytologic atypia with prominent pleomorphism, multiple mitoses, and often necrosis, findings that are usually lacking in clear cell sarcoma. In addition, the nests in clear cell sarcoma are often surrounded by fibrous bands, which are not typically seen in melanoma. Metastatic melanoma usually occurs in elderly patients with a history of a previous diagnosis of a primary melanoma elsewhere, although metastatic melanomas of unknown primary origin do occur in a small percentage of cases.[41,42] Primary dermal melanoma, by definition, occurs in patients without a history of melanoma, but typically presents in sun-damaged skin of the elderly,[41] whereas clear cell sarcoma most often occurs on the distal extremities of young adults patients.

The differential diagnosis also includes rare myoepithelial carcinomas with clear cell features[43] and metastatic clear cell carcinomas to the soft tissue, especially the clear cell type of RCC.[1,28,29] RCC typically shows a prominent vascular component, with numerous small capillary-type vessels surrounding the tumor nests and lobules (see **Fig. 7**). RCC also is usually positive for epithelial markers, including pancytokeratin, CK AE1/3, EMA, and CAM5.2, as well as for RCC antigen and CD10, markers, which are negative in clear

cell sarcoma.[28] Metastatic HCC and adrenal cortical carcinoma can also enter the differential diagnosis, because the cells may show a clear cytoplasmic appearance in many cases, but are often large, pleomorphic-appearing epithelioid cells. Immunohistochemistry shows frequent positivity for inhibin, calretinin, and neuroendocrine markers, including neuron-specific enolase and synaptophysin in adrenal cortical carcinoma.[28] Cytokeratins, including AE1/AE3 and pancytokeratin,

---

Pitfalls
CLEAR CELL SARCOMA

! Some cases can appear similar to epithelial clear cell tumors, such as RCC and HCC. The specific phenotype, however, expressing melanocytic markers and negative for epithelial markers should differentiate clear cell sarcoma from these tumors.

! Metastatic melanoma and rare primary dermal/subcutaneous melanoma can simulate clear cell sarcoma both histologically and immunohistochemically.

! If overly reliant on immunohistochemical findings for melanocytic markers, then clear cell sarcoma may be misdiagnosed as melanoma. Clinical and genetic/molecular correlation are key in making this distinction.

are only positive in less than 40% of cases. Melan-A is often positive, but the tumors are negative for other melanocytic markers, including S100 and HMB-45.[28] HCC also shows a different immunophenotype from PEComa, because HCC expresses cytokeratins, HepPar1, arginase, and glypican 3 and shows canalicular staining for CD10 and polyclonal CEA.[29]

Other sarcomas with clear cell features can also be considered in the differential diagnosis, including liposarcoma, especially well-differentiated cases. The cells lack the distinctive nested or packeted pattern, however, surrounded by prominent fibrous bands of clear cell sarcoma and usually form larger lobules to nodules encompassed by thickened collagenous septae.[1,4] In addition, atypical spindle cells with hyperchromatic-staining nuclei, which are often present in the collagenous septate, and multivacuolated cells with indented hyperchromatic nuclei (lipoblasts) are often present in liposarcoma (although they are not necessary for the diagnosis) and lacking in clear cell sarcoma.[1] Immunohistochemistry often shows positivity for MDM2 and/or CDK2,[4] but negative staining for melanocytic markers (although S100 can be positive in a minority of cases).

OTHER RARE CLEAR CELL TUMORS

Clear cell fibrous papule is a rare cutaneous mesenchymal tumor, which typically presents in adults in the nasolabial region.[44–46] These are benign fibroblastic proliferations associated with a prominent collagenous stroma and increased numbers of telangiectatic blood vessels. The tumors are often larger and more cellular than conventional fibrous papules (angiofibromas), which also occur in the nasolabial region of adults. At low magnification, these lesions are composed of a nodular, dermal-based proliferation of enlarged bland-appearing clear cells with abundant finely granular to clear-staining cytoplasm. Immunophenotypically, the cells are positive for CD68 and NKI/C3 (CD63), with variable FXIIIa staining, but are negative for neural and melanocytic markers, including S100, Melan-A/MART-1, and HMB-45, and negative for epithelial markers, including cytokeratins, EMA, and CEA.[44–47]

Distinctive dermal clear cell mesenchymal neoplasm is a rare cutaneous neoplasm, which has been reported to occur on the extremities of adults.[48,49] It is a superficial dermal-based, nodular proliferation of enlarged clear cells with abundant cytoplasm and vesicular nuclei with prominent nucleoli (Fig. 15). The cells typically lack significant cytologic atypia or pleomorphism and have a low mitotic index, although some cases can show increased atypia and mitotic activity.[48] Given their superficial localization, they can be confused with clear cell fibrous papule and other clear cell cutaneous neoplasms, including tricholemmoma, tricholemmal carcinoma, and clear cell squamous cell carcinoma, but these tumors typically show prominent epidermal attachments and/or overlying carcinoma in situ.[50] By immunohistochemistry, the cells are positive for NKI/C3 and may be positive for CD68 but are negative for CD34 and FXIIIa; smooth muscle markers, including actin and desmin; neural and melanocytic markers, including S100, Melan-A/MART-1,

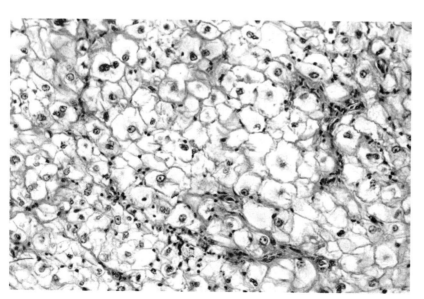

Fig. 15. Distinctive dermal clear cell mesenchymal neoplasm is a rare cutaneous neoplasm, which is composed of enlarged, clear-staining cells with abundant cytoplasm and vesicular nuclei with small nucleoli. (*Courtesy of* A. Lazar, MD, PhD.)

and HMB-45; and epithelial markers, including cytokeratins and EMA.

REFERENCES

1. d'Amore ES, Ninfo V. Clear cell tumors of the somatic soft tissues. Semin Diagn Pathol 1997;14(4):270–80.
2. Montgomery E, Meis J, Ramos A, et al. Clear cell sarcoma of tendons and aponeuroses. A clinicopathologic study of 58 cases with analysis of prognostic factors. Int J Surg Pathol 1992;1:89–100.
3. Folpe AL, Kwiatkowski DJ. Perivascular epithelioid cell neoplasms: pathology and pathogenesis. Hum Pathol 2010;41:1–15.
4. Olofsson A, Willén H, Göransson M, et al. Abnormal expression of cell cycle regulators in FUS-CHOP carrying liposarcomas. Int J Oncol 2004;25(5): 1349–55.
5. Crowson AN, Carlson-Sweet K, Macinnis C, et al. Clear cell atypical fibroxanthoma: a clinicopathologic study. J Cutan Pathol 2002;29(6):374–81.
6. Bonetti F, Pea M, Martignoni G, et al. PEC and Sugar. Am J Surg Pathol 1992;16:307–8.
7. Bonetti F, Pea M, Martignoni G, et al. The perivascular epithelioid cell and related lesions. Adv Anat Pathol 1997;4:343–58.
8. Walsh SN, Sanqueza OP. PEComas: a review with emphasis on cutaneous lesions. Semin Diagn Pathol 2009;26:123–30.
9. Hornick JL, Fletcher CD. Sclerosing PEComa: clinicopathologic analysis of a distinctive variant with a predilection for the retroperitoneum. Am J Surg Pathol 2008;32(4):493–501.
10. Stone CH, Lee MW, Amin MB, et al. Renal angiomyolipoma: further immunophenotypic characterization of an expanding morphologic spectrum. Arch Pathol Lab Med 2001;125:751–8.
11. Chang KL, Folpe AL. Diagnostic utility of microphthalmia transcription factor in malignant melanoma and other tumors. Adv Anat Pathol 2001;8: 273–5.
12. Ahrens WA, Folpe AL. CD1a immunopositivity in perivascular epithelioid cell neoplasms: true expression or technical artifact? A streptavidin-biotin and polymer-based detection system immunohistochemical study of perivascular epithelioid cell neoplasms and their morphologic mimics. Hum Pathol 2011;42(3):369–74.
13. Adachi Y, Horie Y, Kitamura Y, et al. CD1a expression in PEComas. Pathol Int 2008;58:169–73.
14. Folpe AL, Mentzel T, Lehr HA, et al. Perivascular epithelioid cell neoplasms of soft tissue and gynecologic origin: a clincopathologic study of 26 cases and review of the literature. Am J Surg Pathol 2005;29:1558–75.
15. Carvalho FM, Carvalho JP, Maluf FC, et al. A new morphological variant of uterine PEComas with sex-cord-like pattern and WT1 expression: more doubts about the existence of uterine PEComas. Ann Diagn Pathol 2010;14(2):129–32.
16. Sukov WR, Cheville JC, Amin MB, et al. Perivascular epithelioid cell tumor (PEComa) of the urinary bladder: report of 3 cases and review of the literature. Am J Surg Pathol 2009;33(2):304–8.
17. Liegl B, Hornick JL, Fletcher CD. Primary cutaneous PEComa: distinctive clear cell lesions of skin. Am J Surg Pathol 2008;32(4):608–14.
18. Yamashita K, Fletcher CD. PEComa presenting in bone: clinicopathologic analysis of 6 cases and literature review. Am J Surg Pathol 2010;34(11): 1622–9.
19. Folpe AL, Goodman ZD, Ishak KG, et al. Clear cell myomelanocytic tumor of the falciform ligament/ligamentum teres: a novel member of the perivascular epithelioid clear cell family of tumors with a predilection for children and young adults. Am J Surg Pathol 2000;24(9):1239–46.
20. Nese N, Martignoni G, Fletcher CD, et al. Pure epithelioid PEComas (so-called epithelioid angiomyolipoma) of the kidney: a clinicopathologic study of 41 cases: detailed assessment of morphology and risk stratification. Am J Surg Pathol 2011; 35(2):161–75.
21. Tallarigo C, Baldassarre R, Bianchi G, et al. Diagnostic and therapeutic problems in multicentric renal angiomyolipoma. J Urol 1992;148:1880–4.
22. Fine SW, Reuter VE, Epstein JI, et al. Angiomyolipoma with epithelial cysts (AMLEC): a distinct cystic variant of angiomyolipoma. Am J Surg Pathol 2006; 30(5):593–9.
23. Bonetti F, Pea M, Martignoni G, et al. Cellular heterogeneity in Lymphangiomyomatosis of the lung. Hum Pathol 1991;22:727–8.
24. Chan JK, Tsang WY, Pau MY, et al. Lymphangioleiomyomatosis and angiomyolipoma: closely related entities characterized by hamartomatous proliferation of HMB-45 positive smooth muscle. Histopathology 1993;22:445–55.
25. Travis WD, Colby TV, Koss MN, et al. Atlas of nontumor pathology: non-neoplastic disorders of the lower respiratory tract. First Series, Fascicle 2. Washington, DC: American Registry of Pathology; 2002.
26. Martignoni G, Pea M, Reghellin D, et al. PEComas: the past, the present and the future. Virchows Arch 2008;452(2):119–32.
27. Bonetti F, Pea M, Martignoni G, et al. Clear cell ("sugar") tumor of the lung is a lesion strictly related to angiomyolipoma—the concept of a family of lesions characterized by the presence of the perivascular epithelioid cells (PEC). Pathology 1994; 26:230–6.
28. Sangoi AR, Fujiwara M, West RB, et al. Immunohistochemical distinction of primary adrenal cortical

lesions from metastatic clear cell renal cell carcinoma: a study of 248 cases. Am J Surg Pathol 2011;35(5):678–86.

29. Chan ES, Yeh MM. The use of immunohistochemistry in liver tumors. Clin Liver Dis 2010;14(4): 687–703.

30. Weiss SW. Smooth muscle tumors of soft tissue. Adv Anat Pathol 2002;9(6):351–9.

31. Clark MA, Johnson MB, Thway K, et al. Clear cell sarcoma (melanoma of soft parts): the Royal Marsden Hospital experience. Eur J Surg Oncol 2008; 34(7):800–4.

32. Hisaoka M, Ishida T, Kuo TT, et al. Clear cell sarcoma of soft tissue: a clinicopathologic, immunohistochemical, and molecular analysis of 33 cases. Am J Surg Pathol 2008;32(3):452–60.

33. Lyle PL, Amato CM, Fitzpatrick JE, et al. Gastrointestinal melanoma or clear cell sarcoma? Molecular evaluation of 7 cases previously diagnosed as malignant melanoma. Am J Surg Pathol 2008;32(6):858–66.

34. Antonescu CR, Nafa K, Segal NH, et al. EWS-CREB1: a recurrent variant fusion in clear cell sarcoma–association with gastrointestinal location and absence of melanocytic differentiation. Clin Cancer Res 2006;12(18):5356–62.

35. Segal NH, Pavlidis P, Noble WS, et al. Classification of clear-cell sarcoma as a subtype of melanoma by genomic profiling. J Clin Oncol 2003;21(9):1775–81.

36. Antonescu CR, Tschernyavsky SJ, Woodruff JM, et al. Molecular diagnosis of clear cell sarcoma: detection of EWS-ATF1 and MITF-M transcripts and histopathological and ultrastructural analysis of 12 cases. J Mol Diagn 2002;4(1):44–52.

37. Granter SR. Clear cell sarcoma shows immunoreactivity for microphthalmia transcription factor: further evidence for melanocytic differentiation. Mod Pathol 2001;14(1):6–9.

38. Rubin BP, Fletcher JA, Renshaw AA, et al. Clear cell sarcoma of soft parts: report of a case primary in the kidney with cytogenetic confirmation. Am J Surg Pathol 1999;23(5):589–94.

39. Dim DC, Cooley LD, Miranda RN. Clear cell sarcoma of tendons and aponeuroses: a review. Arch Pathol Lab Med 2007;131(1):152–6.

40. Stacchiotti S, Grosso F, Negri T, et al. Tumor response to sunitinib malate observed in clear-cell sarcoma. Ann Oncol 2010;21(5):1130–1.

41. Cassarino DS, Cabral ES, Kartha RV. Swetter SM. Primary dermal melanoma: distinct immunohistochemical findings and clinical outcome compared with nodular and metastatic melanoma. Arch Dermatol 2008;144(1):49–56.

42. Kamposioras K, Pentheroudakis G, Pectasides D, et al. Malignant melanoma of unknown primary site. To make the long story short. A systematic review of the literature. Crit Rev Oncol Hematol 2011;78(2):112–26.

43. Stojsic Z, Brasanac D, Boricic I, et al. Clear cell myoepithelial carcinoma of the skin. A case report. J Cutan Pathol 2009;36(6):680–3.

44. Chiang YY, Tsai HH, Lee WR, et al. Clear cell fibrous papule: report of a case mimicking a balloon cell nevus. J Cutan Pathol 2009;36(3):381–4.

45. Park HS, Cho S, Kim KH, et al. Fibrous papule of the face, clear cell type: a case report. J Eur Acad Dermatol Venereol 2007;21(9):1267–8.

46. Bansal C, Stewart D, Li A, et al. Histologic variants of fibrous papule. J Cutan Pathol 2005;32(6):424–8.

47. Lee AN, Stein SL, Cohen LM. Clear cell fibrous papule with NKI/C3 expression: clinical and histologic features in six cases. Am J Dermatopathol 2005;27(4):296–300.

48. Lazar AJ, Fletcher CD. Distinctive dermal clear cell mesenchymal neoplasm: clinicopathologic analysis of five cases. Am J Dermatopathol 2004;26(4):273–9.

49. Gavino AC, Pitha JV, Bakshi NA. Atypical distinctive dermal clear cell mesenchymal neoplasm arising in the scalp. J Cutan Pathol 2008;35(4):423–7.

50. Cassarino DS, DeRienzo D, Barr RJ. Cutaneous squamous cell carcinoma: a comprehensive clinicopathologic classification–part two. J Cutan Pathol 2006;33(4):261–79.

PRIMITIVE ROUND CELL NEOPLASMS

Khin Thway, FRCPath

KEYWORDS
- Round cell neoplasms • Ewing sarcoma • Alveolar rhabdomyosarcoma
- Poorly differentiated synovial sarcoma • Neuroblastoma

ABSTRACT

Primitive round cell neoplasms (small round cell tumors) of soft tissue are a diverse group of malignant tumors composed of monotonous undifferentiated cells with high nuclear-cytoplasmic ratio. Many occur more frequently, although not exclusively, in childhood. As tumors with primitive round cell morphology are seen in virtually every basic tumor category, the diagnosis of small round cell neoplasms requires the use of ancillary diagnostic techniques: immunohistochemistry and often molecular genetics. The principal tumors in this group include Ewing sarcoma/primitive neuroectodermal tumor, desmoplastic small round cell tumor, alveolar rhabdomyosarcoma, poorly differentiated synovial sarcoma, neuroblastoma, and ganglioneuroblastoma.

OVERVIEW

Primitive round cell neoplasms (small round cell tumors) of soft tissue are a diverse group of malignant tumors composed of monotonous undifferentiated cells with high nuclear-cytoplasmic ratio. Many occur more frequently, although not exclusively, in childhood. As tumors with primitive round cell morphology are seen in virtually every basic tumor category, the diagnosis of small round cell neoplasms requires the use of ancillary diagnostic techniques: immunohistochemistry and often molecular genetics. Tumors often show immunophenotypic overlap but many have distinct chromosomal translocations that produce novel fusion genes resulting in disordered cellular function. Molecular or molecular cytogenetic detection of these fusion genes (usually by fluorescence in situ hybridization [FISH] or reverse transcription-polymerase chain reaction [RT-PCR]) is therefore an essential part of the diagnostic workup of many of these tumors. Genetic studies may provide prognostic information and have an increasing influence on clinical management.

The principal tumors in this group include Ewing sarcoma/primitive neuroectodermal tumor, desmoplastic small round cell tumor, alveolar rhabdomyosarcoma, poorly differentiated synovial sarcoma, neuroblastoma, and ganglioneuroblastoma. Other neoplasms with small round cell morphology include round cell liposarcoma, soft tissue lymphoma (especially lymphoblastic lymphoma), leukemic deposits, small cell carcinoma, and olfactory neuroblastoma. Many can be identified by their clinical setting and by the use of appropriate immunohistochemical panels.

EWING SARCOMA/PRIMITIVE NEUROECTODERMAL TUMOR

OVERVIEW

Ewing sarcoma (ES) and primitive neuroectodermal tumor (PNET), and Ewing-like tumors (Ewing family tumors [EFTs]) are a group of small round cell sarcomas occurring in bone or soft tissue that share common histologic and molecular features, but varying degrees of neuroectodermal differentiation. PNET refers to tumors with evidence of neuroectodermal differentiation by light or electron microscopy or immunohistochemistry, whereas ES is used for tumors lacking this, but it is unclear if this distinction has clinical impact.[1,2] EFTs are characterized by recurrent balanced translocations where the *EWSR1* gene

The author has nothing to disclose.
Department of Histopathology, Royal Marsden Hospital, The Royal Marsden NHS Foundation Trust, 203 Fulham Road, London SW3 6JJ, UK
E-mail address: khin.thway@rmh.nhs.uk

Surgical Pathology 4 (2011) 799–818
doi:10.1016/j.path.2011.08.009
1875-9181/11/$ – see front matter © 2011 Elsevier Inc. All rights reserved.

on chromosome 22 is fused with members of the *ETS* family of genes, leading to the formation of novel fusion oncogenes. The most common gene fusion, t(11;22)(q24;q12) (*EWSR1-FLI1*), is found in up to 90% of tumors. Most patients with ES/PNET are adolescents or adults younger than 30 years, although the age distribution is wide. Tumors can arise anywhere in the skeletal system but especially in long bones. Extraskeletally, tumors can occur at almost any site, but well-documented sites include the paravertebral area, the thoracopulmonary region (Askin tumor), retroperitoneum, abdomen, and extremity deep soft tissue. EFTs are usually very responsive to chemotherapy and radiation, and treatment is typically multimodal in nature. Patients with metastatic or recurrent disease, however, have a disease-free survival rate of less than 20% with conventional chemotherapeutic regimens, necessitating the need for targeted therapies, many of which are being evaluated for ES, including insulin-like growth factor 1-receptor (IGF1R) inhibitors.[3]

GROSS FEATURES

Tumors tend to be fleshy and friable, and hemorrhage and necrosis are common.

MICROSCOPIC FEATURES

Histologically, most tumors comprise sheets of very uniform cells with round or ovoid vesicular

Key Features
EWING SARCOMA AND PNET

- Most commonly occur in children and young adults, although age distribution is wide
- Characterized by translocations involving *EWSR1* and *ETS* family genes
- Neural differentiation in PNET
- Minimal intercellular reticulin

nuclei with fine chromatin, small or inapparent nucleoli, and indistinct cell borders (**Fig. 1**). The amount of cytoplasm is small or scanty, and the cytoplasm is frequently clear with hematoxylin and eosin, because of the presence of glycogen, which may also indent tumor nuclei. Some tumors contain larger, more irregular and pleomorphic cells, often with conspicuous nucleoli, and are referred to as large cell or atypical ES,[4] and, more rarely, cells may be spindled. There is variable rosette formation in PNET, and the most common are Homer-Wright rosettes, where cells are arranged around a central fibrillary core. Rarer are Flexner-Wintersteiner rosettes, which contain a well-defined central lumen. Necrosis is a frequent finding. Tumors can have a pseudoalveolar arrangement and may be divided by fibrous septa.

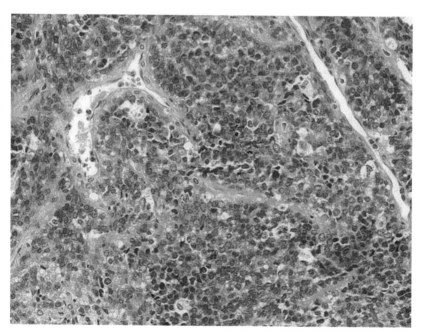

Fig. 1. Ewing sarcoma. The tumor comprises nests and sheets of uniform small cells with round or ovoid vesicular nuclei with fine chromatin, small or inapparent nucleoli, and indistinct cell borders (hemotoxylin-eosin [H&E], original magnification ×200).

Rare and atypical variants of EFT[4] include spindle cell sarcoma-like EFT,[5] "adamantinoma-like" EFT, which has nests of moderately atypical cells with peripheral palisading and a desmoplastic stroma and which typically expresses cytokeratin,[1,2] and sclerosing EFT, which has a prominent hyalinized matrix.[2]

OTHER DIAGNOSTIC TECHNIQUES

More than 90% of EFTs show diffuse membranous expression of CD99 (**Fig. 2**), although this is a nonspecific marker, found in a variety of tumors including those in the differential diagnosis of ES. Nuclear expression of Friend leukemia integration 1 transcription factor (FLI1) is seen in about 70%. ES/PNET can express a wide range of other markers, including S100 protein, cytokeratins, and occasionally desmin.[6] PNET shows variable expression of neural markers, such as neuron-specific enolase (NSE), neurofilament, CD56, chromogranin, and synaptophysin. Caveolin-1 shows membranous and cytoplasmic expression in 95% of cases, including CD99-negative cases,[7] although again is not a specific marker for ES. Cytoplasmic glycogen can be detected with periodic acid-Schiff stain, which is abolished by pretreatment with diastase. Characteristically, there is absence of reticulin fibers between tumor cells (**Fig. 3**). EFTs are characterized by recurrent chromosomal translocations fusing *EWSR1* with members of the *ETS* gene family.[8,9] There are a variety of in-frame *EWSR1-FLI1* fusion transcripts because of variations in the location of the *EWSR1* and *FLI-1* genomic breakpoints. The 2 main ones fuse *EWSR1* exon 7 to *FLI1* exon 6, and *EWSR1* exon 7 to *FLI1* exon 5, and are described as types 1 and 2 respectively. Five percent to 10% of EFTs harbor a variant t(21;22)(q22;q12) fusion (*EWSR1-ERG*). Rare fusions include t(2;22)(q33;q12) (*EWSR1-FEV*), t(7;22)(p22;q12) (*EWSR1-ETV1*), and t(17;22)(q12;q12) (*EWSR1-E1AF*), each accounting for fewer than 1% of cases. The *EWSR1* gene rearrangement can be routinely detected in paraffin-embedded material by FISH using *EWSR1*-specific break-apart probes flanking the common *EWSR1* breakpoints, or the more common fusion transcripts can be identified by RT-PCR. Because of the numerous variant fusions, however, molecular investigations may be negative in morphologically and immunohistochemically typical EFT.

DIAGNOSIS AND DIFFERENTIAL DIAGNOSIS

Extraskeletal mesenchymal chondrosarcoma shows a prominent hemangiopericytic pattern and focal chondroid formation, and lacks a specific translocation. Olfactory neuroblastoma has a lobulated architecture, variable amounts of neurofibrillary matrix, often shows a population of S100 protein–positive sustentacular cells, and is negative for CD99. Small cell osteosarcoma has a similar peak age incidence, but foci of malignant osteoid and sometimes malignant cartilage are discernible, and is CD99 negative. Alveolar

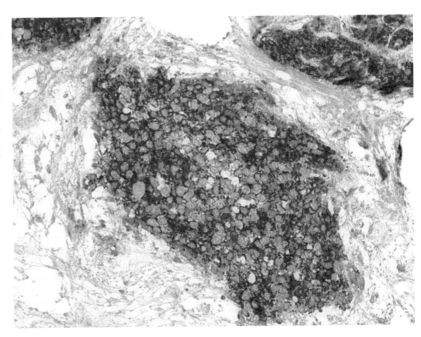

Fig. 2. Ewing sarcoma. Many tumors show diffuse and strong membranous expression of CD99, although this is a nonspecific marker that is also expressed in other small round cells tumors within the differential diagnosis (immunohistochemistry, CD99, original magnification ×200).

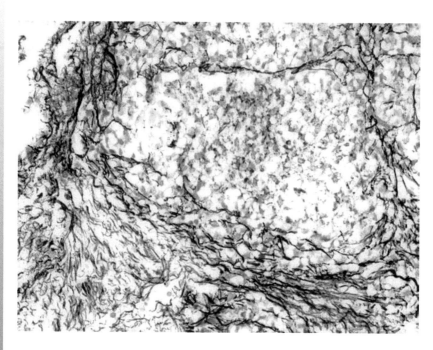

Fig. 3. Ewing sarcoma. The tumor characteristically shows absence of reticulin fibers between cells (reticulin, original magnification ×200).

rhabdomyosarcoma also occurs in teenagers and young adults, but usually has a characteristic nested architecture with central discohesion; is strongly positive for desmin, myogenin, and MyoD1; and harbors specific translocations fusing *FOXO1* with *PAX3* or *PAX7* genes. Desmoplastic small round cell tumor characteristically occurs in the abdomen or pelvis, shows polyphenotypic differentiation, expressing epithelial, muscle, and neural markers, and harbors a specific *EWSR1-WT1* gene fusion. Lymphoma will often show

△△ **Differential Diagnosis**
EWING SARCOMA AND PNET

- Desmoplastic small round cell tumor
- Poorly differentiated synovial sarcoma
- Mesenchymal chondrosarcoma
- Round cell liposarcoma
- Lymphoma
- Neuroblastoma
- Metastatic neuroendocrine carcinoma
- Olfactory neuroblastoma
- Small cell osteosarcoma

(!) **Pitfalls**
EWING SARCOMA AND PNET

! CD99 is a very nonspecific marker that is expressed in many other tumors, including those in the differential diagnosis of ES, such as poorly differentiated synovial sarcoma, mesenchymal chondrosarcoma, lymphoblastic lymphoma, and metastatic carcinoma.

! Lymphoma will often show involvement of lymphoid tissue (lymph node, spleen) and expresses lymphoid immunohistochemical markers.

! The small cell component of extraskeletal mesenchymal chondrosarcoma resembles ES, and its cartilaginous component may not be sampled in a core biopsy. In rare cases of ES, there is divergent differentiation, including chondroid formation, which can resemble mesenchymal chondrosarcoma. Both tumors are CD99 positive, and hence genetic analysis can be required for diagnosis.

! As *EWSR1* can fuse with many different partner genes, it is important to be aware that, even using several RT-PCR assays with different primer pairs, not all fusion transcripts of EFT will be detected, leading to false negative results.

involvement of lymphoid tissue (lymph node, spleen) and express lymphoid immunohistochemical markers.

PROGNOSIS

Survival is currently approximately 75% for patients with localized tumors, although 5-year survival is only about 25% for those presenting with metastatic disease. The most common metastatic sites are lung, bone, and bone marrow. Atypical ES appears to confer a worse clinical outcome.[7] The presence of an *EWSR1-FLI1* rearrangement appears prognostically favorable, and patients with type 1 *EWSR1-FLI1* fusions also appear to have significantly better survival than those with other types of *EWSR1-FLI1* fusions.[10]

DESMOPLASTIC SMALL ROUND CELL TUMOR

OVERVIEW

Desmoplastic small round cell tumor (DSRCT) is an aggressive small round cell neoplasm that predominantly affects children, adolescents, and young adults, with a male preponderance. Its lineage is uncertain, but it shows polyphenotypic differentiation, displaying immunoreactivity for epithelial, muscle, and neural markers. It is characterized by a t(11;22)(p13;q12) translocation that produces the *EWSR1-WT1* fusion oncogene. The tumor characteristically occurs in the abdomen or pelvis, often with widespread serosal involvement.

Occurrence in other sites is rare, but these include the paratesticular region (owing to continuity with the peritoneum via the processus vaginalis), ovary, thoracic cavity, head and neck, and brain. Treatment is by surgical excision and chemotherapy.

GROSS FEATURES

DSRCT commonly forms multiple firm, gritty, white nodules on the peritoneal surface, or can form large bulky masses with hemorrhage and necrosis.

MICROSCOPIC FEATURES

DSRCT is composed of highly cellular sheets of uniform cells with small, round hyperchromatic or vesicular nuclei, inconspicuous nucleoli, and scanty cytoplasm. In smaller numbers of tumors, the cytoplasm is more abundant, with clearing or vacuolation. There is a prominent desmoplastic stromal reaction, dividing the tumor into sharply demarcated or angulated islands (**Fig. 4**), and which consists of spindle fibroblasts and myofibroblasts embedded within collagen. There are frequent mitoses and necrosis is common. Some tumors show focal epithelial differentiation, with glands or pseudoglands. Rosette formation is rarely seen, and some tumors may contain eosinophilic rhabdoid inclusions of intermediate filaments within the cytoplasm. Tumors may also show larger nuclei with atypia, and rarely can consist of predominantly atypical nuclei or have a spindled morphology.[11]

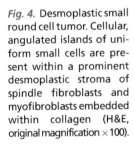

Fig. 4. Desmoplastic small round cell tumor. Cellular, angulated islands of uniform small cells are present within a prominent desmoplastic stroma of spindle fibroblasts and myofibroblasts embedded within collagen (H&E, original magnification ×100).

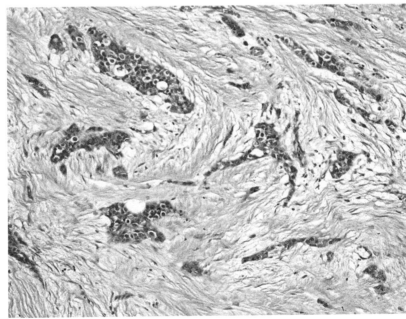

Key Features
DESMOPLASTIC SMALL ROUND CELL TUMOR

- Most commonly arises in children, adolescents, and young adults
- Male predilection
- Abundant fibrous stroma surrounding tumor islands
- Polyphenotypic immunoprofile, with expression of desmin, keratin, and neural markers
- Paranuclear dot-like desmin
- Most tumors immunoreactive for antibodies directed to the carboxyl terminus of WT1

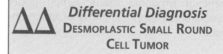

Differential Diagnosis
DESMOPLASTIC SMALL ROUND CELL TUMOR

- Ewing sarcoma
- Alveolar rhabdomyosarcoma
- Metastatic neuroendocrine carcinoma
- Round cell liposarcoma
- Lymphoma/leukemia
- Neuroblastoma

OTHER DIAGNOSTIC TECHNIQUES

Ninety percent of DSRCTs are immunoreactive for antibodies directed to the carboxyl terminus of WT1 (**Fig. 5**).[12,13] DSRCT shows divergent differentiation toward multiple lineages, with coexpression of desmin (which is characteristically dotlike and paranuclear) (**Fig. 6**), cytokeratins, and neural markers.[11,14] Approximately 25% of tumors express CD99. The characteristic *EWSR1-WT1* translocation can be detected in paraffin-embedded material by FISH, using an *EWSR1*-specific break-apart probe, or the *EWSR1-WT1* fusion transcript can be identified by RT-PCR.

DIAGNOSIS AND DIFFERENTIAL DIAGNOSIS

Although ES has cells with a similar morphology, it lacks a prominent desmoplastic stroma. It can express focal cytokeratin, but lacks WT1 expression and very rarely shows focal desmin expression. Many cases show strong CD99 expression (although this is also seen in a smaller proportion of DSRCTs) and most tumors harbor characteristic translocations involving *EWSR1* and the ETS family of transcription factors. Alveolar rhabdomyosarcoma also occurs in young patients, but occurs chiefly in the extremities, head and neck, and trunk and typically shows diffuse and strong expression of desmin and skeletal muscle–specific markers and harbors specific *PAX3/7-FOXO1* gene fusions. Endometrial stromal sarcoma occurs in older

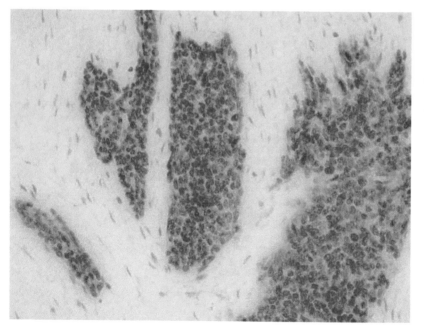

Fig. 5. Ninety percent of desmoplastic small round cell tumors are immunoreactive for antibodies directed to the carboxyl terminus of WT1 (immunohistochemistry, WT1, original magnification ×200).

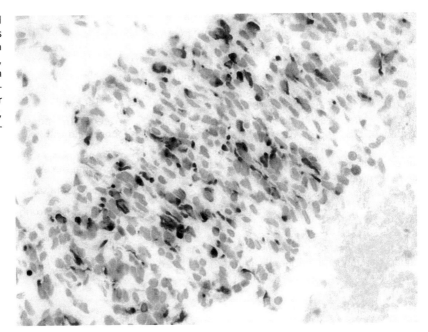

Fig. 6. Desmoplastic small round cell tumor shows divergent differentiation toward multiple lineages, and expression of desmin is characteristically dot-like and paranuclear (immunohistochemistry, desmin, original magnification ×200).

women; usually strongly expresses CD10, estrogen receptors, and progesterone receptors; and also harbors characteristic translocations. Metastatic small cell carcinoma occurs in an older population, comprises cells with nuclear moulding and stippled chromatin pattern, and does not express desmin or WT1.

PROGNOSIS

DSRCT has a very poor prognosis, with nearly uniformly fatal outcome and reported overall 3-year and 5-year survivals of 44% and 15%.[15] Patients often have widespread peritoneal involvement at presentation, and there is frequent local recurrence. Sites of metastasis include liver,

lung, and lymph nodes. Multimodal therapy, including aggressive surgical resection, has been shown to improve survival in patients with DSRCT.[15]

ALVEOLAR RHABDOMYOSARCOMA

OVERVIEW

This is a primitive malignant tumor showing partial differentiation toward skeletal muscle. It accounts for approximately 30% of rhabdomyosarcomas (RMS)[16] (which are the most common soft tissue sarcomas in children, constituting approximately 7% of childhood cancers) and is an aggressive neoplasm. Alveolar rhabdomyosarcoma (ARMS) predominantly affects adolescents and young adults and is rare in those older than 45 years. It typically presents as a rapidly growing extremity mass, but can also occur in the head and neck or trunk. ARMS is consistently associated with characteristic chromosomal translocations in about 60% to 70% of tumors: t(2;13)(q35;q14) and the rarer t(1;13)(q36;q14). These 2 subsets are histologically indistinguishable. These fuse 2 genes, each encoding transcription factors. *FOXO1* on chromosome 13 is a member of the forkhead transcription factor family, whereas *PAX3* or *PAX7* on chromosomes 2 and 1, respectively, belong to the paired box family of transcription factors. These generate, respectively, *PAX3-FOXO1* and *PAX7-FOXO1* fusion genes that code for chimeric proteins that act as aberrant

> **Pitfalls**
> **DESMOPLASTIC SMALL ROUND CELL TUMOR**
>
> ! Some DSRCTs express CD99, and can be mistaken for ES, particularly if the characteristic stromal pattern is not sufficiently represented on biopsy.
>
> ! The dot keratin can also cause confusion with metastatic small cell carcinoma or even Merkel cell carcinoma, but these occur in an older population. Evidence of visceral primary site might be apparent for small cell carcinoma, many cases of which also express TTF1.

transcription factors, which are hypothesized to generate novel transcriptional programs in an unknown target cell.[17] The remaining cases of histologic ARMS do not have detectable translocations. These might be accounted for by variant fusions with other genes, and rarer fusions, such as t(2;2) and t(2;8) (PAX3-NCOA1 and PAX3-NCOA2), are described.[18] It is possible that some ARMS represent truly fusion-negative cases,[19] and expression profiling studies have indicated that these are biologically and clinically more similar to embryonal RMS (ERMS) than fusion-positive ARMS.[20,21]

GROSS FEATURES

Tumors are fleshy, infiltrative masses. The cut surface is tan and frequently hemorrhagic and necrotic.

MICROSCOPIC FEATURES

ARMS comprises sheets and nests of small to intermediate-sized cells with round or ovoid hyperchromatic nuclei and scant cytoplasm. Frequently there is central necrosis and cellular discohesion. When viable cells are preserved at the periphery of tumor islands, the morphology resembles the histologic appearances of pulmonary alveoli (Fig. 7). Fibrous septa are commonly interspersed (Fig. 8). Rhabdomyoblasts can be seen in some cases, but are not as common as in ERMS. Tumor giant cells are quite commonly seen, with nuclei

Key Features
ALVEOLAR RHABDOMYOSARCOMA

- Predominantly occurs in adolescents and young adults

- Deep soft tissues of extremities, head and neck, and trunk

- Alveolar spaces formed by central loss of cohesion of cells

- Fibrous septa separate tumor nests

- Diffuse and strong desmin, myogenin, and MyoD1 in most cases

- Characteristic PAX-FOXO1 balanced translocations t(2;13)(q35;q14) and t(1;13)(p36;q14) are diagnostic

arranged in peripheral "wreathlike" distributions and copious eosinophilic cytoplasm. Rarely, tumors show clear cell morphology owing to cytoplasmic glycogen[22] and may mimic lipoblasts, although lack nuclear indentation. Although tumor cells have a generally uniform appearance, there may be areas of pleomorphism, although cellular spindling is lacking, unlike in embryonal RMS. The solid variant of ARMS has similar cellular features but lacks the characteristic architecture, although small nests with the typical appearances of ARMS may be found with thorough sampling

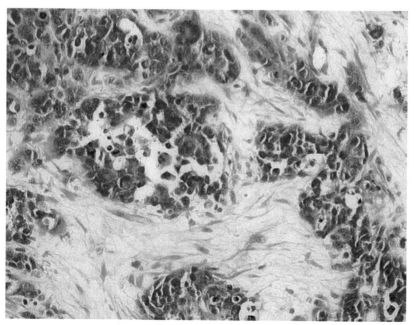

Fig. 7. Alveolar rhabdomyosarcoma. This tumor comprises nests of small to intermediate-sized cells with round or ovoid hyperchromatic nuclei and scant cytoplasm. There is central necrosis with viable cells preserved at the periphery of tumor islands, reminiscent of the histologic appearances of pulmonary alveoli (H&E, original magnification ×400).

Fig. 8. Alveolar rhabdo-myosarcoma. Fibrous septa are commonly interspersed between tumor nests (H&E, original magnification ×40).

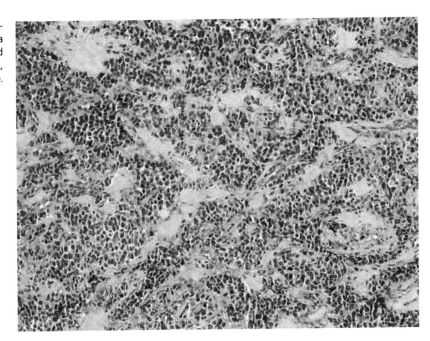

and examination. Some tumors show mixed embryonal and alveolar morphology, where areas resembling ERMS, such as spindled cells and myxoid stroma, are present, but these tumors are thought to behave in a similar fashion to ARMS and are classified as such. The histologic appearances of ARMS do not predict the presence or type of gene fusion, although a solid architecture is more associated with fusion negativity.

OTHER DIAGNOSTIC TECHNIQUES

Desmin expression is typically strongly positive in most cells (**Fig. 9**). There is also expression of myogenin (**Fig. 10**) and MyoD1, which are intranuclear myogenic transcriptional regulatory proteins expressed at early stages of skeletal muscle differentiation, and are the most sensitive and specific markers for skeletal muscle differentiation. There is nuclear positivity, often in a large proportion of tumor nuclei, and the proportion of cells with strong nuclear myogenin expression tends to be greater in ARMS than ERMS.[23,24] Smooth muscle actin is occasionally expressed, and tumors can variably express neuroendocrine markers, particularly CD56. ARMS has 2 characteristic translocations, t(2;13)(q35;q14) and t(1;13)(p36;q14), that juxtapose either the *PAX3* or *PAX7* genes with the *FOXO1* gene. The genetic breakpoints can be detected by FISH, and the fusion transcripts by RT-PCR in paraffin-embedded material. Approximately 20% of ARMS do not harbor

a detectable *PAX-FOXO1* fusion, and tend to be associated with a solid alveolar architecture.[25]

DIAGNOSIS AND DIFFERENTIAL DIAGNOSIS

ERMS can be highly cellular, with ovoid or rounded cells, and can be mistaken for ARMS, particularly as some ARMS lack characteristic alveolar architecture. ERMS generally occurs in a younger population (children younger than 10 years) and may occur in sites unusual for ARMS, such as the urogenital region, whereas is rare in the limbs. Desmin and myogenin expression tend to be less diffuse than for ARMS, and it does not harbor

 Differential Diagnosis
ALVEOLAR
RHABDOMYOSARCOMA

- Embryonal rhabdomyosarcoma
- Ewing sarcoma
- Poorly differentiated synovial sarcoma
- Extrarenal rhabdoid tumor
- Neuroblastoma
- Olfactory neuroblastoma
- Lymphoma/leukemia

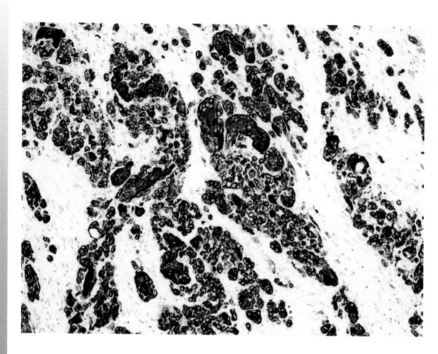

Fig. 9. Alveolar rhabdomyosarcoma shows strong and diffuse desmin expression. Note the multinucleate tumor giant cells that are also interspersed (immunohistochemistry, desmin, original magnification ×100).

PAX-FOXO1 fusions. Olfactory neuroblastoma has a lobulated architecture, with variable amounts of neurofibrillary matrix, often shows a population of S100 protein–positive sustentacular cells, and is positive for neuroendocrine markers. Extrarenal rhabdoid tumor occurs most often in younger children and infants, and is composed of larger cells, with eccentric nuclei and more abundant cytoplasm, that express keratin but are negative for integrase interactor 1 (INI1) and desmin.

PROGNOSIS

ARMS is an aggressive neoplasm shown to have a 5-year event-free survival rate of 45% (in contrast to 70% in ERMS), and may present primarily with

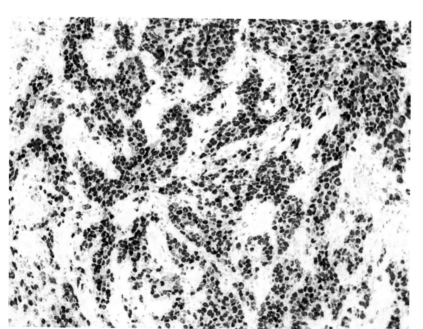

Fig. 10. Alveolar rhabdomyosarcoma also shows strong nuclear expression of skeletal muscle markers myogenin (shown here) and MyoD1, which is typically more diffuse than that seen in the embryonal subtype of rhabdomyosarcoma (immunohistochemistry, myogenin, original magnification ×40).

Pitfalls
ALVEOLAR
RHABDOMYOSARCOMA

! Widespread metastatic disease within nodes and marrow on biopsy (often with a solid pattern of infiltration) can resemble lymphoma or leukemia. The cells of ARMS are negative for CD45 and diffusely positive for desmin and myogenin.

! The head and neck is a common site for ARMS, and the tumor may resemble olfactory neuroblastoma, which occurs at specific sites in the sinonasal tract, but is strongly positive for neuroendocrine markers and is negative for desmin.

! ES and DSRCT also occur in young patients, but both harbor characteristic gene fusions involving *EWSR1* and members of the ETS family of transcription factors (ES) or *WT1* (DSRCT). The desmin expression in DSRCT is frequently dotlike and paranuclear. ES can rarely express desmin, but this is not of the diffuse nature seen in ARMS, which also shows strong nuclear expression of myogenin and MyoD1.

widespread nodal or bony metastases. Accurately distinguishing ARMS from ERMS is therefore crucial for treatment and prognostication. For patients with metastatic disease, those with *PAX7-FOXO1* appear to have a better prognosis than those with *PAX3-FOXO1*,[26] although fusion status is not associated with outcome differences in patients with localized disease.

POORLY DIFFERENTIATED SYNOVIAL SARCOMA

OVERVIEW

Synovial sarcoma is a soft tissue neoplasm that occurs most frequently in adolescents and young adults, is characterized by a specific reciprocal translocation (X;18)(p11;q11), and shows variable epithelial differentiation. It accounts for approximately 5% to 10% of all soft tissue sarcomas, and approximately 20% of synovial sarcomas are poorly differentiated. Synovial sarcoma can occur at any anatomic site, although about 90% occur in the extremities and a subset occurs in the head and neck region. Poorly differentiated synovial sarcoma (PDSS) tends to occur more proximally than classical synovial sarcoma, and is composed of sheets of rounded or ovoid cells with increased mitotic activity, focal necrosis, and

high proliferation index (Ki67),[27] and resembles small round cell tumors, such as ES or lymphoma.

GROSS FEATURES

Tumors tend to be circumscribed tan or white masses, with a soft cut surface. Focal hemorrhage and necrosis are common.

MICROSCOPIC FEATURES

Tumors comprise sheets of uniform rounded cells with overlapping ovoid nuclei, scanty cytoplasm, and indistinct cell boundaries (**Fig. 11**). More rarely, tumors may have larger cells or those with rhabdoid morphology with abundant eccentric cytoplasm. Mitotic figures are prominent.

OTHER DIAGNOSTIC TECHNIQUES

PDSS shares a similar immunophenotype to classical synovial sarcoma. Tumors show focal but generally strong expression of epithelial membrane antigen and pancytokeratins such as AE1/AE3 (**Fig. 12**), as well as CK7 and CK19. Almost all cases show nuclear expression of TLE1,[28] a very sensitive but not wholly specific marker that may also be expressed in some solitary fibrous tumors and hemangiopericytomas, nerve sheath tumors, and a small number of Ewing sarcomas.[29,30] Like conventional synovial sarcomas, there is usually also diffuse expression of bcl-2,[31] with variable numbers of tumors expressing CD99,[32] CD56,[33] calponin (**Fig. 13**), or focal S100 protein.[34] CD34 is virtually always negative. There is a nested reticulin pattern. More than 90% of synovial sarcomas harbor a balanced reciprocal chromosomal

Key Features
POORLY DIFFERENTIATED
SYNOVIAL SARCOMA

- Can arise in any site, but tends to occur more proximally

- Nuclear overlapping

- A hemangiopericytic vascular pattern is commonly present

- Virtually all tumors show diffuse nuclear expression of TLE1

- There is focal expression of epithelial membrane antigen and cytokeratins, and variable CD99 and S100 protein expression

- The specific chromosomal translocation t(X;18)(p11;q11) is diagnostic

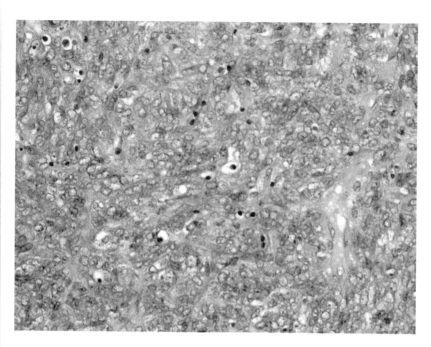

Fig. 11. Poorly differentiated synovial sarcoma. Tumors comprise sheets of uniform rounded cells with overlapping ovoid nuclei, scanty cytoplasm, and indistinct cell boundaries (H&E, original magnification ×400).

translocation t(X;18)(p11.q11) in which the *SS18* gene is juxtaposed with variants *SSX1*, *SSX2*,[35] or very rarely *SSX4*[36] of the *SSX* gene. Poorly differentiated synovial sarcoma has been shown to have a distinct gene expression signature.[37–39] Synovial sarcomas generally show a modest response to conventional chemotherapeutic regimens, and targeted therapies are required. In vitro and xenograft research on synovial sarcoma cell lines have identified some critical pathways that are potentially targetable, and possible future therapeutic strategies include anti-IGF1R pathway agents, antiangiogenic agents, and anti-Bcl-2/proapoptotic agents.[40]

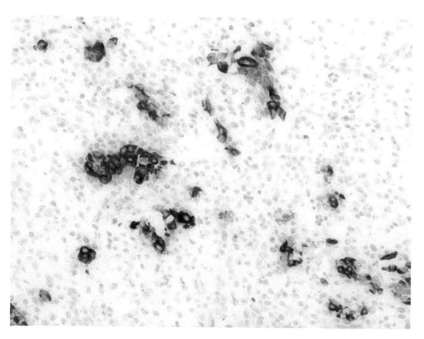

Fig. 12. Poorly differentiated synovial sarcoma. There is focal expression of pancytokeratin (immunohistochemistry, pancytokeratin, original magnification x200).

Fig. 13. Poorly differentiated synovial sarcoma.
Calponin expression is a
frequent finding (immu-
nohistochemistry, calpo-
nin, original magnification
×400).

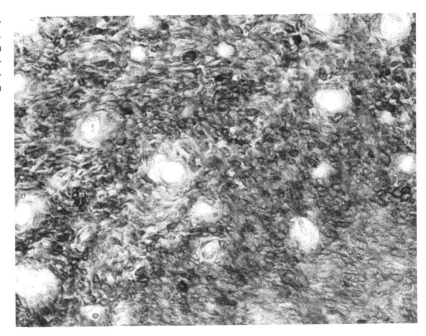

DIAGNOSIS AND DIFFERENTIAL DIAGNOSIS

Tranducin-like enhancer of split 1 (TLE1) is highly sensitive but not wholly specific for synovial sarcoma, and is helpful in excluding the tumor when the result is negative. ES/PNET and alveolar RMS each have characteristic gene fusions that be detected by FISH or RT-PCR. Both small cell and Merkel cell carcinoma occur in older adults. Small cell carcinoma shows nuclear moulding; necrosis and mitoses are frequent; and many express cyto-keratin (often in a dot distribution), TTF1, chromog-ranin, and synaptophysin. Merkel cell carcinoma expresses CK20 in a perinuclear dotlike distribu-tion, and expresses neurofilament. Metastatic endometrial stromal sarcoma frequently shows diffuse positivity for estrogen and progesterone receptors and CD10, and also has specific translo-cations detectable routinely by RT-PCR.

PROGNOSIS

PDSS is associated with a worse prognosis than the conventional type. Other adverse prognostic factors include age older than 40 years, larger tumor size (>5 cm), and high disease stage and grade.

 Differential Diagnosis
POORLY DIFFERENTIATED
SYNOVIAL SARCOMA

- Ewing sarcoma
- Alveolar rhabdomyosarcoma
- Small cell carcinoma
- Merkel cell carcinoma
- Endometrial stromal sarcoma

 Pitfalls
POORLY DIFFERENTIATED
SYNOVIAL SARCOMA

! Poorly differentiated synovial sarcoma can resemble ES, which can also express cytokera-tins focally and is also CD99 positive. The nuclei of PDSS are less regular than those of ES, and also appear to overlap, and tumors express TLE1 but not FLI1.

! Small cell carcinoma can also mimic PDSS, but may show nuclear moulding. Cytokeratin expression is more diffuse (and often dotlike) and it often expresses TTF1.

NEUROBLASTOMA AND GANGLIONEUROBLASTOMA

OVERVIEW

Neuroblastoma and ganglioneuroblastoma are malignant childhood tumors derived from primordial neural crest cells that migrate from the spinal cord to populate the developing sympathetic ganglia and adrenal medulla. Neuroblastic tumors show a spectrum of differentiation and biologic behavior corresponding to points along the pathway of neuroblastic maturation. Ganglioneuroma is a well-differentiated and benign tumor, whereas ganglioneuroblastoma shows moderate differentiation and neuroblastoma is the least differentiated, with primitive neuroblasts showing a variable degree of ganglionic differentiation.

Neuroblastoma is the third most common childhood malignant tumor, after hematolymphoid and central nervous system neoplasms, but the most common solid tumor of infancy. The presenting age is between approximately 18 and 21 months, with most cases diagnosed by 5 years, but the tumor can occur very rarely in adults. There is a slight male predilection, a higher incidence in whites than African Americans,[41] and most cases are sporadic, although familial cases with autosomal dominant inheritance are described.

Neuroblastomas and ganglioneuroblastomas generally follow the distribution of the sympathetic ganglia. Most neuroblastomas arise in the retroperitoneum, about half of these occurring in the adrenal gland, and other sites include the mediastinum, and cervical and sacral regions.[42] In addition to a mass, there is a range of nonspecific presenting signs and symptoms, including fever, weight loss, anemia, and watery diarrhea. Patients can also present with syndromes, such as "myoclonus-opsoclonus," thought to be caused by an autoimmune response against cross-reactive proteins of tumor and neuronal cells,[43] or the "blueberry muffin baby," which occurs because of cutaneous metastases. Most patients have elevated levels of urinary catecholamines and their metabolites.

Ganglioneuroblastoma shows a degree of differentiation intermediate between ganglioneuroma and neuroblastoma. It is composed of ganglion cells seen in varying stages of maturation, mixed with immature neuroblasts. The proportions and distributions of ganglion cells and neuroblasts vary, and the tumor has a range of morphology and behavior. Tumors show a distribution similar to that of ganglioneuroma and occur most commonly in the retroperitoneum or mediastinum.

GROSS FEATURES

Grossly, neuroblastomas are lobulated or multinodular fleshy masses, with a soft yellow to white cut surface, often showing hemorrhage, necrosis, or calcification, and sometimes cyst formation. Ganglioneuroblastomas are lobulated masses, often with a heterogeneous cut surface. There are firm, whitish areas corresponding to ganglioneuromatous areas with soft hemorrhagic regions consistent with poorly differentiated neuroblastomatous areas. Gritty white calcified areas are a fairly common finding.

MICROSCOPIC FEATURES

Neuroblastoma consists of nests, lobules, or sheets of cells of medium to large size (**Fig. 14**). Nuclei are ovoid or rounded, and are hyperchromatic, with even or clumped chromatin. The cytoplasm is amphophilic and fairly minimal, and there is delicate, pale-staining neurofibrillary matrix resembling neuropil that is present in variable amounts. Nuclear crushing and streaking because of artifact is relatively common.

Several classification systems exist for neuroblastoma. Tumors are divided into undifferentiated, poorly differentiated, and differentiating subtypes, according to the percentage of cells with ganglionic differentiation. Differentiating neuroblastoma contains more than 5% cells with ganglionic differentiation, although the amount of Schwannian stroma must be less than 50% of the tumor (in contrast to ganglioneuroblastomas). The poorly differentiated form shows less than 5% of differentiating cells and minimal or no Schwannian stroma. Undifferentiated neuroblastoma shows no ganglionic differentiation and minimal or no Schwannian stroma.

Key Features
NEUROBLASTOMA AND
GANGLIONEUROBLASTOMA

- Occur in infants and children in first 2 years of life, with most tumors diagnosed by 5 years
- Commonest extracranial solid tumor in children
- Tumors follow distribution of the sympathetic ganglia
- *MYCN* amplification associated with a worse prognosis

Fig. 14. Neuroblastoma. This tumor comprises nests and lobules of medium to large cells with rounded nuclei and minimal amphophilic cytoplasm, as well as variable amounts of delicate, pale-staining neurofibrillary matrix resembling neuropil (H&E, original magnification × 100).

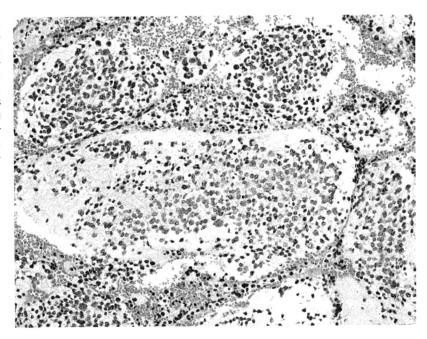

In tumors showing ganglionic differentiation, ganglion cells are enlarged polygonal cells with round vesicular nuclei with prominent nucleoli and moderate or large amounts of amphophilic cytoplasm (**Fig. 15**). Rosettes may be identifiable, ranging from those in more primitive, morule-like cell clusters to well-formed Homer-Wright rosettes, in which the neuritic processes of neuroblasts are arranged around a central point. A large cell variant of neuroblastoma comprises large neuroblasts with sharply delineated nuclear membranes and prominent nucleoli, and appears to be more aggressive in behavior.[44] A pleomorphic/anaplastic variant is described, which contains cells with prominent

Fig. 15. Neuroblastoma. In tumors showing ganglionic differentiation, ganglion cells are enlarged polygonal cells with round vesicular nuclei with prominent nucleoli and moderate or large amounts of amphophilic cytoplasm (H&E, original magnification ×400).

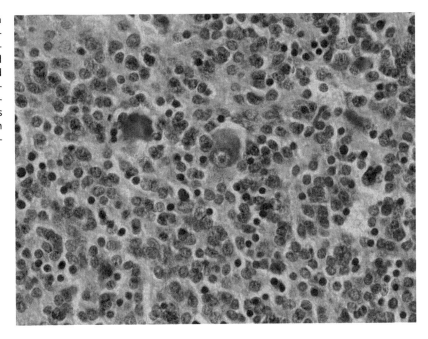

cellular pleomorphism, including bizarre cells, but the clinical significance of this variant is uncertain.[45] Neuroblastoma may mature into ganglioneuroma, occurring either secondary to treatment or spontaneously.

Ganglioneuroblastomas contain areas of ganglioneuromatous stroma along with neuroblastoma-like areas of primitive neuroblasts, and are subclassified according to the arrangement and proportion of these areas. Nodular ganglioneuroblastoma comprises well-demarcated cellular nodules of neuroblastoma alongside large areas of typical ganglioneuroma. Intermixed ganglioneuroblastoma is composed of microscopic nests of neuroblastoma within ganglioneuromatous stroma. In both nodular and intermixed subtypes, there is greater than 50% Schwannian stroma. Ganglion cells are polygonal, with moderate to abundant amphophilic cytoplasm, round to ovoid vesicular nuclei, and prominent nuclei. They vary in maturation and may appear atypical or dysplastic, and binucleate or trinucleate forms may be present. Stromal characteristics can vary, from a delicate, pale-staining fibrillary array of tumor cell neurites to a more collagenous network containing large numbers of Schwann cells. There is sometimes calcification and rarely pigmentation, owing to the presence of neuromelanin, which is confirmed ultrastructurally.[46]

OTHER DIAGNOSTIC TECHNIQUES

Strong positivity for NSE is a characteristic, although not specific, finding in neuroblastoma,

as expression is often found in other small round cell tumors including PNET. NB84 is strongly expressed by virtually all neuroblastomas (Fig. 16). This antibody recognizes an uncharacterized antigen of 57 kD in neuroblastoma,[47] but is not entirely specific, and is expressed in other small round cell tumors including small cell osteosarcomas and ES. Other markers for which there is strong expression include CD56, neurofilament protein, PGP9.5, chromogranin, and synaptophysin. Neuroblastomas are negative for CD99, cytokeratins, and muscle and leucocytic markers. Approximately 25% of cases of neuroblastoma show amplification of the *MYCN* oncogene. Loss of heterozygosity at chromosomes 1p36 and 11q23 can also be found.

The neuroblastic component of ganglioneuroblastoma expresses NB84 and markers of neuroectodermal differentiation. The ganglion cells are positive for NSE, neurofilament protein, and CD56. S100 protein is expressed by stromal Schwann cells, although it is negative within ganglion cells.

DIAGNOSIS AND DIFFERENTIAL DIAGNOSIS

Neuroblastoma can be difficult to detect in bone marrow trephine biopsies, as cells can resemble hematopoietic precursors, and are often crushed. Immunohistochemistry with a panel comprising NSE, NF, CD56, and NB84 is a sensitive method for detecting metastatic neuroblastoma. ES/PNET, desmoplastic small round cell tumor, and alveolar RMS affect older patient populations, and each

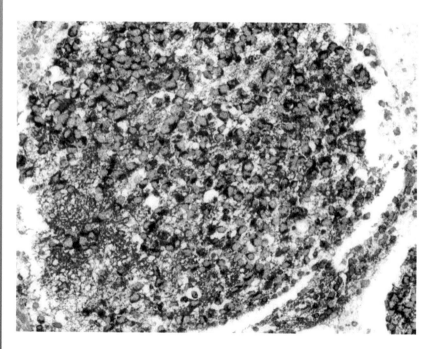

Fig. 16. NB84 is strongly expressed by virtually all neuroblastomas (immunohistochemistry, NB84, original magnification ×200).

Differential Diagnosis
NEUROBLASTOMA AND
GANGLIONEUROBLASTOMA

- Ewing sarcoma/PNET
- Alveolar rhabdomyosarcoma
- Lymphoma/leukemia

Pitfalls
NEUROBLASTOMA AND
GANGLIONEUROBLASTOMA

! NB84 is expressed in other small round cell tumors including small cell osteosarcoma, ES/PNET, desmoplastic small round cell tumor, and rhabdomyosarcoma.

! Core biopsies may not be representative of the entire tumor, and may underrepresent the amount of neuroblastic elements within ganglioneuroblastoma.

have characteristic gene fusions that can be detected by FISH or RT-PCR. The cells of lymphoma and leukemia have a more dispersed appearance and are positive for their respective hematolymphoid markers, such as CD45, CD20, CD3, or TdT.

PROGNOSIS

The behavior of neuroblastoma varies widely among patients, ranging from spontaneous regression in a small percentage to rapid progression with widespread metastases and death. Because of the heterogeneity in biologic behavior, risk estimation of each patient is required to decide appropriate management. Current trials stratify patients by clinical parameters (eg, patient age and disease stage), and for molecular markers, such as *MYCN* oncogene amplification and loss of chromosome 1p.[48] The presence of *MYCN* amplification is associated with a worse prognosis, as are loss of heterozygosity at 1p and 11q. The clinical stage

and histologic subtype appear to be the most important factors influencing overall survival.[49]

ROUND CELL LIPOSARCOMA

Myxoid-round cell liposarcoma is the second most frequent liposarcoma, after the well differentiated/dedifferentiated subtype. It most commonly affects younger adults, and occurs most frequently in the deep soft tissues of the extremities. Histologically it comprises sheets and patternless distributions of uniform cells with round or ovoid nuclei with minimal or small amounts of myxoid stroma (**Fig. 17**). The prominent vascular network of delicate, curvilinear thin-walled vessels characteristic of myxoid liposarcoma is much less prominent or

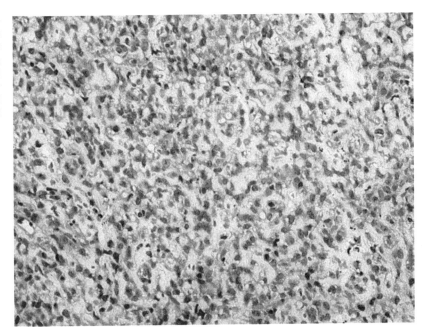

Fig. 17. Round cell liposarcoma. This tumor is composed of patternless distributions of uniform cells with round or ovoid nuclei with minimal or small amounts of myxoid stroma (H&E, original magnification ×200).

inconspicuous in round cell liposarcoma. Tumors harbor characteristic translocations, most frequently t(12;16)(q13;p11) in more than 90% of cases, which fuse the *DDIT3* and *FUS* genes, or the rarer t(12;22)(q13;q12), fusing *DDIT3* and *EWSR1* genes. Round cell liposarcoma can express variable S100 protein but generally is not immunoreactive for other markers.

The tumor can metastasize to other soft tissue sites, as well as to the lungs.

LYMPHOMA AND TUMORS OF HEMOPOIETIC CELLS

Lymphomas can involve the soft tissue by extension from adjacent nodes or as part of systemic disease. Primary soft tissue lymphoma is rare, but can arise in the extremities or trunk of older adults.[50] Most are diffuse large B-cell lymphomas, but other non-Hodgkin lymphomas can also occur. Diagnosis is by expression of the relevant panels of lymphoid markers (including TdT for lymphoblastic lymphoma), and absence of expression of antigens expressed in other lineages. Granulocytic sarcoma (extramedullary myeloid tumor) can form a soft tissue mass (chloroma) in patients with acute or chronic myeloid leukemia. The tumor comprises sheets of immature myeloid cells with distinct nuclear membranes, small nucleoli, and minimal to moderate amounts of cytoplasm. The cells express myeloperoxidase, CD117, CD43, CD68, and lysozyme. Mastocytosis can occur in the skin or, very rarely, as a soft tissue mass. The mast cells are positive for toluidine blue, and express CD117.

REFERENCES

1. Lazar A, Abruzzo LV, Pollock RE, et al. Molecular diagnosis of sarcomas: chromosomal translocations in sarcomas. Arch Pathol Lab Med 2006;130(8): 1199–207.
2. Ordonez JL, Osuna D, Herrero D, et al. Advances in Ewing's sarcoma research: where are we now and what lies ahead? Cancer Res 2009;69(18):7140–50.
3. Olmos D, Martins AS, Jones RL, et al. Targeting the insulin-like growth factor 1 receptor in Ewing's sarcoma: reality and expectations. Sarcoma 2011;2011: 402508.
4. Nascimento AG, Unii KK, Pritchard DJ, et al. A clinicopathologic study of 20 cases of large-cell (atypical) Ewing's sarcoma of bone. Am J Surg Pathol 1980;4(1):29–36.
5. Folpe AL, Goldblum JR, Rubin BP, et al. Morphologic and immunophenotypic diversity in Ewing family tumors: a study of 66 genetically confirmed cases. Am J Surg Pathol 2005;29(8):1025–33.
6. Parham DM, Dias P, Kelly DR, et al. Desmin positivity in primitive neuroectodermal tumors of childhood. Am J Surg Pathol 1992;16(5):483–92.
7. Llombart-Bosch A, Machado I, Navarro S, et al. Histological heterogeneity of Ewing's sarcoma/PNET: an immunohistochemical analysis of 415 genetically confirmed cases with clinical support. Virchows Arch 2009;455(5):397–411.
8. Delattre O, Zucman J, Melot T, et al. The Ewing family of tumors—a subgroup of small-round-cell tumors defined by specific chimeric transcripts. N Engl J Med 1994;331(5):294–9.
9. Arvand A, Denny CT. Biology of EWS/ETS fusions in Ewing's family tumors. Oncogene 2001;20(40): 5747–54.
10. de Alava E, Kawai A, Healey JH, et al. EWS-FLI1 fusion transcript structure is an independent determinant of prognosis in Ewing's sarcoma. J Clin Oncol 1998;16(4):1248–55.
11. Ordonez NG. Desmoplastic small round cell tumor: I: a histopathologic study of 39 cases with emphasis on unusual histological patterns. Am J Surg Pathol 1998;22(11):1303–13.
12. Gerald WL, Miller HK, Battifora H, et al. Intra-abdominal desmoplastic small round-cell tumor. Report of 19 cases of a distinctive type of high-grade polyphenotypic malignancy affecting young individuals. Am J Surg Pathol 1991;15(6):499–513.
13. Antonescu CR, Gerald WL, Magid MS, et al. Molecular variants of the EWS-WT1 gene fusion in desmoplastic small round cell tumor. Diagn Mol Pathol 1998;7(1):24–8.
14. Ordonez NG. Desmoplastic small round cell tumor: II: an ultrastructural and immunohistochemical study with emphasis on new immunohistochemical markers. Am J Surg Pathol 1998;22(11): 1314–27.
15. Lal DR, Su WT, Wolden SL, et al. Results of multimodal treatment for desmoplastic small round cell tumors. J Pediatr Surg 2005;40(1):251–5.
16. Newton WA Jr, Gehan EA, Webber BL, et al. Classification of rhabdomyosarcomas and related sarcomas. Pathologic aspects and proposal for a new classification—an Intergroup Rhabdomyosarcoma Study. Cancer 1995;76(6):1073–85.
17. Mercado GE, Barr FG. Fusions involving PAX and FOX genes in the molecular pathogenesis of alveolar rhabdomyosarcoma: recent advances. Curr Mol Med 2007;7(1):47–61.
18. Sumegi J, Streblow R, Frayer RW, et al. Recurrent t(2;2) and t(2;8) translocations in rhabdomyosarcoma without the canonical PAX-FOXO1 fuse PAX3 to members of the nuclear receptor transcriptional coactivator family. Genes Chromosomes Cancer 2010;49(3):224–36.
19. Barr FG, Qualman SJ, Macris MH, et al. Genetic heterogeneity in the alveolar rhabdomyosarcoma

subset without typical gene fusions. Cancer Res 2002;62(16):4704–10.

20. Davicioni E, Finckenstein FG, Shahbazian V, et al. Identification of a PAX-FKHR gene expression signature that defines molecular classes and determines the prognosis of alveolar rhabdomyosarcomas. Cancer Res 2006;66(14):6936–46.

21. Williamson D, Missiaglia E, de Reynies A, et al. Fusion gene-negative alveolar rhabdomyosarcoma is clinically and molecularly indistinguishable from embryonal rhabdomyosarcoma. J Clin Oncol 2010; 28(13):2151–8.

22. Boman F, Champigneulle J, Schmitt C, et al. Clear cell rhabdomyosarcoma. Pediatr Pathol Lab Med 1996;16(6):951–9.

23. Morotti RA, Nicol KK, Parham DM, et al. An immunohistochemical algorithm to facilitate diagnosis and subtyping of rhabdomyosarcoma: the Children's Oncology Group experience. Am J Surg Pathol 2006;30(8):962–8.

24. Morgenstern DA, Rees H, Sebire NJ, et al. Rhabdomyosarcoma subtyping by immunohistochemical assessment of myogenin: tissue array study and review of the literature. Pathol Oncol Res 2008; 14(3):233–8.

25. Parham DM, Qualman SJ, Teot L, et al. Correlation between histology and PAX/FKHR fusion status in alveolar rhabdomyosarcoma: a report from the Children's Oncology Group. Am J Surg Pathol 2007; 31(6):895–901.

26. Sorensen PH, Lynch JC, Qualman SJ, et al. PAX3-FKHR and PAX7-FKHR gene fusions are prognostic indicators in alveolar rhabdomyosarcoma: a report from the children's oncology group. J Clin Oncol 2002;20(11):2672–9.

27. van de Rijn M, Barr FG, Xiong QB, et al. Poorly differentiated synovial sarcoma: an analysis of clinical, pathologic, and molecular genetic features. Am J Surg Pathol 1999;23(1):106–12.

28. Jagdis A, Rubin BP, Tubbs RR, et al. Prospective evaluation of TLE1 as a diagnostic immunohistochemical marker in synovial sarcoma. Am J Surg Pathol 2009;33(12):1743–51.

29. Terry J, Saito T, Subramanian S, et al. TLE1 as a diagnostic immunohistochemical marker for synovial sarcoma emerging from gene expression profiling studies. Am J Surg Pathol 2007;31(2):240–6.

30. Matsuyama A, Hisaoka M, Iwasaki M, et al. TLE1 expression in malignant mesothelioma. Virchows Arch 2010;457(5):577–83.

31. Pilotti S, Mezzelani A, Azzarelli A, et al. bcl-2 expression in synovial sarcoma. J Pathol 1998;184(3):337–9.

32. Dei Tos AP, Wadden C, Calonje E, et al. Immunohistochemical demonstration of glycoprotein p30/32mic2 (CD99) in synovial sarcoma. A potential cause of diagnostic confusion. Appl Immunohistochem 1995;3:168–73.

33. Miettinen M, Cupo W. Neural cell adhesion molecule distribution in soft tissue tumors. Hum Pathol 1993; 24(1):62–6.

34. Fisher C, Schofield J. S100 protein positive synovial sarcoma. Histopathology 1991;19:375–7.

35. Crew AJ, Clark J, Fisher C, et al. Fusion of SYT to two genes, SSX1 and SSX2, encoding proteins with homology to the Kruppel-associated box in human synovial sarcoma. EMBO J 1995;14(10): 2333–40.

36. Agus V, Tamborini E, Mezzelani A, et al. Re: a novel fusion gene, SYT-SSX4, in synovial sarcoma. J Natl Cancer Inst 2001;93(17):1347–9.

37. Nakayama R, Mitani S, Nakagawa T, et al. Gene expression profiling of synovial sarcoma: distinct signature of poorly differentiated type. Am J Surg Pathol 2010;34(11):1599–607.

38. van de Rijn M, Barr FG, Collins MH, et al. Absence of SYT-SSX fusion products in soft tissue tumors other than synovial sarcoma. Am J Clin Pathol 1999; 112(1):43–9.

39. Tamborini E, Agus V, Perrone F, et al. Lack of SYT-SSX fusion transcripts in malignant peripheral nerve sheath tumors on RT-PCR analysis of 34 archival cases. Lab Invest 2002;82(5):609–18.

40. Jones KB, Haldar M, Schiffman JD, et al. Of mice and men: opportunities to use genetically engineered mouse models of synovial sarcoma for preclinical cancer therapeutic evaluation. Cancer Control 2011;18(3):196–203.

41. Stiller CA, Parkin DM. International variations in the incidence of neuroblastoma. Int J Cancer 1992; 52(4):538–43.

42. DeLorimier AA, Bragg KU, Linden G. Neuroblastoma in childhood. Am J Dis Child 1969;118(3): 441–50.

43. Korfei M, Fuhlhuber V, Schmidt-Woll T, et al. Functional characterisation of autoantibodies from patients with pediatric opsoclonus-myoclonus-syndrome. J Neuroimmunol 2005;170(1–2):150–7.

44. Tornoczky T, Kalman E, Kajtar PG, et al. Large cell neuroblastoma: a distinct phenotype of neuroblastoma with aggressive clinical behavior. Cancer 2004;100(2):390–7.

45. Cozzutto C, Carbone A. Pleomorphic (anaplastic) neuroblastoma. Arch Pathol Lab Med 1988;112(6): 621–5.

46. Mullins JD. A pigmented differentiating neuroblastoma: a light and ultrastructural study. Cancer 1980;46(3):522–8.

47. Thomas JO, Nijjar J, Turley H, et al. NB84: a new monoclonal antibody for the recognition of neuroblastoma in routinely processed material. J Pathol 1991;163(1):69–75.

48. Fischer M, Spitz R, Oberthur A, et al. Risk estimation of neuroblastoma patients using molecular markers. Klin Padiatr 2008;220(3):137–46.

49. Burgues O, Navarro S, Noguera R, et al. Prognostic value of the International Neuroblastoma Pathology Classification in Neuroblastoma (Schwannian stroma-poor) and comparison with other prognostic factors: a study of 182 cases from the Spanish Neuroblastoma Registry. Virchows Arch 2006; 449(4):410–20.

50. Lanham GR, Weiss SW, Enzinger FM. Malignant lymphoma. A study of 75 cases presenting in soft tissue. Am J Surg Pathol 1989;13(1):1–10.

DERMAL AND SUBCUTANEOUS PLEXIFORM SOFT TISSUE NEOPLASMS

Hillary Elwood, MD[a],*, Janis Taube, MD, MSc[b]

KEYWORDS

- Plexiform fibrohistiocytic tumor • Cellular neurothekeoma • Dermal nerve sheath myxoma
- Plexiform schwannoma • Plexiform neurofibroma

ABSTRACT

This article presents an overview of soft tissue tumors that have a plexiform histomorphology. The more commonly encountered entities, including plexiform fibrohistiocytic tumor, cellular neurothekeoma, dermal nerve sheath myxoma, plexiform schwannoma, and plexiform neurofibroma, are discussed in detail, and other tumors are noted. Information on clinical features, microscopic findings, ancillary studies, differential diagnosis, and prognosis is provided for each entity.

OVERVIEW

"Plexiform" is used as both a macroscopic and microscopic descriptor in pathology. Macroscopically, it is often applied to lesions that show a multinodular gross appearance or those lesions with a so-called "bag of worms" pattern, with multiple entwined tumor nodules. It is used in microscopic histomorphology to describe lesions with multiple discrete tumor bundles ramifying through the tissue, resembling an interwoven network or plexus. Tumors with microscopic plexiform features do not necessarily have a plexiform gross appearance and vice versa. In general, many soft tissue tumors may adopt a plexiform pattern (including tumors encountered again in other articles of this issue). Although most of these plexiform soft tissue tumors are benign, even those that are histologically bland can occasionally recur at the site of origin. Of the lesions described in this article, only one, the plexiform fibrohistiocytic tumor, has the potential for metastasis. What follows is a clincopathologic description of soft tissue tumors that exhibit plexiform histology with an emphasis on the more commonly encountered entities.

PLEXIFORM FIBROHISTIOCYTIC TUMOR

Plexiform fibrohistiocytic tumor (PFHT) was first described in 1988 in a case series by Drs Enzinger and Zhang.[1] It occurs predominantly in children and young adults on the upper extremities, especially the forearm, shoulder, wrists, and fingers.[1] Early case series described a female predominance,[1,2] but subsequent series indicate an equal sex distribution.[3] Clinically, the tumor usually presents as a slow-growing, small, painless, dermal or subcutaneous mass that slowly enlarges over months to years. PFHT is the only plexiform soft tissue tumor that has shown the possibility for metastasis. It is considered a tumor of intermediate biologic potential, with local recurrence common and rare reports of lymph node or lung metastasis.[4]

The authors have nothing to disclose.
[a] Department of Pathology, The Johns Hopkins Hospital, Path 401, 600 North Wolfe Street, Baltimore, MD 21287, USA
[b] Departments of Dermatology and Pathology, The Johns Hopkins Hospital, 600 North Wolfe Street, Baltimore, MD 21287, USA
* Corresponding author.
E-mail address: Helwood2@jhmi.edu

Key Features
PLEXIFORM FIBROHISTIOCYTIC TUMOR

- Occurs mainly in children and young adults

- Most commonly involves the upper extremities

- Infiltrative plexiform lesion usually located at the dermal-subcutaneous junction

- Often biphasic: nodules of mononuclear histiocytelike cells and multinucleate giant cells (both usually CD68 positive), fascicles of elongated spindle cells (usually smooth muscle actin positive)

- Three subtypes described based on proportions of each component

- Local recurrence in 12.5% to 37.5% of cases

- Rare metastasis (lymph nodes and lung)

- No correlation between clinical, histologic or genetic factors and propensity for metastasis

GROSS AND MICROSCOPIC FEATURES

On gross examination, PFHT is usually a multinodular, poorly circumscribed mass, most often situated at the dermal-subcutaneous junction, although it can occur entirely in the dermis or in the subcutaneous tissue. It rarely exceeds a size of 3 cm. Microscopic examination reveals an infiltrating multinodular tumor composed of 2 elements in varying proportions (Fig. 1). One element is the well-delineated nodules of mononuclear histiocytelike cells with associated multinucleated osteoclastlike giant cells; the other element is fascicles of elongated fibroblastlike spindle cells. Based on the relative amounts of these 2 components, 3 histologic subtypes have been identified: fibrohistiocytic, fibroblastic, or mixed. The histologic subtype does not have a prognostic significance, thus the importance lies simply in recognition and appropriate classification of the lesion as a PFHT. The fibrohistiocytic subtype is composed predominantly of mononuclear histiocytelike cell nodules with varying amounts of associated giant cells (Figs. 2 and 3). The fibroblastic subtype is composed mainly of interlaced short and long fascicles of fibroblastlike spindle cells associated with variable amounts of hyalinized collagen (Figs. 4 and 5); however, focal areas of fibrohistiocytelike cells and giant cells can also usually be found in the fibroblastic subtype. The mixed subtype is composed of both patterns in relatively equal proportion. In the original description, most cases exhibited fibrohistiocytic or mixed patterns.[1] In cases with fibrohistiocytic nodules, a lymphocytic infiltrate often surrounds those structures (Figs. 6 and 7). Cellular atypia is rare in these lesions. Mitotic activity may be seen, but is usually less than 4 per high-power field (HPF). Recurrent lesions may show an increased

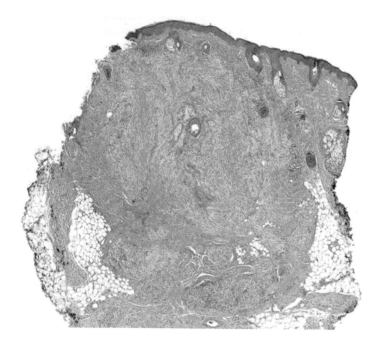

Fig. 1. Plexiform fibrohistiocytic tumor. Infiltrating multinodular tumor centered at the dermal-subcutaneous junction (hematoxylin-eosin stain [H&E], original magnification ×20).

Fig. 2. Plexiform fibro-histiocytic tumor. Circumscribed nodules of mononuclear histiocyte-like cells characteristic of the fibrohistiocytic component (H&E, original magnification ×40).

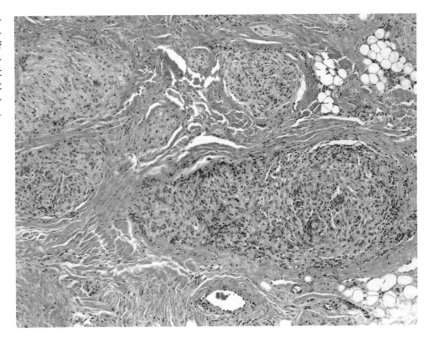

mitotic activity when compared with the original tumor.[1] Occasional osseous metaplasia has been documented, particularly in the fibroblastic subtype.[1,2] Vascular invasion has been observed in 10% to 20% of cases.[4] Microhemorrhage, adnexal sparing, and focal myxoid change have also been described.[3]

ANCILLARY STUDIES

Immunohistochemical studies show little specificity; however, CD68 is positive in the histiocyte-like cells and multinucleate giant cells and smooth muscle actin (SMA) is typically positive in the spindled fibroblastlike cells. Tumor cells are

Fig. 3. Plexiform fibro-histiocytic tumor. Fibro-histiocytic nodules with associated multinucleated osteoclastlike giant cells (H&E, original magnification ×64).

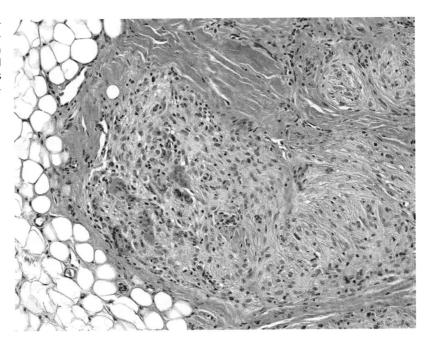

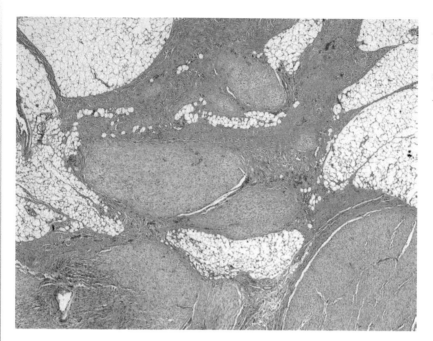

Fig. 4. Plexiform fibrohistiocytic tumor. Fibroblastic variant showing bundles of spindles cells set in a fibrous stroma (H&E, original magnification ×10).

uniformly negative for keratin, desmin, HMB-45, S-100, factor XIIIa, beta-catenin, and CD34. Two PFHTs with clonal chromosome aberrations have been reported but no consistent genetic abnormalities have been identified.[5,6]

DIFFERENTIAL DIAGNOSIS

The classic morphology of plexiform cellular nodules at the dermal-epidermal junction should immediately lead one to consider the diagnosis

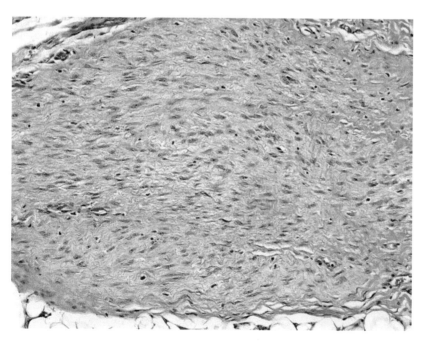

Fig. 5. Plexiform fibrohistiocytic tumor. Fibroblastic variant with fibroblastlike spindle cells (H&E, original magnification ×64).

Fig. 6. Plexiform fibrohistiocytic tumor. Superficial (*A*) and deep (*B*) views of the same tumor showing the multinodular appearance with involvement of deep dermis and subcutaneous tissue and prominent associated lymphocytic response (H&E, original magnification ×10).

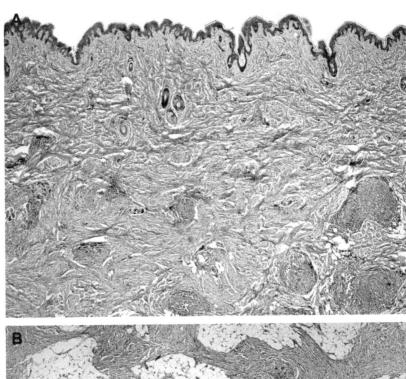

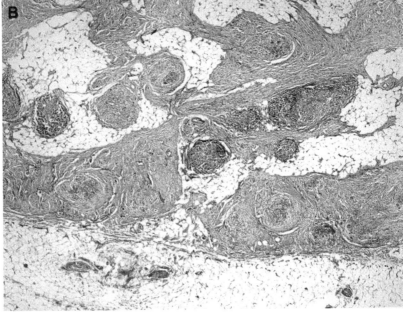

of PFHT; however, the histologic variants, particularly the purely fibroblastic variant, can pose diagnostic difficulty. For those lesions entirely composed of spindle cells (the fibroblastic subtype), the differential may include fibromatosis and myofibroma. In those cases, careful examination of the lesion for focal areas of more typical fibrohistiocytic aggregates and giant cells can be helpful. Fibromatosis does not contain giant cells and is uniformly cellular with long parallel fascicles,

as opposed to the plexiform nodules of fibroblastic PFHT. Myofibroma is multinodular and may contain giant cells but is distinguished by whorled lobules of myofibroblasts with central smaller cells in a hemangiopericytomatous pattern.

The subtypes of PFHT with pronounced histiocytelike nodules and giant cells, particularly those tumors with associated lymphocytic infiltrate, can sometimes resemble a granulomatous process. The absence of necrosis and the presence of

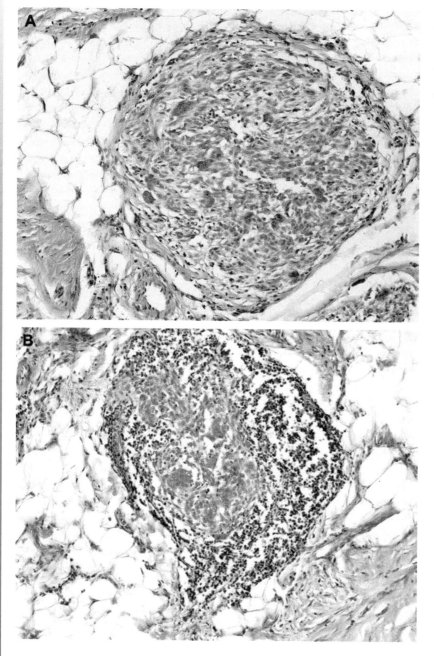

Fig. 7. Plexiform fibrohistiocytic tumor. Nodules with prominent giant cells (*A*) and lymphocytes (*B*) demonstrating how on biopsy these might be confused with a granulomatous process (H&E, original magnification ×64).

a fibroblastic component are helpful in confirming the diagnosis of PFHT. Tumors of the fibrohistiocytic subtype that contain increased giant cells might also be confused with giant cell tumor of soft parts or less likely a superficial undifferentiated pleomorphic sarcoma with prominent osteoclastlike giant cells. Giant cell tumor of soft parts is multinodular and often occurs on the upper arm like PFHT; however, it does not have the infiltrative pattern of PFHT. Giant cell tumor of soft parts also

often shows peripheral osteoid or metaplastic bone formation, a feature not seen in PFHT. A giant cell–rich undifferentiated pleomorphic sarcoma differs from PFHT in that it shows marked cytologic atypia and increased mitotic activity.

Additional differential diagnoses include fibrous hamartoma of infancy (FHI) and lipofibromatosis, which can also involve the extremities of children. Yet, both of these tumors are rarely plexiform, they do not contain giant cells, and they have

Pitfalls
PLEXIFORM FIBROHISTIOCYTIC TUMOR

! On biopsy, inflamed nodules of histiocytelike cells and giant cells may resemble a granulomatous process

! Broad histologic differential diagnosis (varies by predominant histologic component)

Key Features
CELLULAR NEUROTHEKEOMA

- Dermal to subcutaneous lesion with multinodular or nested infiltrative pattern
- Epithelioid to spindled lesional cells
- Focal SMA, CD68 positivity
- S100 negative
- Rarely recur

a variable lesional adipose tissue component. Cellular neurothekeoma enters the differential for superficial PFHT as well, and many investigators consider cellular neurothekeoma and PFHT to be closely related or potentially the same neoplasm (see discussion in the Cellular Neurothekeoma section later in this article).

PROGNOSIS

PFHT has a local recurrence rate estimated between 12.5% and 37.5%.[1,2] Two patients in the original case series developed regional lymph node metastases; subsequent case series showed 1 case of regional lymph nodes metastasis and 3 cases of pulmonary metastases.[2] Only one death from systemic metastatic PFHT has been reported.[7] The tumor is considered as an intermediate-grade (rarely metastasizing) tumor in the World Health Organization 2002 classification.[4] No clinical, histologic, or genetic factors have been identified that correlate with prognosis. Wide local reexcision after diagnosis is the most recommended clinical approach.

CELLULAR NEUROTHEKEOMA

Cellular neurothekeoma (CN), a benign cutaneous tumor of uncertain histogenesis, was originally described in 1980 by Gallager and Helwig.[8] At the time, these tumors were thought to be of nerve sheath differentiation, and, indeed, many considered CN to be a cellular variant of nerve sheath myxoma. The relationship, or lack thereof, between dermal nerve sheath myxoma and CN has been debated for some time; however, a recent study by Sheth and colleagues[9] that evaluated gene expression profiles of both lesions, suggests that neurothekeomas may be of fibrohistiocytic origin as opposed to peripheral nerve sheath origin. Clinically, the tumor typically presents in the first 3 decades of life as an asymptomatic, superficial, slow-growing, solitary papule or nodule on the extremities or head and neck area, more often occurring in women.[10]

GROSS AND MICROSCOPIC FEATURES

Macroscopic examination most often shows an ill-defined, infiltrative lesion occupying the dermis with occasional extension into the subcutis. Microscopically, the tumor has a multinodular or nested architecture and is composed of epithelioid to spindle cells with large ovoid nuclei and abundant eosinophilic cytoplasm (**Figs. 8–12**). Pseudonuclear inclusions may be seen. Some tumors may show focal to prominent myxoid areas. Typically, there is a "Grenz" zone separating the tumor from the overlying epidermis. Most tumors will show some degree of cellular pleomorphism; osteoclastic giant cells are seen in fewer than half of cases. Additionally and not uncommonly, a brisk mitotic rate and atypical mitotic figures are seen. Perineural and vascular invasion have been reported.[10,11]

ANCILLARY STUDIES

These tumors are focally positive for SMA and CD68, and diffusely positive for S100A6 and NKI-C3.[12,13] Tumor cells are negative for S100, cytokeratin, glial fibrillary acidic protein (GFAP), HMB-45, Mart-1, and endomysial antibodies (EMA). Although S100A6 and NKI-C3 are positive, they are not specific for the diagnosis of neurothekeoma.[12,13]

DIFFERENTIAL DIAGNOSIS

CN may be related to PFHT.[14] The 2 entities can be especially difficult to distinguish when PFHT involves a superficial subcutaneous or deep dermal location. Indeed, the 2 entities seem to have more in common than they do differences, with both tumors occurring on the head and neck or the extremities of young adults, both showing identical immunolabeling and similar plexiform morphology, and both having giant cells and spindle cells. The 2 differences that have been

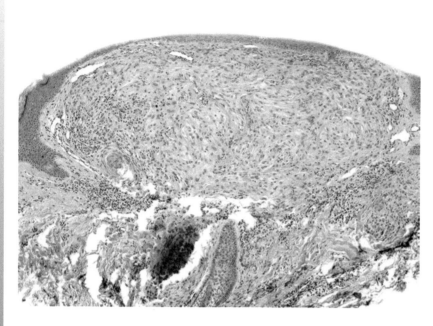

Fig. 8. Cellular neurothekeoma. Vaguely multinodular tumor in the superficial dermis without involvement of the overlying epidermis (H&E, original magnification ×64).

emphasized are the superficial location of CN and its benign prognosis (less likely to recur, no chance of metastasis). Additional molecular investigation and further studies are needed to determine whether these are unique entities or just superficial and deep variants of the same tumor. For now, CN can be distinguished from PFHT by the superficial location, the epithelioid lesional cells, and the lack of biphasic architecture (ie, fibrohistiocytic and fibroblastic components).

Also closely related to CN are the superficial fibrohistiocytic lesions, such as dermatofibromas/fibrous histiocytomas, which can demonstrate similar molecular signatures.[9] Classic dermatofibromas

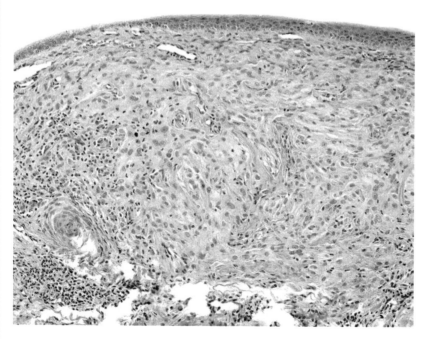

Fig. 9. Cellular neurothekeoma. Tumor composed of epithelioid cells with abundant eosinophilic cytoplasm (H&E, original magnification ×64).

Fig. 10. Cellular neuro-thekeoma. Multinodular appearance of tumor in deep dermis (H&E, original magnification ×20).

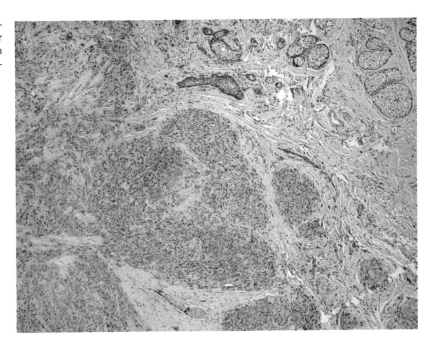

can be distinguished by the irregular fascicles extending through the dermis as compared with the more nested architecture of CN. A pilar leiomyoma, particularly the epithelioid variant, may also resemble CN and can be distinguished by broader, more elongate nuclei and by strong staining for SMA and desmin.

The differential diagnosis for CN, given its histology and superficial location, can also include a specific subset of melanocytic lesions including Spitz nevus, deep penetrating nevus, plexiform spindle-cell nevus, and the fascicular variant of cellular blue nevi. Spitz nevus in particular can enter the differential, as it tends to arise in the

Fig. 11. Cellular neuro-thekeoma. Epitheliod to spindle cells comprise the tumor (H&E, original magnification ×64).

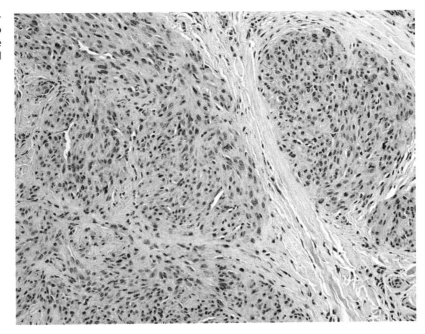

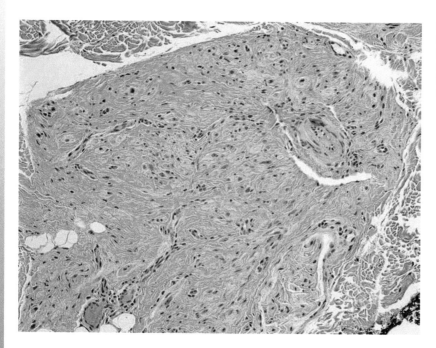

Fig. 12. Cellular neurothekeoma. Nodule with extensive collagen deposition showing scattered tumor cells (H&E, original magnification ×64).

same demographic (head and neck of children and adolescents) as CN. Unlike CN, all of these nevi would show diffuse staining for S100 protein and some positivity for melanocytic markers. Additionally, all but the blue nevus would likely show a junctional melanocytic component, whereas CN does not involve the epidermis.

CNs showing a prominent myxoid background may also be confused with dermal nerve sheath myxoma (DNSM). The first clue to separating the 2 is demographics: CN tends to occur on the head and neck and extremities of young adults and almost never occurs on hands or fingers. In contrast, DNSM mostly arises on the distal extremities, including the hands and fingers, of young to middle-aged adults, and rarely occurs on the head and neck. Microscopically, CNs usually have irregular margins, whereas most DNSMs are sharply demarcated with fibrous bands separating myxoid nodules. The cells of DNSM are usually bland spindle to stellate cells, whereas lesional cells of CN are spindled to epithelioid and can show cellular atypia. Immunohistochemistry can be helpful, as DNSM is consistently positive for S-100 and GFAP, both usually negative in CN.

PROGNOSIS

If incompletely excised, CN may recur in at the prior site of resection. Location seems to be a predictor of recurrence, with incompletely excised lesions of the head and neck being the most likely to recur.[10] Of note, atypical histologic features, such as pleomorphism or brisk mitotic activity, are not predictive of recurrence. There have been no reports of metastasis or malignant transformation of this tumor.

DERMAL NERVE SHEATH MYXOMA

DNSM is a peripheral nerve sheath tumor that was originally described by Harkin and Reed in 1969.[15] As discussed previously, these were initially considered to be related to CNs, but recent studies have shown them to be genetically distinct entities, with molecular profiles closely aligning those of dermal schwannomas.[9] DNSM typically arises on the extremities of young to middle-aged adults with a peak incidence in the fourth decade of life and no gender predilection. The tumor is slow growing and painless and often involves the hands or fingers.[16]

GROSS AND MICROSCOPIC FEATURES

DNSM is usually a well-demarcated dermal tumor composed of nodules of sparsely cellular myxoid stroma usually separated by fibrous bands (**Figs. 13 and 14**). The tumor cells are variably shaped Schwann cells, ranging from epithelioid to spindled to stellate in morphology (**Figs. 15 and 16**); occasionally these cells may have a vacuolated or ring-shaped appearance that superficially resembles lipomatous cells. Often the lesional cells are arranged within the myxoid matrix in

Fig. 13. Dermal nerve sheath myxoma. Well-demarcated dermal tumor with nodules of myxoid stroma separated by fibrous bands (H&E, original magnification ×10).

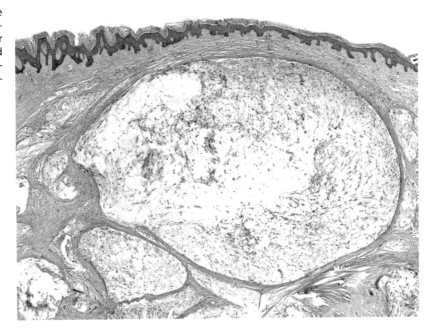

corded or syncytial-like aggregates. Mitotic figures are infrequent to absent and atypia is generally lacking.

ANCILLARY STUDIES

Lesional cells are positive for S100 and GFAP and show limited to no reactivity for EMA and CD34.

DIFFERENTIAL DIAGNOSIS

Both CNs (discussed previously) and plexiform neurofibromas with prominent myxoid changes enter the differential diagnosis. Plexiform neurofibroma is generally more cellular and composed of spindle cells with wavy nuclei, often with associated mast cells.

Fig. 14. Dermal nerve sheath myxoma. Multinodular dermal tumor composed of numerous myxoid nodules of varying size (H&E, original magnification ×10).

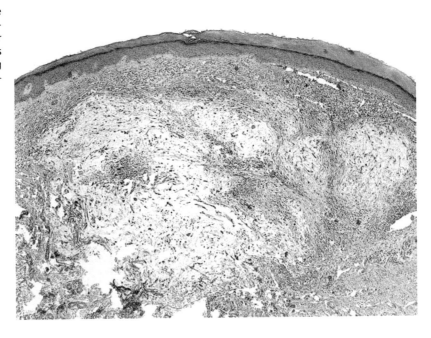

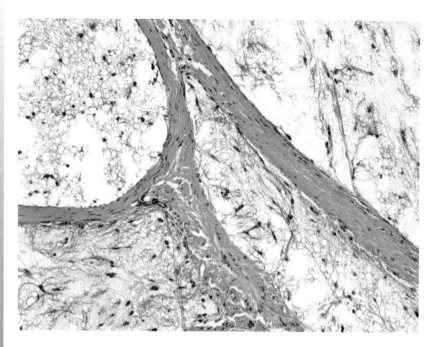

Fig. 15. Dermal nerve sheath myxoma. Tumor nodules are composed of sparsely cellular myxoid stroma containing variably shaped plump to spindled to stellate cells (H&E, original magnification ×64).

Focal cutaneous mucinosis and ganglion cysts may show some resemblance to DNSM, but they are negative for S100, do not contain the same stellate cellular component, and do not show the plexiform or nodular growth pattern of DNSM. Superficial acral fibromyxoma is a dermal tumor that commonly presents on the fingers and can show abundant myxoid matrix; these tumors are less well demarcated than DNSM and can further be distinguished by CD34 immunolabeling and absence of S100 expression.

PROGNOSIS

DNSM commonly recurs locally at the site of prior excision. In the most recent case series, nearly

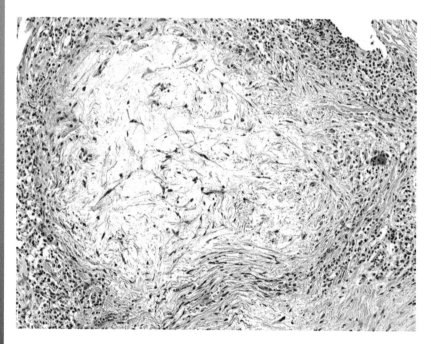

Fig. 16. Dermal nerve sheath myxoma. Spindled to stellate tumor cells in myxoid stroma (H&E, original magnification ×64).

50% of the cases showed recurrent disease, over a long time interval ranging from between 1 year and 27 years later.[16] Complete local excision with negative margins is recommended. No malignant transformation from DNSM has been described.

PLEXIFORM SCHWANNOMA

The plexiform variant of schwannoma was first described in an abstract in 1978 by Harkin, and colleagues[17] in a case series of benign peripheral nerve sheath tumors composed of Schwann cells arranged in a plexiform pattern. Subsequent case reports and studies have revealed that the plexiform variant accounts for approximately 4% of all schwannomas.[18] Like conventional schwannomas, plexiform schwannomas (PS) most commonly occur as a solitary, asymptomatic, slow-growing nodule in the superficial soft tissues, most commonly of the head and neck area and on the extremities of young adults.[18] A deep-seated variant of PS has been described, typically occurring in the soft tissues of the extremities or in the pelvis of women.[19] Additionally, there are rare reports of viscerally occurring PS in the gastrointestinal tract.[20]

GROSS AND MICROSCOPIC FEATURES

On gross examination, these tumors are round to elongate multinodular masses with a white-tan to pink cut surface. Microscopic examination shows a nodular proliferation of bland, dominantly spindle-shaped Schwann cells surrounded by a rim of perineurial cells, and contained within a thin, fibrous capsule (Fig. 17). Like other types of schwannomas, the plexiform variant can show both Antoni A and Antoni B zones. Antoni A areas are defined by compact, often palisaded areas of

---

> ### Key Features
> #### PLEXIFORM SCHWANNOMA
>
> - Plexiform variant accounts for 4% of all schwannomas
>
> - Predilection for flexor surface of extremities and head and neck of young adults
>
> - Often cellular, may lack Antoni B and Verocay bodies
>
> - Diffuse uniform S100 expression useful in diagnosis
>
> - Rare association with NF2

increased cellularity. The cells themselves are spindled or fusiform cells with eosinophilic cytoplasm and hyperchromatic, elongated nuclei (Fig. 18). In contrast, the Antoni B areas, if present, are less ordered and less cellular and demonstrate a loose matrix and large, irregular vessels. Verocay bodies, formed by the alignment of 2 compact rows of nuclei separated by cell processes, may be evident in the Antoni A areas but are less typically found in plexiform schwannomas in comparison with their usual-type counterparts (Fig. 19). Some tumors may have a lymphoid cuff beneath the capsule.

In further contrast to typical schwannomas, plexiform schwannomas frequently demonstrate noticeably increased cellularity, occasionally qualifying them as so-called "cellular variants" (Fig. 20). The more cellular plexiform schwannomas predominantly exhibit Antoni A morphology, lack Verocay bodies, and can have an increased mitotic rate, which is usually less than 4 per 10 HPF, although there have been reports as high as 34 per 10 HPF.[19] Deep-seated variants of plexiform schwannomas may also show necrosis or degenerative changes.

ANCILLARY STUDIES

Plexiform schwannomas, like all schwannoma variants, are diffusely positive for S100 and variably positive for GFAP. Most tumors will demonstrate EMA positivity at the periphery of the nodule, reflecting the presence of the perineurium.

DIFFERENTIAL DIAGNOSIS

Plexiform neurofibroma (NF) in particular should be distinguished from plexiform schwannoma (PS), given the syndromic association as well as potential for malignant transformation of plexiform NF. Most plexiform NFs are hypocellular with a myxoid background, which easily distinguishes them from PS; however, some plexiform NFs may show more cellular areas with palisading, bringing schwannoma firmly into the differential. In those instances, the pattern of S100 immunolabeling may be helpful. Although both plexiform schwannomas and plexiform neurofibromas show S100 positivity, plexiform schwannomas typically exhibit a diffuse uniform staining, whereas neurofibromas show scattered patchy staining. Additionally, specific distribution of EMA expression may be helpful in that it often highlights the encapsulated nature of PS in contrast to the focal EMA expression in scattered perineural cells within neurofibromas.

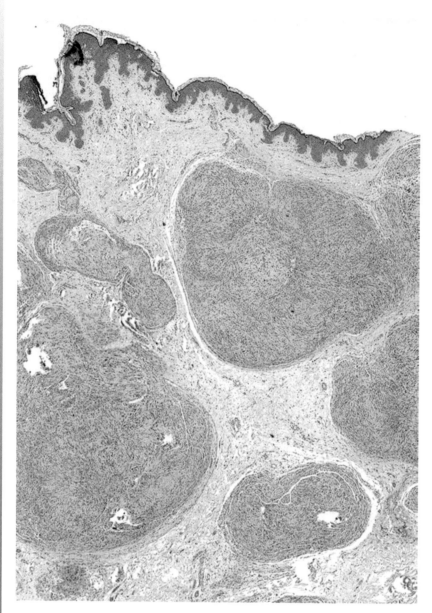

Fig. 17. Plexiform schwannoma. The tumor forms multiple cellular nodules in the superficial and deep dermis (H&E, original magnification ×10).

Other entities that may enter the differential diagnosis for PS are CN, palisaded encapsulated neuroma (PEN), and malignant peripheral nerve sheath tumors (MPNSTs). MPNSTs can show a multinodular pattern, and have increased mitotic activity and prominent cellularity that can resemble a cellular PS. In those instances, sampling of the lesion to look for an underlying benign component of MPNST can be helpful, as can S100 immunolabeling, which typically is patchy in MPNSTs. In cutaneous locations, CN may enter the differential, particularly those that show myxoid areas resembling Antoni B areas; the absence of other features of schwannoma is

Fig. 18. Plexiform schwannoma. Similar histology as conventional schwannoma with Antoni A and B areas (H&E, original magnification ×20).

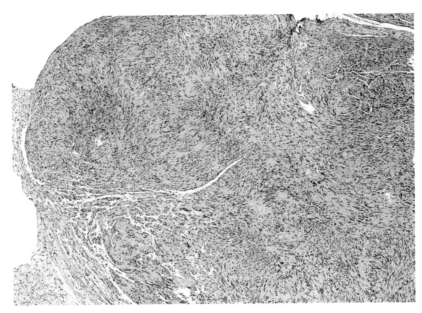

helpful to distinguish between these lesions. PEN can also show a plexiform pattern in cutaneous tissues but is distinguished by the presence of axons, a less uniform Schwann cell composition, and clefting between the tumor fascicles.

Benign nerve sheath tumors with features of both perineurioma and schwannoma may also demonstrate plexiform morphology. Hybrid schwannomas/perineuriomas architecturally resemble perineurioma with a storiform to whorled growth pattern, and often

Fig. 19. Plexiform schwannoma. Verocay bodies can be seen in the tumor nodules (H&E, original magnification ×64).

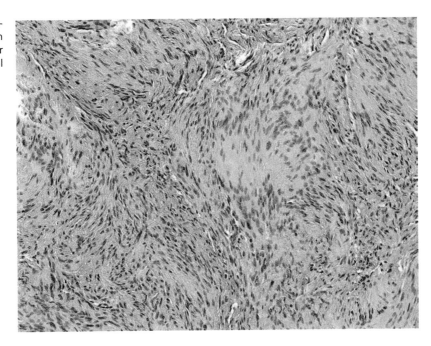

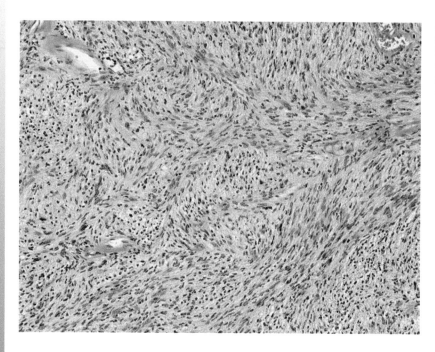

Fig. 20. Plexiform cellular schwannoma. Cellular variant with interlacing fascicles of spindle cells in an Antoni A pattern (H&E, original magnification ×64).

lacking the typical Antoni A and B areas of schwannoma (**Fig. 21**); however, the dominant cytologic features are those of Schwann cells, namely spindle cells containing plump, wavy nuclei and pale cytoplasm (**Fig. 22**). Equal amounts of staining for S100 and EMA confirm the dual lineages and can aid in distinguishing this lesion from a pure plexiform schwannoma (**Figs. 23** and **24**).[21]

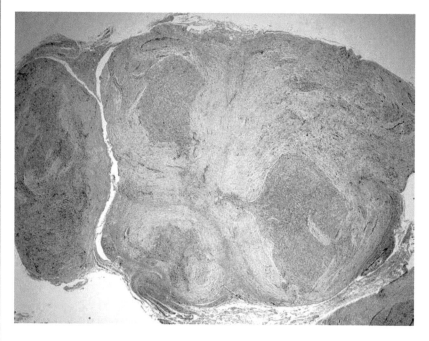

Fig. 21. Hybrid schwannoma/perineurioma. Example of hybrid tumor with plexiform pattern (H&E, original magnification ×20).

Fig. 22. Hybrid schwannoma/perineurioma. High-power views (*A*, *B*) of cytologic morphology (H&E, original magnification *A*: ×40A; *B*: ×64).

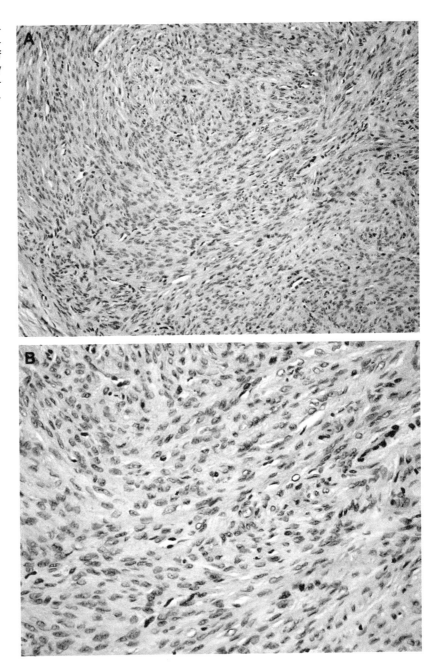

PROGNOSIS

Although most cases of PS are sporadic, there are rare cases of PS occurring in the setting of neurofibromatosis type 2 (NF2) or schwannomatosis.[21] In these instances, the tumors more commonly occur as multiple lesions; it is postulated that the presence of 2 or more plexiform schwannomas, particularly in young patients, should prompt the clinician to consider a workup for NF2.

Plexiform schwannomas follow a benign clinical course, and complete surgical excision is curative.

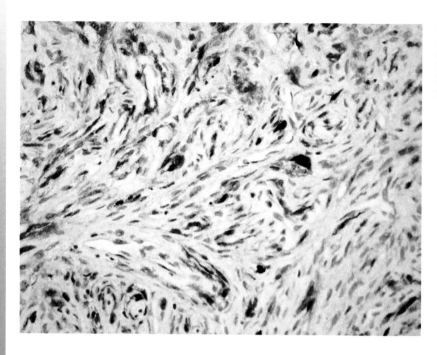

Fig. 23. Hybrid schwannoma/perineurioma. S100 staining highlights the Schwann cells in this hybrid tumor (original magnification ×64).

The tumors tend to recur at sites of incomplete resection.[22,23] Plexiform schwannoma occurring in infants or young children show the most propensity to recur, often exhibiting troubling histologic features (high mitotic rate, increased cellularity) but these findings are not indicative of aggressive behavior.[24] There have been no reports of metastases from plexiform schwannomas.

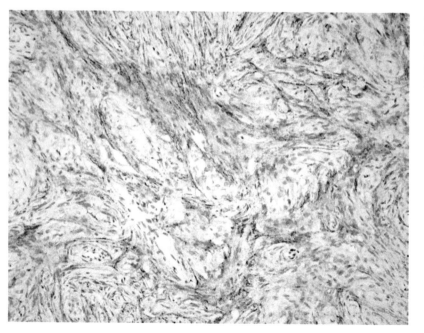

Fig. 24. Hybrid schwannoma/perineurioma. EMA staining confirms the dual lineage nature of this lesion (original magnification ×40).

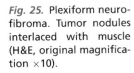

Key Features
PLEXIFORM NEUROFIBROMA

- Virtually pathognomonic for neurofibromatosis type 1

- Spindle-cell proliferation with wavy nuclei

- No high-grade pleomorphism, necrosis, or brisk mitotic activity

- Mast cells common

- Patchy S100 positivity

- Risk for malignant transformation

PLEXIFORM NEUROFIBROMA

Plexiform NF, a variant of conventional neurofibroma, is a multinodular benign peripheral nerve sheath tumor seen almost exclusively in patients with neurofibromatosis type 1 (NF1). NF1, an autosomal dominant condition caused by mutation of the NF1 gene on chromosome 17, has protean manifestations including multiple neurofibromas, café au lait spots, and Lisch nodules of the iris. Plexiform NF is considered virtually pathognomonic for NF1 and is present in approximately 50% of patients with NF1[25,26]; it has very rarely been described in patients without NF1. Neurofibromas usually develop in early childhood and demonstrate a variable growth rate, occurring as superficial or deep lesions. The dermal or subcutaneous lesions are often described as having a "bag of worms" or twisted rope–like sensation on palpation. The larger lesions can involve deep nerves at any site but commonly involve the limbs, pelvis, or retroperitoneum and can be associated with overlying redundant skin folds, hyperpigmentation, and hypertrichosis.[27,28]

GROSS AND MICROSCOPIC FEATURES

The diagnosis of plexiform NF is generally reserved for lesions that show both a multinodular gross appearance and a well-developed plexiform microscopic pattern. On gross examination, plexiform NFs replace portions of peripheral nerves, converting them into a thick tortuous mass of tumor nodules. This tortuous mass, when viewed microscopically, shows multiple nerves expanded by tumor cut in various planes of section (Fig. 25). The tumor nodules are composed of delicate spindle cells with indistinct cytoplasmic membranes and wavy nuclei embedded in a loose background (Figs. 26 and 27). The surrounding stroma can by myxoid, edematous, or fibrotic and often contains variable numbers of mast cells. The overall cellularity is variable, ranging from densely cellular to loosely arranged foci. In the more cellular areas, nuclear palisading may occur, but true Verocay bodies are not characteristic of this lesion.

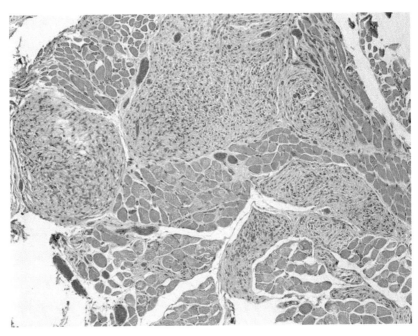

Fig. 25. Plexiform neurofibroma. Tumor nodules interlaced with muscle (H&E, original magnification ×10).

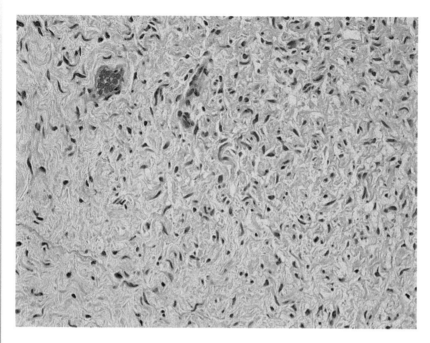

Fig. 26. Plexiform neuro-fibroma. Typical spindle tumor cells with indistinct cytoplasmic membranes and wavy nuclei embedded in a loose background (H&E, original magnification ×100).

Plexiform NF may have scattered atypical cells but it lacks brisk mitotic activity, necrosis, or high-grade nuclear pleomorphism; the presence of any of these latter features should raise the possibility of malignant transformation. In long-standing lesions, the tumor may spill out of the nerves into the soft tissue, resulting in both plexiform and diffuse growth within the same tumor (**Fig. 28**).

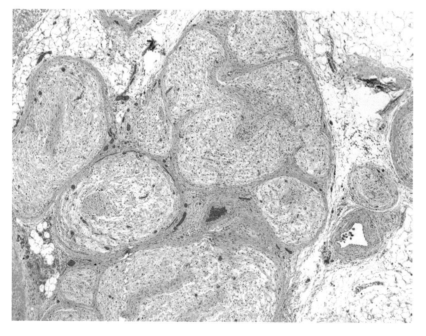

Fig. 27. Plexiform neurofibroma. Multinodular tumor with prominent myxoid change (H&E, original magnification ×10).

Fig. 28. Plexiform neurofi-broma. Tumor spilling out into soft tissue showing both plexiform and diffuse areas (H&E, original magnification ×20).

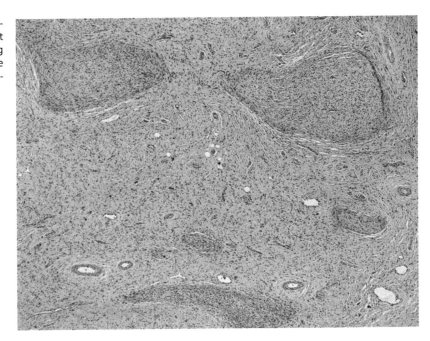

ANCILLARY STUDIES

Plexiform NFs variably express S-100 and EMA depending on the predominant cell type in the tumor. As such, the tumor typically has patchy positivity for S100 (highlighting the Schwann cells) and scattered positivity for EMA (perineural cells) throughout the tumor. This is in contrast to plexiform schwannoma, which shows diffuse S100 positivity and peripheral EMA positivity.

DIFFERENTIAL DIAGNOSIS

Plexiform schwannoma clearly enters the differential for plexiform NF, particularly for the plexiform NF with increased cellular density (see previous discussion of plexiform schwannoma for useful tips in distinguishing the 2 entities). PFHT, particularly the fibroblastic subtype, can sometimes

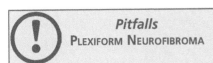

Pitfalls
PLEXIFORM NEUROFIBROMA

! Plexiform NF can have cellular areas with palisading that resemble a plexiform schwannoma. S100 immunostain can be helpful to distinguish the 2 entities; S100 should be diffusely positive in schwannoma and focal or patchy positive in neurofibroma.

resemble NF and can be distinguished by focal areas of typical fibrohistiocytelike and giant cells, as well as the lack of S100 staining.

PROGNOSIS

As previously mentioned, plexiform NF is a marker for NF1. Additionally, it is associated with the possibility of malignant transformation.[25–29]

DIFFUSE NEUROFIBROMA

Although plexiform NF can show areas of diffuse architecture, there are also diffuse variants of neurofibroma. Diffuse NF does not have a plexiform histology but is noted here for comparison to plexiform NF. Diffuse neurofibroma is an uncommon variant of neurofibroma that occurs most commonly on the head and neck area of children and young adults. It presents as a plaquelike elevation of skin, and the overlying epidermis may be hyperpigmented. It is unclear how often these types of neurofibroma are associated with NF1.[28]

Grossly, the entire subcutis and deep dermis is thickened by a firm, gray-white, ill-defined lesion. Microscopic examination shows an infiltrative tumor involving dermis and subcutaneous tissues composed of spindled Schwann cells with short, round contours (**Fig. 29**). The lesion extends through the soft tissue, preserving the normal adnexal structures (**Fig. 30**). Round eosinophilic

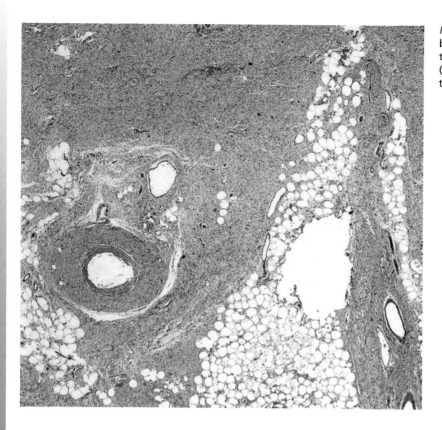

Fig. 29. Diffuse neurofibroma permeating through the subcutaneous tissue (H&E, original magnification ×10).

accumulations termed Wagner-Meissner bodies are often found in these lesions.

As mentioned previously, plexiform NF can show areas with a diffuse pattern of growth.

Additionally, dermatofibrosarcoma protuberans (DFSP) shows the same pattern of growth and adnexal sparing as diffuse NF; when the histomorphology is similar, immunohistochemistry is useful

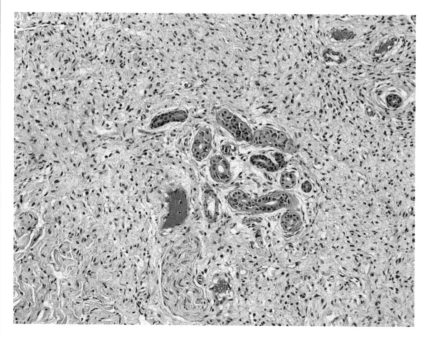

Fig. 30. Diffuse neurofibroma extending around adnexal structures (H&E, original magnification ×64).

to distinguish the 2 entities (CD34 positivity in DFSP, patchy S100 in diffuse NF). Desmoplastic melanoma can also enter the differential; these generally occur in a much older demographic and may show an intraepidermal melanocytic component. The presence of lymphoid aggregates, perineural or vascular invasion, rare atypical cells, or strong S100 immunoexpression may also help distinguish desmoplastic melanoma.

OTHER TUMORS WITH PLEXIFORM PATTERNS

Two additional rare tumors are defined by a plexiform pattern: plexiform xanthomatous tumor and ossifying plexiform tumor. Plexiform xanthomatous tumor (PXT) has been described exclusively in young to middle-aged men and most commonly occurs on the knee and elbow.[29] PXT has a distinctive plexiform arrangement of epithelioid and xanthomatous cells in the dermis and subcutis that are positive for CD68. There have been rare reports of recurrence of this tumor.[29] Ossifying plexiform tumor is a rare dermal tumor, described only 3 times in the literature and each time occurring on the digits of adult women. The tumor is composed of fascicles of epithelioid to spindle cells in a loose myxoid stroma that contains large irregular mature bone in the center.[30,31] Some investigators have suggested that this tumor is an ossifying variant of cellular neurothekeoma.[30]

Plexiform variants exist for several soft tissue tumors in addition to those already discussed. A plexiform variant of leiomyoma has been described in the esophagus and in the female genital tract.[32] A plexiform granular cell tumor exists, composed of fascicles of granular cells, usually in the deep dermis, and differing slightly from traditional granular cell tumors by the lack of a marked overlying epidermal hyperplasia.[33] Other soft tissue tumors may show a vaguely multinodular appearance or may even have distinctly plexiform areas, including ossifying fibromyxoid tumor and giant cell tumor of soft tissue (of low malignant potential). In the superficial and deep dermis, plexiform variants of melanocytic variants have also been described, including plexiform Spitz nevus, spindle-cell nevus, cellular blue nevus, and congenital melanocytic with plexiform growth.[34]

REFERENCES

1. Enzinger FM, Zhang R. Plexiform fibrohistiocytic tumor presenting in children and young adults. Am J Surg Pathol 1988;12(11):818–26.

2. Remstein E, Arndt CA, Nascimento AG. Plexiform fibrohistiocytic tumor: clinicopathologic analysis of 22 cases. Am J Surg Pathol 1999;23(6):662–70.

3. Moosavi C, Jha P, Fanburg-Smith JC. An update on plexiform fibrohistiocytic tumor and addition of 66 new cases from the Armed Forces Institute of Pathology. Ann Diagn Pathol 2007;11:313–9.

4. Nascimento AG, Dal Cin P. Plexiform fibrohistiocytic tumor. In: Fletcher C, Unni K, Mertens F, editors. Pathology and Genetics of Tumours of soft tissue and bone. Lyons (France): IARC; 2002. p. 116–7.

5. Smith S, Fletcher CD, Smith MA, et al. Cytogenetic analysis of a plexiform fibrohistiocytic tumor. Cancer Genet Cytogenet 1990;48:31–4.

6. Redlich GC, Montgomery KD, Allgood GA, et al. Plexiform fibrohistiocytic tumor with a clonal cytogenetic anomaly. Cancer Genet Cytogenet 1999;108:141–3.

7. Salomao DR, Nascimento AG. Plexiform fibrohistiocytic tumor with systemic metastasis. Am J Surg Pathol 1997;21:469–76.

8. Gallager RL, Helwig EB. Neurothekeoma—a benign cutaneous tumor of neural origin. Am J Clin Pathol 1980;74:759–64.

9. Sheth S, Li X, Binder S, et al. Differential gene expression profiles of neurothekeomas and nerve sheath myxomas by microarray analysis. Mod Pathol 2011;24:343–54.

10. Hornick JL, Fletcher CD. Cellular neurothekeoma: detailed characterization in a series of 133 cases. Am J Surg Pathol 2007;31(3):329–40.

11. Fetsch JF, Laskin WB, Hallman JR, et al. Neurothekeoma: an analysis of 178 tumors with detailed immunohistochemical data and long-term patient follow-up information. Am J Surg Pathol 2007;31(7):1103–14.

12. Plaza JA, Torres-Cabala C, Evans H, et al. Immunohistochemical expression of S100A6 in cellular neurothekeoma: clinicopathologic and immunohistochemical analysis of 31 cases. Am J Dermatopathol 2009; 31(5):419–22.

13. Sachdev R, Sundram UN. Frequent positive staining with NKI/C3 in normal and neoplastic tissues limits its usefulness in the diagnosis of cellular neurothekeoma. Am J Clin Pathol 2006;126(4):554–63.

14. Jaffer S, Ambrosini-Spaltra A, Mancini AM, et al. Neurothekeoma and plexiform fibrohistiocytic tumor: mere histologic resemblance or histogenetic relationship? Am J Surg Pathol 2009;33(6):905–13.

15. Harkin JC, Reed RJ. Solitary benign nerve sheath tumors. In: Firminger HI, editor. Atlas of tumor pathology, tumors of the peripheral nervous system, 2nd series. Washington, DC: Armed Forces Institute of Pathology; 1969. p. 60–4.

16. Fetsch JF, Laskin WB, Miettinen M. Nerve sheath myxoma: a clinicopathologic and immunohistochemical analysis of 57 morphologically distinctive, S-100 protein- and GFAP-positive, myxoid peripheral nerve sheath tumors with a predilection for the

extremities and a high local recurrence rate. Am J Surg Pathol 2005;29(12):1615–24.

17. Harkin JC, Arrington J, Reed R. Benign plexiform schwannoma; a lesion distinct from plexiform neurofibroma [abstract]. J Neuropathol Exp Neurol 1978;37:622.

18. Berg JC, Scheithauer BW, Spinner RJ, et al. Plexiform schwannoma: a clinicopathologic overview with emphasis on the head and neck region. Hum Pathol 2008;39:633–40.

19. Agaram NP, Prakash S, Antonescu CR. Deepseated plexiform schwannoma. Am J Surg Pathol 2005;29(8):1042–8.

20. Miettinen M, Shekitka KM, Sobin LH. Schwannomas in the colon and rectum: a clinicopathologic and immunohistochemical study of 20 cases. Am J Surg Pathol 2001;25:846–55.

21. Hornick JL, Bundock EA, Fletcher CD. Hybrid schwannoma/perineurioma. Am J Surg Pathol 2009;33(10):1554–61.

22. Ko JY, Kim JE, Kim YH, et al. Cutaneous plexiform schwannomas in a patient with neurofibromatosis type 2. Ann Dermatol 2009;21(4):402–5.

23. Woodruff JM, Funkhouser JW, Marshall ML, et al. Plexiform (multinodular) schwannoma. Am J Surg Pathol 1983;7:691–7.

24. Woodruff JM, Scheithauer BW, Kurtkaya-Yapcer O, et al. Congenital and childhood plexiform cellular schwannoma: a troublesome mimic of malignant peripheral nerve sheath tumor. Am J Surg Pathol 2003;27(10):1321–9.

25. Jett K, Friedman JM. Clinical and genetic aspects of neurofibromatosis 1. Genet Med 2010;12(1):1–11.

26. Tucker T, Friedman JM, Friedrich RE, et al. Longitudinal study of neurofibromatosis 1 associated plexiform neurofibromas. J Med Genet 2009;46:81–5.

27. Woodruff JM. Pathology of tumors of the peripheral nerve sheath in type 1 neurofibromatosis. Am J Med Genet 1999;89:23–30.

28. Weiss SW, Goldblum JR. Benign tumors of peripheral nerves. In: Weiss SW, Goldblum JR, editors. Soft tissue tumors. St Louis (MO): Mosby; 2001. p. 1126–37.

29. Michal M, Fanburg-Smith JC. Plexiform xanthomatous tumor: a report of 20 cases in 12 patients. Am J Surg Pathol 2002;26(10):1302–11.

30. Rooney MT, Nascimento AG, Tung R. Ossifying plexiform tumor. Report of a cutaneous ossifying lesion with histologic features of neurothekeoma. Am J Dermatopathol 1994;16(2):189–92.

31. Walsh SN, Sangueza OP. Ossifying plexiform tumor: report of two new cases. Am J Dermatopathol 2008;30(1):73–6.

32. Jaroszewski DE, Lam-Himlin D, Gruden J, et al. Plexiform leiomyoma of the esophagus. Ann Diagn Pathol 2011, in press.

33. Aldabaugh B, Azmi F, Vadmal M, et al. Plexiform pattern in cutaneous granular cell tumors. J Cutan Pathol 2009;36:1174–6.

34. Abbas O, Bhawan J. Cutaneous plexiform lesions. J Cutan Pathol 2010;37:613–23.

MYXOID NEOPLASMS

Muhammad I. Zulfiqar, MD[a], Umer N. Sheikh, MD[a],
Elizabeth A. Montgomery, MD[b],*

KEYWORDS

- Myxoid neoplasms • Cutaneous myxoma • Intramuscular myxoma • Benign lesions
- Malignant neoplasms

ABSTRACT

Myxoid tumors of soft tissue constitute a heterogeneous group of neoplasms characterized by the presence of a myxoid stromal matrix, which appears on H&E as an amorphous material and may be confused with edema. Superficial myxoid lesions in general are benign and deep ones are malignant. Grossly, they have a variable gelatinous quality and overlapping histologic features that may present diagnostic difficulties for pathologists. Most are sporadic neoplasms, with only a small percentage arising in patients with hereditary disorders. Discussed are key features of classic myxoid lesions, histologic features, characteristic clinical presentations, immunohistochemical patterns, cytogenetic analysis, and differential diagnosis.

SUPERFICIAL ACRAL FIBROMYXOMA

OVERVIEW

Superficial acral fibromyxomas (SAFs) present in young adults with no gender predilection. They are slow growing, asymptomatic, and usually involve the fingers and toes.[1]

GROSS FEATURES OF SUPERFICIAL ACRAL FIBROMYXOMA

SAFs are dome shaped, polypoid, or verrucoid in appearance, and are smaller than 5 cm. They are soft to firm in consistency and have a gelatinous or solid, off-white cut surface.

LIGHT MICROSCOPIC FEATURES OF SUPERFICIAL ACRAL FIBROMYXOMA

These tumors are moderately cellular, consisting of stellate to spindled fibroblastic cells (**Figs. 1–3**). The stroma ranges from myxoid to collagenous with numerous slender vessels. Scattered multinucleated cells are found in about half of the cases. Only slight nuclear pleomorphism is detected and mitoses are usually sparse and not atypical. The pattern of growth ranges from pushing to infiltrative. With the exception of the presence of mast cells (see **Fig. 3**B), there is minimal inflammation. Immunohistochemically, most cases are positive for CD34, whereas epithelial membrane antigen (EMA) and CD99 are detected in some cases.[2]

SAFs are distinguished from a variety of other soft tissue tumors. Fibrous histiocytomas lack abundant myxoid matrix. SAFs commonly express CD34, which is rarely found in true fibrous histiocytomas. Dermatofibrosarcoma protuberans (DFSP) is a superficial, exophytic mass involving the trunk or the proximal portion of an extremity. The hands and feet are usually not affected. Some examples of DFSP may contain abundant myxoid matrix, have diminished storiform architecture or an accentuated vasculature, and show immunoreactivity for CD34; however, they are distinguished from SAF by the presence of small areas with monotonous, tight storiform architecture, a more infiltrative growth pattern, and a lack of reactivity for epithelial membrane antigen (EMA). The acquired (digital) fibrokeratoma is a solitary hyperkeratotic projection with a collarette of slightly raised skin and a central, normocellular to mildly

[a] Department of Pathology, St John Hospital and Medical Center, 22101 Moross Road, CCB-SB, Detroit, MI 48236, USA
[b] Department of Pathology, The Johns Hopkins Medical Institutions, 401 North Broadway, Weinberg 2242, Baltimore, MD 21231-2410, USA
* Corresponding author.
E-mail address: emontgom@jhmi.edu

Surgical Pathology 4 (2011) 843–864
doi:10.1016/j.path.2011.08.012
1875-9181/11/$ – see front matter © 2011 Elsevier Inc. All rights reserved.

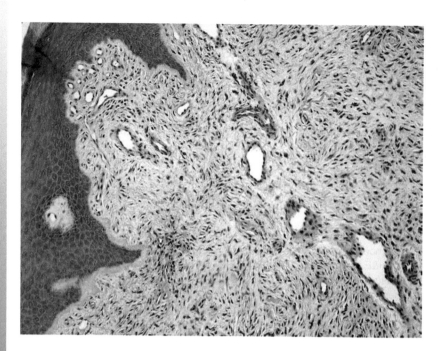

Fig. 1. Superficial acral fibromyxoma. Tumor with overlying nail bed (hemotoxylin-eosin [H&E], original magnification ×20).

hypercellular connective tissue core with interwoven thick collagen bundles, predominantly oriented in the vertical axis of the lesion and in continuity with the underlying dermis. Sclerosing perineurioma has a strong predilection for the fingers and palms of young adults. This process contains abundant dense collagen and variable numbers of small epithelioid and spindled cells with corded, trabecular, and whorled (onion bulb–like) growth patterns. The tumor cells are immunoreactive for EMA, glucose transporter 1 (GLUT1), and claudin 1, but lack expression for CD34.

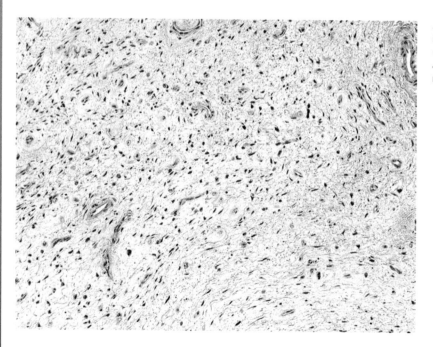

Fig. 2. Superficial acral fibromyxoma. Tumor showing hyperchromatic cells and vessels (H&E, original magnification ×20).

Fig. 3. Superficial acral fibromyxoma. Tumor cells are stellate to spindled (*A*). Interspersed mast cells are present (*B*). (H&E, original magnification, *A*, ×20; *B*, ×100.)

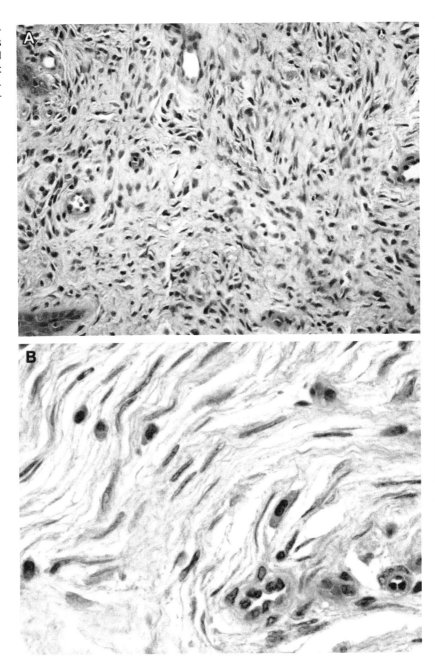

Superficial angiomyxoma (cutaneous myxoma) is a benign soft tissue tumor of the dermis and subcutis that occurs over a wide age range and is weakly linked to Carney complex. This lesion has a multinodular configuration and contains abundant stromal mucin that forms pools and peripheral acellular cleftlike spaces. The lesional cells have mildly pleomorphic nuclei with smudgy chromatin, and cytoplasmic-nuclear invaginations. CD34 expression is present. Acral myxoinflammatory fibroblastic sarcoma is an uncommon soft tissue tumor with incidence in mid-adult life. The process has a predilection for the hands, feet, wrists, and ankles. This entity differs from

Key Features
SUPERFICIAL ACRAL FIBROMYXOMA

1. Predilection for soft tissue of fingers or toes.

2. Stellate to spindled fibroblastic cells in a myxoid to collagenous stroma with minimum pleomorphism and mitotic activity.

3. CD34 immunoreactivity.

Pitfalls
SUPERFICIAL ACRAL FIBROMYXOMA

! The location and expression of CD34 could suggest epithelioid sarcoma but these tumors lack keratin expression.

! The lesional cells can be hyperchromatic and are thus concerning for a sarcoma.

SAF by involvement of the subcutis and deep soft tissues, multinodular growth pattern, and stellate and spindle-shaped cells with large pleomorphic, vesicular nuclei, and prominent inclusionlike nucleoli. A substantial inflammatory component is also seen, consisting of lymphocytes, granulocytes, histiocytes, and plasma cells. CD34 immunoreactivity may be present, but EMA expression is absent.

DIAGNOSIS OF SUPERFICIAL ACRAL FIBROMYXOMA

SAF presents in young adults with no gender predilection. These tumors are slow-growing, asymptomatic, smaller than 5-cm, dome-shaped, polypoid, or verrucoid lesions involving the fingers and toes. They are soft to firm in consistency with a gelatinous or solid, off-white cut surface. Microscopically, they are moderately cellular, consisting of fibroblastic cells in a myxoid stroma with numerous slender blood vessels. Scattered multinucleated cells and mast cells are present. Nuclear pleomorphism and mitoses are rare. The tumor cells stain for CD34.

Differential Diagnosis
SUPERFICIAL ACRAL FIBROMYXOMA

1. Fibrous histiocytoma

2. Dermatofibrosarcoma protuberans

3. Digital fibrokeratoma

4. Sclerosing perineurioma

5. Superficial angiomyxoma (cutaneous myxoma)

6. Acral myxoinflammatory fibroblastic sarcoma

PROGNOSIS OF SUPERFICIAL ACRAL FIBROMYXOMA

The tumors are slowing growing and asymptomatic. Although they can recur locally, there is no tendency for metastasis.[1]

CUTANEOUS MYXOMAS

OVERVIEW

Cutaneous myxomas (CMs) commonly present as solitary lesions unassociated with Carney complex. Multiple lesions, with or without associated Carney complex, are the second most common presentation of CM.[3] As an aside, Carney complex consists of pigmented skin lesions, endocrine disorders, psammomatous melanocytic schwannomas, and myxomatous tumors. This contrasts with Carney syndrome, consisting of gastric epithelioid gastrointestinal stromal tumors, pulmonary chondroma, and extra-adrenal paraganglioma.

Sporadic lesions present as solitary, painless, slow-growing nodules primarily involving the trunk and lower limbs, followed by head and neck and upper extremity. They present in middle age with a male predominance, although they have been reported in genital regions of both sexes.[4] Syndromic lesions are multiple and usually involve the eyelid.[5]

GROSS FEATURES OF CUTANEOUS MYXOMA

CMs are polypoid or pedunculated skin lesions consisting of poorly circumscribed soft, lobulated nodules, ranging in size from 1 to 5 cm, involving the subcutis and occasionally deeper muscle. The cut surface is mucoid or gelatinous and gray to white. Incomplete collagenous bands traverse the cut surface, resulting in a nodular configuration.

LIGHT MICROSCOPIC FEATURES OF CUTANEOUS MYXOMA

The process extends into both the dermis and subcutaneous fat, but occasionally only one location is affected. The tumor consists of multiple, variably cellular nodules composed of bland-appearing, spindled to stellate-shaped, and occasionally multinucleated cells scattered haphazardly throughout an angiomyxoid stroma (**Figs. 4** and **5**). There are often prominent intralesional neutrophils. The stromal matrix contains abundant hyaluronic acid that forms microcysts within the nodules and cleftlike spaces at the interface of the nodules with the surrounding tissue. Thin, wavy collagen fibers course through the stroma. The vascular component consists of small to medium-sized, thin-walled, nonarborizing vessels. Mitotic activity is negligible. Other features include perivascular hyalinization, fibrin and hemosiderin deposition, and interstitial hemorrhage. Epithelial structures, representing entrapped adnexal glands, may be seen (see **Fig. 4**). Immunohistochemically, these tumors show reactivity for vimentin, CD34, muscle-specific actin, alpha-smooth muscle actin, and factor XIIIa, and S-100 protein.[4]

CM must be distinguished from several superficial lesions. Focal cutaneous mucinosis lacks the neutrophils, lobular growth pattern, and elaborate vasculature seen in CM. Aggressive angiomyxoma is a deep-seated tumor of the genital region, which only focally involves the skin, lacks neutrophils, and contains ectatic, nonarborizing vessels. Myxoid neurofibromas lack the well-developed vasculature of myxoma and contain wavy, comma-shaped cells that express S-100 protein. Myxoid dermatofibrosarcoma protuberans are more

Key Features
CUTANEOUS MYXOMA

1. Vaguely lobular, poorly circumscribed, gelatinous mass.

2. Bland-appearing spindled cells in abundant myxoid matrix, nonarborizing vasculature, prominent neutrophils, and entrapped adnexal structures.

3. Immunoreactivity for vimentin, CD34, muscle-specific actin, alpha-smooth muscle actin, factor XIIIa, and S-100.

infiltrative, CD34-positive lesions that show at least small areas of more typical dermatofibrosarcoma.

DIAGNOSIS OF CUTANEOUS MYXOMA

CM may or may not be associated with Carney complex. The sporadic lesions are most common, and present as solitary, painless, slow-growing polypoid or pedunculated nodules involving the trunk, legs, head, and neck of middle-aged men. Syndromic lesions are multiple and usually involve the eyelid. They range in size from 1 to 5 cm, and involve the subcutis or deeper muscle. The cut surface is mucoid or gelatinous and gray to white. The tumor consists of multiple, variably cellular nodules composed of bland-appearing, spindled

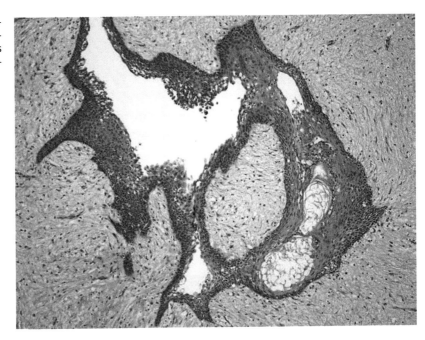

Fig. 4. Cutaneous myxoma. Tumor with entrapped adnexal structures (H&E, original magnification ×10).

to stellate-shaped, and occasionally multinucleated cells scattered haphazardly throughout an angiomyxoid stroma. There are prominent intralesional neutrophils. The stroma is hyaluronic and acid-rich, forming microcysts within the nodules. Small to medium-sized, thin-walled, nonarborizing vessels course through the stroma. Mitotic activity is negligible. Entrapped adnexal glands may be seen. The tumor cells show reactivity for CD34, muscle-specific actin, alpha-smooth muscle actin, factor XIIIa, and S-100 protein.

PROGNOSIS OF CUTANEOUS MYXOMA

Although benign, local recurrences are common, especially in lesions with entrapped epithelial structures.[3]

INTRAMUSCULAR MYXOMA

OVERVIEW

Intramuscular myxomas (IMs) have a peak incidence in middle-aged women. They develop in the deep skeletal muscle of thigh, pelvic girdle, shoulder, and arms.[6,7] They present as slow-growing, painless masses. Multiple lesions may be associated with fibrous dysplasia of bone.[8]

GROSS FEATURES OF INTRAMUSCULAR MYXOMA

IM presents as a well-demarcated tumor with an oval or lobular shape. The size ranges from 5 to 10 cm. The cut surface has a soft mucoid consistency and gray-white color, with thin, traversing

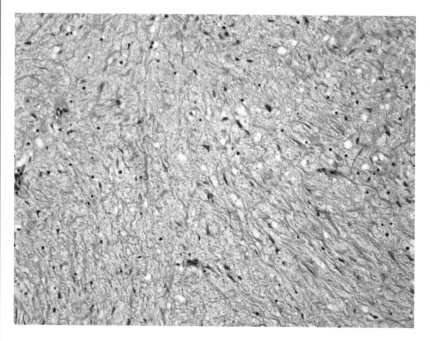

Fig. 5. Cutaneous myxoma. Tumor cells are bland and small with interspersed larger cells (H&E, original magnification ×20).

fibrous trabeculae and small mucin-filled cysts. The tumor can be seen infiltrating the surrounding skeletal muscle, splaying apart individual muscle fibers.

LIGHT MICROSCOPIC FEATURES OF INTRAMUSCULAR MYXOMA

The tumor is characterized by scattered, bland spindled and stellate-shaped cells, sparse small vessels, and numerous thin collagen fibers suspended in a richly myxoid stromal matrix (**Figs. 6** and **7**). The matrix is Alcian blue positive and hyaluronidase sensitive. The tumor cells have a small nucleus and scant amount of pale, occasionally vacuolated, eosinophilic cytoplasm. Ill-defined cytoplasmic processes, continuous with delicate strands of collagen, run haphazardly throughout the tumor. Mitotic activity is virtually nonexistent. Occasionally, residual atrophic skeletal muscle fibers, foamy histiocytes, and mast cells are identified within the myxoid matrix. Small, nonarborizing, capillary-sized vessels are scattered throughout the matrix. At the periphery of the lesion, atrophic skeletal muscle fibers adjacent to the tumor are separated by edema fluid or infiltrating tumor. Fat cells are commonly interspersed in the skeletal muscle. The term "cellular myxoma" is used when it shows greater cellularity and abundant collagen accompanied by a greater number of blood vessels; but, even cellular lesions lack the mitotic activity, cytologic atypia, branching

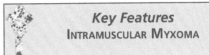

Key Features
INTRAMUSCULAR MYXOMA

1. Skeletal muscle–associated masses with mucoid consistency and gray-white cut surface.

2. Bland spindled and stellate-shaped cells in a myxoid matrix.

3. Nonarborizing capillary-sized vessels scattered throughout the matrix.

vascular network, and necrosis characteristic of a sarcoma.[6,7]

Several lesions must be distinguished from IM. Myxoid nodular fasciitis is usually much smaller, more superficially located, and shows focal areas of increased cellularity with short, randomly arranged fascicles of bland myofibroblasts. Myxoid variants of desmoid fibromatosis occur within the abdomen, and contain a well-developed, thin-walled, nonarborizing vasculature and at least focal areas of typical fibromatosis. Myxoid liposarcoma is typically intramuscular like IM but contains an extremely well-developed, arborizing, capillary-sized vasculature and easily identifiable lipoblasts. Myxofibrosarcoma (myxoid malignant fibrous histiocytoma) is usually more superficial than IM and has a well-developed, thick-walled vasculature and contains hyperchromatic, pleomorphic tumor

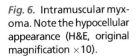

Fig. 6. Intramuscular myxoma. Note the hypocellular appearance (H&E, original magnification ×10).

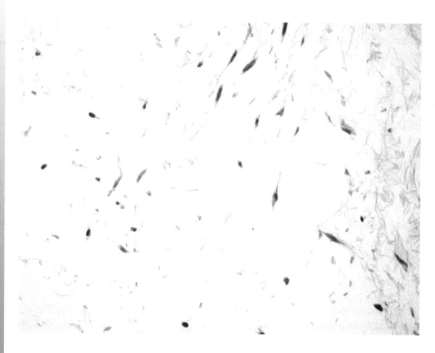

Fig. 7. Intramuscular myxoma. The lesion is composed of bland spindle cells that are essentially devoid of mitotic activity (H&E, original magnification ×40).

cells. Extraskeletal myxoid chondrosarcoma is composed of cords and chains of small eosinophilic cells embedded in a dense-appearing myxoid matrix, often with abundant hemorrhage, but with relatively few blood vessels.

DIAGNOSIS OF INTRAMUSCULAR MYXOMA

IM presents in the deep skeletal muscle of thigh, pelvic girdle, shoulder, and arms of middle-aged women as a slow-growing, painless mass. They are 5 to 10 cm in size and lobular with a soft mucoid consistency and gray-white cut surface. The tumor is intimately associated with skeletal muscle. The tumor is composed of scattered, bland spindled and stellate-shaped cells, sparse small vessels, and numerous thin collagen fibers suspended in a richly myxoid stromal matrix. The matrix is Alcian blue positive and hyaluronidase sensitive. The tumor cells have a small nucleus and scant amount of pale, vacuolated, eosinophilic cytoplasm. Mitotic activity is absent. Occasionally, residual atrophic skeletal muscle fibers, foamy histiocytes, and mast cells are identified in the myxoid matrix. Simple nonarborizing capillary-sized vessels are scattered throughout the matrix. Immunohistochemically, the tumor cells express vimentin and rarely smooth muscle actin.

PROGNOSIS OF INTRAMUSCULAR MYXOMA

IMs are benign tumors and local recurrence is rare.

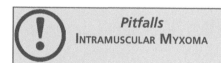

△△ Differential Diagnosis
INTRAMUSCULAR MYXOMA

1. Myxoid nodular fasciitis
2. Myxoid variants of desmoid fibromatosis
3. Myxoid liposarcoma
4. Myxofibrosarcoma (myxoid malignant fibrous histiocytoma)
5. Extraskeletal myxoid chondrosarcoma

! Pitfalls
INTRAMUSCULAR MYXOMA

! In needle biopsy specimens, small foci of low-grade fibromyxoid sarcomas can be indistinguishable from IM.

MYXOID LIPOSARCOMA

OVERVIEW

Myxoid liposarcomas (MLs) present in the fourth to fifth decade as a painless, soft tissue mass. Men are affected more than women. The tumors have a predilection for the deep soft tissue of the thigh. These tumors are also discussed in the article "Liposarcomas" by Singhi and Montgomery elsewhere in this issue.

GROSS FEATURES OF MYXOID LIPOSARCOMA

MLs are large tumors (larger than 10 cm). They are usually well-circumscribed, lobulated, multinodular lesions that may appear encapsulated. The cut surface varies from gelatinous and tan-white to opaque and yellow with focal hemorrhage. The round cell component, which signifies hypercellular areas, may impart a fleshy appearance.

LIGHT MICROSCOPIC FEATURES OF MYXOID LIPOSARCOMA

ML is characterized by a delicate plexiform capillary network present throughout the lesion (Fig. 8). They are low to moderately cellular and are composed of small, uniform, spindled to oval tumor cells arranged as cords and clusters in a richly myxoid ground substance often featuring mucin pooling. The tumor cells cluster around the blood vessels and the periphery of tumor nodules. They are monotonous appearing with scant cytoplasm, uniform dark-staining nuclei, and indistinct nucleoli. Because MLs are translocation-associated sarcomas, they have essentially no nuclear pleomorphism and no abnormal mitoses. Scattered to numerous lipoblasts can be identified that are most often monovacuolated and tend to cluster around vessels or at the periphery of the lesion. Foci of mature-appearing fat may be found. Immunohistochemically, the tumor cells stain for S-100 protein.[9,10] Most myxoid/round cell liposarcomas demonstrate the t12;16(q13;p11) chromosomal translocation, which results in *CHOP-FUS* or, less commonly, *CHOP-EWS* rearrangement.[11,12]

The key contenders in the differential diagnosis of myxoid liposarcoma are intramuscular myxoma and myxofibrosarcoma. Low-grade myxofibrosarcomas are superficial neoplasms (dermis and subcutis) composed of moderately pleomorphic atypical stromal cells and pseudolipoblasts (contain cytoplasmic mucin) associated with thick-walled, arborizing blood vessels. True lipoblasts are absent. There is no specific genetic alteration and there is no S-100 immunoreactivity. Extraskeletal myxoid chondrosarcomas (EMCs) are composed of uniform round to oval cells with eosinophilic cytoplasm in a hypovascular myxoid stroma. The tumor cells tend to organize in strands and cords, and cluster at the periphery of the nodules. Lipoblasts are absent in EMCs. They demonstrate consistent translocations t(9;22)(q22;q12), t(9;17)(q22;q11),

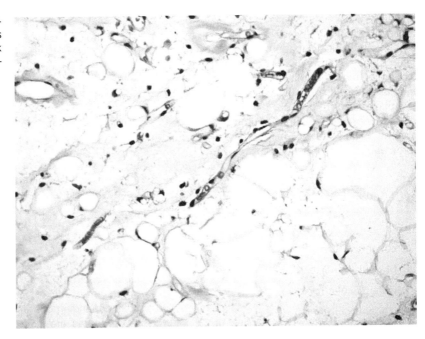

Fig. 8. Myxoid liposarcoma. Several lipoblasts and rich capillary network (H&E, original magnification ×40).

Key Features
Myxoid Liposarcoma

1. Large (larger than 10 cm), well-circumscribed, gelatinous mass.

2. Low to moderately cellular, composed of uniform small spindled and oval tumor cells in a richly myxoid matrix with scattered monovacuolated lipoblasts. No nuclear pleomorphism or mitoses.

3. A t(12;16)(q13;p11) chromosomal translocation resulting CHOP-FUS or CHOP-EWS rearrangement.

Pitfalls
Myxoid Liposarcoma

! Remember to consider lipoblastoma in pediatric patients.

or t(9;15)(q22;q21). Immunohistochemically, they show positivity for vimentin, and S-100 protein. They express endocrine markers, including synaptophysin, neuron-specific enolase (NSE), and occasionally chromagranin, which are not seen in MLs. MLs are more cellular and vascular than intramuscular myxomas. The immunophenotype for MLs (S-100+, CD34−) is different from intramuscular myxomas (S-100−, CD34+). Lipoblastomas are lesions of babies and young children and are further discussed in the article "Liposarcomas" by Singhi and Montgomery elsewhere in this issue, which is wholly devoted to adipose tissue lesions.

DIAGNOSIS OF MYXOID LIPOSARCOMA

ML presents in young adult men as a painless mass in the deep soft tissue of the thigh. Tumors are typically larger than 10 cm, and well-circumscribed, lobulated, multinodular lesions that may appear encapsulated. The cut surface varies from gelatinous and tan-white to opaque and yellow with focal hemorrhage. The round cells, signifying hypercellular areas, may impart a fleshy appearance. MLs are characterized by a delicate plexiform capillary network present throughout the lesion. They are low to moderately cellular and composed of small, uniform, spindled to oval tumor cells arranged as cords and clusters in a richly myxoid stroma. The

Differential Diagnosis
Myxoid Liposarcoma

1. Low-grade myxofibrosarcoma

2. Myxoid chondrosarcoma

3. Intramuscular myxoma

4. Lipoblastoma

tumor cells are monotonous appearing with scant cytoplasm, uniform dark-staining nuclei, and indistinct nucleoli. There is no nuclear pleomorphism and no abnormal mitoses. Scattered to numerous monovacuolated lipoblasts can be identified. Foci of mature-appearing fat may also be found. The tumor cells stain for S-100 protein. Most myxoid/round cell liposarcomas demonstrate the t(12;16) (q13;p11) chromosomal translocation, which results in CHOP-FUS or less commonly CHOP-EWS rearrangement.

PROGNOSIS FOR MYXOID LIPOSARCOMA

Approximately 30% of the patients develop distant metastasis, often to lungs but MLs have a propensity to metastasize to retroperitoneum, soft tissue, and skeleton. Histologic grade, cellularity, and the percentage of round cell component (cellular myxoid liposarcoma) predict the risk for metastasis.[13] A fraction of more than 5% to 25% cellular areas has been suggested as prognostic cutoff.[9,10]

MYXOFIBROSARCOMA (MYXOID MALIGNANT FIBROUS HISTIOCYTOMA)

OVERVIEW

Myxofibrosarcomas present in older men in the sixth to eighth decade of life. They are located in the subcutaneous fat of lower extremities and limb girdles and present as slow-growing painless nodules.

GROSS FEATURES OF MYXOFIBROSARCOMA

Myxofibrosarcoma grows along fibrous septa, forming gelatinous nodules. Large tumors are located in the deep soft tissue, form single masses, and may become partially necrotic and/or hemorrhagic.

LIGHT MICROSCOPIC FEATURES OF MYXOFIBROSARCOMA

Myxofibrosarcomas demonstrate a broad histologic spectrum. They are variably myxoid with the extent of myxoid areas ranging from 10% to 50% depending on the study. Low-grade myxofibrosarcomas are predominantly myxoid (Fig. 9)

Fig. 9. Myxofibrosarcoma. The lesion is richly vascular at low power (H&E, original magnification ×4).

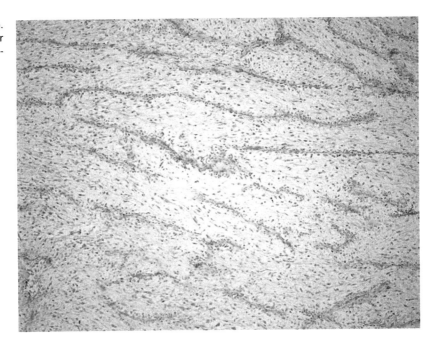

and hypocellular, and contain distinctive curvilinear vessels. The tumor cells are large, spindled to stellate, with hyperchromatic nuclei and varying degrees of nuclear pleomorphism. They aggregate around blood vessels. Vacuolated cells containing acid mucin resembling lipoblasts can be found. Mitotic figures are rarely found. High-grade lesions show greater cellularity, nuclear pleomorphism, multinucleated giant cells, necrosis, and mitotic figures, including abnormal mitoses, but myxoid foci are still recognizable (**Figs. 10** and **11**). Immunohistochemically, the tumor cells stain diffusely for vimentin and occasionally for smooth muscle actin. They are negative for S-100 protein, and CD68, with variable CD34 expression. No specific genetic abnormality has been described.[14,15]

Fig. 10. Myxofibrosarcoma. The tumor cells have pleomorphic nuclei (H&E, original magnification ×20) even though the vascular pattern is reminiscent of that of myxoid liposarcoma.

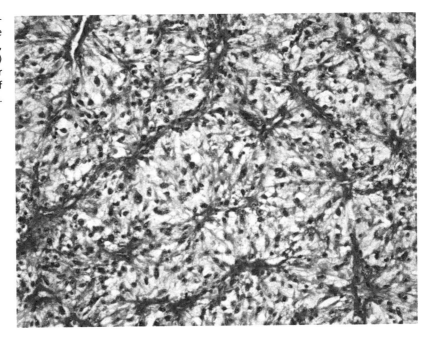

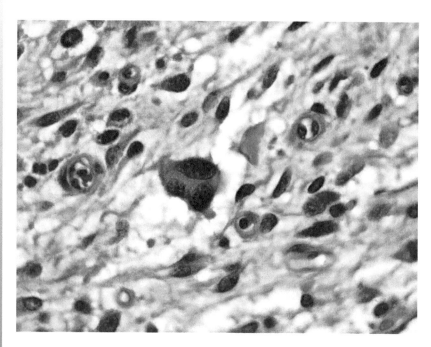

Fig. 11. Myxofibrosarcoma. The tumor cells have pleomorphic nuclei (H&E, original magnification ×40).

The differential diagnosis of myxofibrosarcoma includes a host of benign and malignant lesions. Myxoma, nodular fasciitis, and low-grade fibromyxoid sarcoma occur in young to middle-aged adults, and lack cellular atypia and hyperchromatic nuclei. Neurofibromas and perineurioma are positive for S-100 protein and EMA, respectively. Desmoid tumors have a uniform appearance, lack myxoid nodules and pleomorphic nuclei, and have a fascicular growth pattern. They are reactive for smooth muscle actin and focally reactive for desmin. Low-grade malignant peripheral nerve sheath tumors show focal S-100 positivity. The myxoid variant of dermatofibrosarcoma shows CD34 positivity. Leiomyoma, schwannoma, and stromal sarcoma cause confusion when giant rosettes are present but can easily be excluded on immunohistochemical grounds.

DIAGNOSIS OF MYXOFIBROSARCOMA

Myxofibrosarcomas present in older men as slow-growing and painless gelatinous nodules proliferating along the fibrous septa in the subcutaneous fat of lower extremities and limb girdles. They may also be located in the deep soft tissue, where they form large masses. They demonstrate a variable admixture of myxoid and cellular areas. The

Key Features
MYXOFIBROSARCOMA

1. Gelatinous nodules in the subcutaneous fat of lower extremities.

2. Large, spindled to stellate cells with hyperchromatic nuclei and varying degrees of nuclear pleomorphism. Curvilinear blood vessels.

3. Positive staining for vimentin and smooth muscle actin.

Differential Diagnosis
MYXOFIBROSARCOMA

1. Myxoma

2. Nodular fasciitis

3. Low-grade fibromyxoid sarcoma

4. Neurofibroma and perineurioma

5. Deep fibromatoses (desmoid tumors)

6. Low-grade malignant peripheral nerve sheath tumor

7. Myxoid variant of dermatofibrosarcoma

tumor cells are large, spindled to stellate, with hyperchromatic nuclei and varying degrees of nuclear pleomorphism. They aggregate around blood vessels. Vacuolated cells containing acid mucin resembling lipoblasts are found. Mitotic figures are rarely found. High-grade lesions show greater cellularity, nuclear pleomorphism, multinucleated giant cells, necrosis, and mitotic figures, including abnormal mitoses, but myxoid foci are still recognizable. The tumor stains diffusely for vimentin and occasionally for smooth muscle actin. They are negative for S-100 protein, and CD68 with variable CD34. No specific genetic abnormality has been described.

PROGNOSIS OF MYXOFIBROSARCOMA

The likelihood of metastasis is related to the depth of the lesion and is inversely proportional to the amount of myxoid change. Recurrence occurs in 50% of cases, regardless of grade. Metastasis

Pitfalls
MYXOFIBROSARCOMA

! These are easily confused with myxoid liposarcoma. Remember that myxoid liposarcomas have uniform nuclei and are usually deep, whereas myxofibrosarcoma is usually superficial and has pleomorphic nuclei.

occurs in 20% to 35% of intermediate-grade and high-grade lesions to lungs, bone, and lymph nodes.

EXTRASKELETAL MYXOID CHONDROSARCOMA

OVERVIEW

Extraskeletal myxoid chondrosarcomas (EMCs) present as painless or minimally painful, slow-growing masses in the deep soft tissue of extremities in adults. There is a slight male predominance.[16–18]

GROSS FEATURES OF EXTRASKELETAL MYXOID CHONDROSARCOMAS

EMCs are larger than 5 cm, and appear lobulated with a gray, soft, and gelatinous cut surface.[16]

LIGHT MICROSCOPIC FEATURES OF EXTRASKELETAL MYXOID CHONDROSARCOMAS

These tumors demonstrate a nodular or nodular/lobular growth pattern (**Fig. 12**). The tumor nodules are separated by strands of eosinophilic collagen and are composed of cords, clusters, or nests of uniform oval to spindle cells. The tumor cells are plump with eosinophilic cytoplasm surrounding a central nucleus (**Fig. 13**). The nucleus is dark staining and lacks a visible nucleolus. Mitotic figures are rarely seen. The stromal matrix is

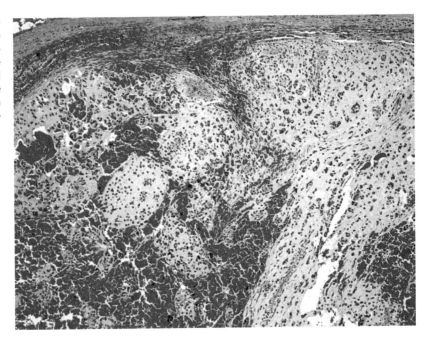

Fig. 12. Extraskeletal myxoid chondrosarcoma. The tumor consists of small uniform cells and lacks the vascular pattern of myxoid liposarcoma. Note the background hemosiderin (H&E, original magnification ×4).

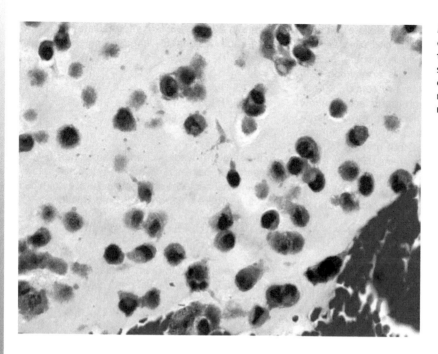

Fig. 13. Extraskeletal myxoid chondrosarcoma. The tumor consists of small spindled to rounded eosinophilic cells in a myxoid matrix (H&E, original magnification ×100).

basophilic, hypovascular, and foamy. It stains with Alcian blue at pH 4.0 and 1.0 because of the presence of chondroitin sulphates. Hyaline cartilage is not found in extraskeletal myxoid chondrosarcoma. The low-grade tumors are less cellular and higher-grade tumors typically show greater cellularity with less extracellular matrix (**Fig. 14**).

The tumor cells in the matrix-poor tumors can be larger, with a high nuclear/cytoplasmic ratio and visible eosinophilic nucleoli. Mitotic figures are readily found.[16] Rarely, dedifferentiation to a high-grade sarcoma occurs.[18] Additionally, a subset of cases has zones of solid sheets of small, round uniform cells (see **Fig. 14**). Immunohistochemically,

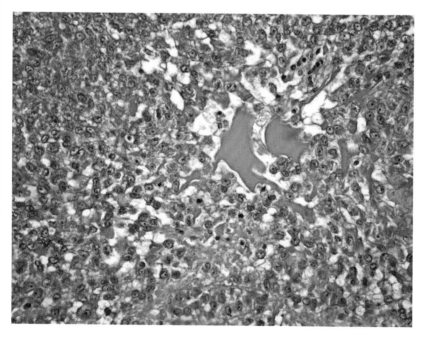

Fig. 14. This lesion is an example of the cellular form of myxoid chondrosarcoma (H&E, original magnification ×40).

Key Features
MYXOID CHONDROSARCOMA

1. Large (larger than 5 cm), lobulated tumors with a gray, soft, and gelatinous cut surface

2. Uniform oval or spindle cells with a dark-staining central nucleus and small amount of eosinophilic cytoplasm in a basophilic foamy stroma. No hyaline cartilage.

3. Diffuse staining for vimentin

4. A t(9;22)(q22–31;q11–12) translocation, resulting in the *EWSR1-NR4A3* fusion

Pitfalls
MYXOID CHONDROSARCOMA

! Because of their bland appearance, these lesions can be confused with cutaneous mixed tumors. Myxoid chondrosarcomas tend to be deeper and have prominent hemosiderin deposition and lack keratin expression.

the tumor cells are uniformly vimentin positive and focally positive for S-100, NSE, and synaptophysin.[19–21] Most tumors exhibit a t(9;22)(q22–31; q11–12) translocation, resulting in the *EWSR1-NR4A3* fusion.[20]

The differential diagnosis of myxoid chondrosarcoma includes several chondroid lesions. In soft tissue chondroma and soft tissue osteosarcoma, the matrix is hyaline cartilage, whereas in EMC the matrix is cartilagelike. Osseous chondrosarcoma with soft tissue extension, when myxoid, may be confused with EMC; however, appropriate clinical and radiological information helps differentiate between the two. Myoepithelioma and ossifying fibromyxoid tumor are rare soft tissue tumors that may exhibit areas similar to EMC.

DIAGNOSIS OF EXTRASKELETAL MYXOID CHONDROSARCOMA

EMCs present as painless or minimally painful, slow-growing masses in the deep soft tissue of extremities in adults, with a slight male predominance. They are larger than 5 cm, lobulated, with a gray, soft, and gelatinous cut surface. The tumor nodules are separated by strands of eosinophilic

Differential Diagnosis
EXTRASKELETAL MYXOID
CHONDROSARCOMA

1. Soft tissue chondroma

2. Soft tissue osteosarcoma

3. Osseous chondrosarcoma

4. Myoepithelioma

5. Ossifying fibromyxoid tumor

collagen and are composed of cords, clusters, or nests of uniform oval to spindle cells. The tumor cells have a small amount of eosinophilic cytoplasm surrounding a central nucleus. The nucleus is dark staining and lacks a visible nucleolus. Mitotic figures are rarely seen. The stromal matrix is basophilic, hypovascular, and foamy. Hyaline cartilage is not found in EMCs. Rarely, dedifferentiation to a high-grade sarcoma occurs. Tumor cells stain uniformly for vimentin and focally for S-100, NSE, and synaptophysin. Most tumors exhibit a t(9;22)(q22–31;q11–12) translocation, resulting in the *EWSR1-NR4A3* fusion.

PROGNOSIS FOR EXTRASKELETAL MYXOID CHONDROSARCOMA

Extraskeletal myxoid chondrosarcomas have a high incidence of local recurrence, prolonged survival after metastasis, and a high rate of death owing to tumor. The prognosis depends on clinical features and not on histologic grade. Older age, large tumor size, and tumor location in the proximal extremity or limb girdle are adverse prognostic factors. Five-year survival rate is greater than 90%; however, 10-year and 15-year disease-free survival rates are lower because of metastasis.[16]

LOW-GRADE FIBROMYXOID SARCOMA

OVERVIEW

Low-grade fibromyxoid sarcomas (LGFMS) present in young adults of either sex as a well-demarcated mass in the deep soft tissues of extremities, trunk, and, rarely, viscera.[22]

GROSS FEATURES OF LOW-GRADE FIBROMYXOID SARCOMA

LGFMS are well-demarcated, lobulated tumors. The cut surface is fibrous or fibromyxoid, glistening-white, and bearing resemblance to a uterine leiomyoma.

LIGHT MICROSCOPIC FEATURES OF LOW-GRADE FIBROMYXOID SARCOMA

These tumors consist of spindle-shaped cells forming sweeping fascicles or whorls, in a focally collagenous and myxoid background (Fig. 15). The cells have pale eosinophilic cytoplasm and deceptively bland, ovoid, or tapered nuclei (Fig. 16), with 1 or 2 small nucleoli and occasional nuclear inclusions. Mitotic figures are rare, and there is no necrosis. Curvilinear or plexiform vessels resembling those seen in a myxoid liposarcoma are readily visible in the myxoid areas. Although grossly well circumscribed, the tumor often infiltrates the surrounding tissues on microscopic examination. Some tumors contain clusters of large rosettes (Fig. 17), consisting of cores of hyalinized collagen surrounded by rounded, epithelioid tumor cells. When numerous, the lesion is called hyalinizing spindle cell tumor with giant rosettes. Fifteen percent to 20% of low-grade fibromyxoid sarcomas contain intermediate-grade or high-grade, densely cellular areas resembling conventional fibrosarcoma. Recurrent tumors tend to be more cellular and mitotically active. Low-grade fibromyxoid sarcoma cells focally express smooth muscle actin and rarely CD34 or desmin. They are generally negative for S-100 protein and EMA.[22–24] A significant proportion of cases demonstrate a t(7;16)(q33;p11) reciprocal translocation. This results in a *FUS-CREB3L2* fusion in more than 95% of cases and *FUS-*

CREB3L1 fusion in 1% of cases.[25,26] These tumors form a spectrum with sclerosing epithelioid fibrosarcoma (see "Epithelioid Lesions" by Andrea T. Deyrup elsewhere in this issue). Preliminary evidence suggests that sclerosing epithelioid fibrosarcoma can be viewed as the high-grade form of low-grade fibromyxoid sarcoma, akin to the relationship between myxoid and round cell liposarcoma (discussed in the article "Liposarcomas" by Singhi and Montgomery elsewhere in this issue).[27]

The differential diagnosis of LGFMS is lengthy. Neurofibroma is S-100 positive. Perineuroma is EMA, claudin-1, GLUT1, and often CD34 positive; however, EMA and claudin-1 positivity can be seen in low-grade fibromyxoid sarcoma and genetic analysis can be required to make a diagnosis in some cases, although MUC4 reportedly is quite specific for these tumors and may supplant the need for such genetic analysis.[28] Deep fibromatoses (desmoid tumors) are uniform, lack myxoid nodules, have a fascicular growth pattern, and are usually reactive for smooth muscle actin and focally for desmin. In contrast to LGFMS, they display beta catenin nuclear labeling.[29] Malignant peripheral nerve sheath tumor is focally S-100 positive and features wavy "bullet-shaped" nuclei (and is illustrated in "Spindle Cell Sarcomas" by Cyril Fisher elsewhere in this issue). Dermatofibrosarcoma (myxoid variant) is CD34 positive. Myxofibrosarcoma has a subcutaneous location and shows a greater degree of nuclear pleomorphism.

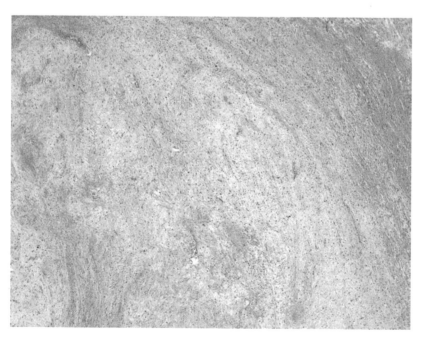

Fig. 15. Low-grade fibromyxoid sarcoma. The tumor demonstrates a swirling architecture (H&E, original magnification ×4).

When giant rosettes are present, leiomyoma, schwannoma, and metastatic low-grade endometrial stromal sarcoma must be considered but can easily be excluded on immunohistochemical grounds.

DIAGNOSIS OF LOW-GRADE FIBROMYXOID SARCOMA

LGFMS presents in young adults of either sex as a well-demarcated mass in the deep soft tissues of extremities, trunk, and, rarely, viscera. The cut surface is fibrous or fibromyxoid, and glistening-white resembling a uterine leiomyoma. The tumor cells are spindle shaped, forming sweeping fascicles or whorls, in a myxoid and focally collagenous stroma. The cells have pale eosinophilic cytoplasm and deceptively bland, ovoid, or tapered nuclei with 1 or 2 small nucleoli and occasional nuclear inclusions. Mitotic figures are rare, and there is no necrosis. Curvilinear or plexiform vessels resembling those seen in a myxoid liposarcoma are readily seen. Some tumors contain clusters of large rosettes, consisting of cores of hyalinized collagen surrounded by rounded, epithelioid-looking tumor cells. A few tumors contain cellular areas resembling conventional fibrosarcoma. The tumor cells focally express smooth muscle actin and rarely CD34 or desmin. MUC4 has emerged as a promising marker for

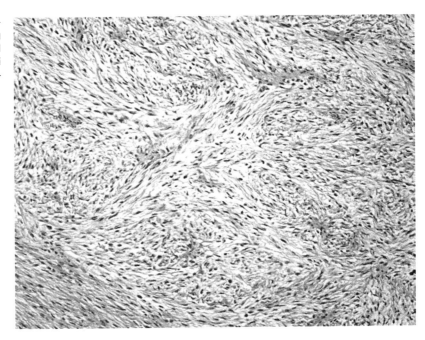

Fig. 16. Low-grade fibromyxoid sarcoma. Swirling pattern of fibrous and myxoid areas. The nuclei are uniform (H&E, original magnification ×20).

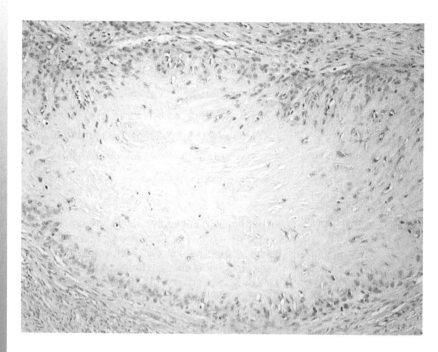

Fig. 17. Low-grade fibro-myxoid sarcoma. A hyaline rosette is present in a cellular area of the tumor (H&E, original magnification ×20).

these tumors. They are generally negative for S-100 and EMA. A significant proportion of tumors demonstrate a t(7;16)(q33;p11) translocation, resulting in *FUS-CREB3L2* or *FUS-CREB3L1* fusion transcript.

PROGNOSIS FOR LOW-GRADE FIBROMYXOID SARCOMA

LGFMS is a low-grade sarcoma with metastatic potential. The 5-year overall survival is greater than 95% if the initial tumor is adequately resected, with a local recurrence rate of 9% to 21%.[27] Deep lesions present with late metastases mostly to lungs. Adverse prognostic factors include positive margin status and high-grade areas.

Pitfalls
LOW-GRADE FIBROMYXOID SARCOMA

! Desmoid fibromatoses can be difficult to separate from low-grade fibromyxoid sarcomas on small biopsies; beta-catenin, MUC4, and genetic analysis can be used in doubtful cases.

MYXOINFLAMMATORY FIBROBLASTIC SARCOMA (INFLAMMATORY MYXOHYALINE TUMOR)

OVERVIEW

Myxoinflammatory fibroblastic sarcomas (MIFS) present over a wide age range, affecting both sexes as painless masses involving the hands and feet.

GROSS FEATURES OF MYXOINFLAMMATORY FIBROBLASTIC SARCOMA

MIFSs are infiltrative, multinodular tumors that typically appear as poorly circumscribed, friable masses of white-tan tissue. Most cases are relatively small with a median size of 3 cm.

LIGHT MICROSCOPIC FEATURES OF MYXOINFLAMMATORY FIBROBLASTIC SARCOMA

MIFSs show an admixture of hyalinized, inflammatory, and myxoid areas (Fig. 18). They are characterized by an admixture of dense inflammation and stroma that varies from myxoid to hyalinized. The tumor cells form sheets and foci of epithelioid spindle cells. The inflammatory cells consist of neutrophils, eosinophils, lymphocytes, and histiocytes in variable numbers. Scattered within the

Fig. 18. Myxoinflammatory fibroblastic sarcoma. The tumor has a hyalinized appearance with an inflammatory background (H&E, original magnification ×10).

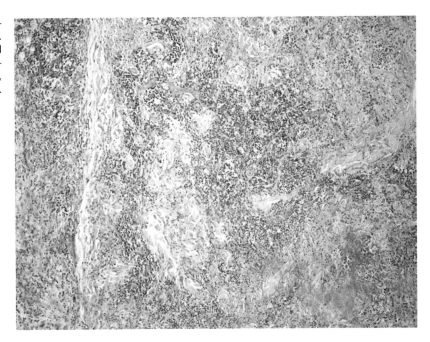

hyalinized and myxoid zones are aggregates of bizarre-appearing tumor cells, with giant macronucleoli, reminiscent of cytomegalovirus (CMV)-infected cells or Reed-Sternberg cells (**Fig. 19**). Mitotic figures are typically sparse. Small foci of necrosis are occasionally seen. Some lesions contain foamy histiocytes, giant cells, and hemosiderin. Immunohistochemically, the neoplastic cells routinely express vimentin and focal CD68. The tumor cells are positive for CD34 in roughly 25% of cases. They lack expression for S-100, desmin, actin, NSE, EMA, CD15, CD30, and CD45. CMV and Epstein-Barr virus (EBV) are not detected.[30,31] The tumors show a consistent t(1;10) with rearrangements of *TGFBR3* and *MGEA5*.[32]

Fig. 19. Myxoinflammatory fibroblastic sarcoma. These tumors contain fibroblasts with large nucleoli that are reminiscent of the nucleoli encountered in Reed-Sternberg cells (H&E, original magnification ×40).

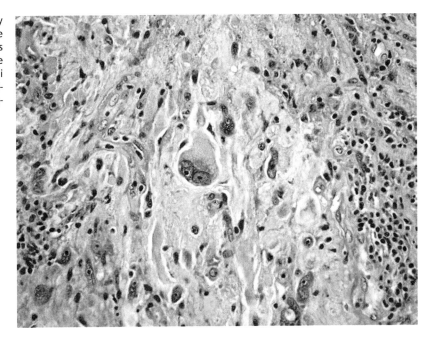

Key Features
MYXOINFLAMMATORY FIBROBLASTIC SARCOMA

1. Poorly circumscribed, friable, fibrous to myxoid masses with a median size of 3 cm.

2. Hyalinized and myxoid areas containing bizarre tumor cells with giant macronuclei, pseudolipoblasts, mixed inflammatory infiltrate, and infrequent mitoses.

3. Positive staining for vimentin and focal CD68.

Pitfalls
MYXOINFLAMMATORY FIBROBLASTIC SARCOMA

! These tumors can be mistaken for infectious lesions.

MIFS can be mistaken for a variety of lesions. Myxofibrosarcoma (myxoid malignant fibrous histiocytoma) is typically larger and more proximally located, occurs in older adults, and shows a well-developed arborizing vasculature, which is absent in MIFS. Inflammatory and infectious lesions lack the clearly malignant cells seen in MIFS, as well as the distinctive admixture of hyalinized and myxoid zones. Giant cell tumors of tendon sheath lack the prominent cytologic atypia and the acute inflammatory cells seen in MIFS. Inflammatory myofibroblastic tumors usually occur in much younger patients, contain fascicles of relatively bland myofibroblasts, and seldom occur in distal locations. Soft tissue Hodgkin lymphoma is extremely rare, and the cells of MIFS lack CD30 and CD15 expression, seen in Reed-Sternberg cells.

DIAGNOSIS OF MYXOINFLAMMATORY FIBROBLASTIC SARCOMA

MIFS affects both sexes and presents over a wide age range as painless, infiltrative, and multinodular tumors involving the hands and feet. The median size is 3 cm. The tumors demonstrate an admixture of dense inflammation and stroma that varies from myxoid to hyalinized. The tumor cells form sheets and foci of epithelioid spindle cells. The inflammatory cells consist of neutrophils, eosinophils, lymphocytes, and histiocytes in variable numbers. Scattered within the hyalinized and myxoid zones are aggregates of bizarre-appearing tumor cells, with giant macronucleoli, reminiscent of CMV-infected cells or Reed-Sternberg cells. Mitotic figures are typically sparse. Small foci of necrosis are occasionally seen. The neoplastic cells routinely express vimentin and focal CD68. They are positive for CD34 in roughly 25% of cases. They lack expression for S-100, desmin, actin, NSE, EMA, CD15, CD30, and CD45. CMV and EBV are not detected. The tumors show a consistent t(1;10) with rearrangements of *TGFBR3* and *MGEA5,* which they share with hemosiderotic fibrohistiocytic lipomatous tumor.[32]

PROGNOSIS FOR MYXOINFLAMMATORY FIBROBLASTIC SARCOMA

MIFS is considered a low-grade sarcoma, with significant potential for aggressive local recurrence, sometimes necessitating amputation, and limited potential for lymph node and distant metastases. Exceptional cases of MIFS show histologic progression to high-grade sarcoma.

Differential Diagnosis
MYXOINFLAMMATORY FIBROBLASTIC SARCOMA

1. Myxofibrosarcoma

2. Infectious and inflammatory lesions

3. Giant cell tumors of tendon sheath

4. Inflammatory myofibroblastic tumor

5. Hodgkin lymphoma

REFERENCES

1. Al-Daraji WI, Miettinen M. Superficial acral fibromyxoma: a clinicopathological analysis of 32 tumors including 4 in the heel. J Cutan Pathol 2008;35(11):1020–6.

2. Fetsch JF, Laskin WB, Miettinen M. Superficial acral fibromyxoma: a clinicopathologic and immunohistochemical analysis of 37 cases of a distinctive soft tissue tumor with a predilection for the fingers and toes. Hum Pathol 2001;32(7):704–14.

3. Allen PW, Dymock RB, MacCormac LB. Superficial angiomyxomas with and without epithelial components. Report of 30 tumors in 28 patients. Am J Surg Pathol 1988;12(7):519–30.

4. Fetsch JF, Laskin WB, Tavassoli FA. Superficial angiomyxoma (cutaneous myxoma): a clinicopathologic study of 17 cases arising in the genital region. Int J Gynecol Pathol 1997;16(4):325–34.

5. Carney JA. Carney complex: the complex of myxomas, spotty pigmentation, endocrine overactivity, and schwannomas. Semin Dermatol 1995;14(2):90–8.

6. Kindblom LG, Stener B, Angervall L. Intramuscular myxoma. Cancer 1974;34(5):1737–44.

7. Nielsen GP, O'Connell JX, Rosenberg AE. Intramuscular myxoma: a clinicopathologic study of 51 cases with emphasis on hypercellular and hypervascular variants. Am J Surg Pathol 1998;22(10):1222–7.

8. Wirth WA, Leavitt D, Enzinger FM. Multiple intramuscular myxomas. Another extraskeletal manifestation of fibrous dysplasia. Cancer 1971;27(5): 1167–73.

9. Kilpatrick SE, Doyon J, Choong PF, et al. The clinicopathologic spectrum of myxoid and round cell liposarcoma. A study of 95 cases. Cancer 1996;77(8): 1450–8.

10. Smith TA, Easley KA, Goldblum JR. Myxoid/round cell liposarcoma of the extremities. A clinicopathologic study of 29 cases with particular attention to extent of round cell liposarcoma. Am J Surg Pathol 1996;20(2):171–80.

11. Antonescu CR, Elahi A, Healey JH, et al. Monoclonality of multifocal myxoid liposarcoma: confirmation by analysis of TLS-CHOP or EWS-CHOP rearrangements. Clin Cancer Res 2000;6(7):2788–93.

12. Tallini G, Akerman M, Dal Cin P, et al. Combined morphologic and karyotypic study of 28 myxoid liposarcomas. Implications for a revised morphologic typing (a report from the CHAMP Group). Am J Surg Pathol 1996;20(9):1047–55.

13. Spillane AJ, Fisher C, Thomas JM. Myxoid liposarcoma—the frequency and the natural history of nonpulmonary soft tissue metastases. Ann Surg Oncol 1999;6(4):389–94.

14. Weiss SW, Enzinger FM. Myxoid variant of malignant fibrous histiocytoma. Cancer 1977;39(4):1672–85.

15. Mentzel T, Calonje E, Wadden C, et al. Myxofibrosarcoma. Clinicopathologic analysis of 75 cases with emphasis on the low-grade variant. Am J Surg Pathol 1996;20(4):391–405.

16. Meis-Kindblom JM, Bergh P, Gunterberg B, et al. Extraskeletal myxoid chondrosarcoma. A reappraisal of its morphologic spectrum and prognostic factors based on 117 cases. Am J Surg Pathol 1999;23: 636–50.

17. Enzinger FM, Shiraki M. Extraskeletal myxoid chondrosarcoma. An analysis of 34 cases. Hum Pathol 1972;3(3):421–35.

18. Antonescu CR, Argani P, Erlandson RA, et al. Skeletal and extraskeletal myxoid chondrosarcoma: a comparative clinicopathologic, ultrastructural, and molecular study. Cancer 1998;83:1504–21.

19. Domanski HA, Carlén B, Mertens F, et al. Extraskeletal myxoid chondrosarcoma with neuroendocrine differentiation: a case report with fine-needle aspiration biopsy, histopathology, electron microscopy, and cytogenetics. Ultrastruct Pathol 2003;27(5):363–8.

20. Goh YW, Spagnolo DV, Platten M, et al. Extraskeletal myxoid chondrosarcoma: a light microscopic, immunohistochemical, ultrastructural and immuno-ultrastructural study indicating neuroendocrine differentiation. Histopathology 2001;39:514–24.

21. Okamoto S, Hisaoka M, Ishida T, et al. Extraskeletal myxoid chondrosarcoma: a clinicopathologic, immunohistochemical, and molecular analysis of 18 cases. Hum Pathol 2001;32(10):1116–24.

22. Folpe AL, Lane KL, Paull G, et al. Low-grade fibromyxoid sarcoma and hyalinizing spindle cell tumor with giant rosettes: a clinicopathologic study of 73 cases supporting their identity and assessing the impact of high-grade areas. Am J Surg Pathol 2000;24(10):1353–60.

23. Evans HL. Low-grade fibromyxoid sarcoma. A report of 12 cases. Am J Surg Pathol 1993;17(6):595–600.

24. Billings SD, Giblen G, Fanburg-Smith JC. Superficial low-grade fibromyxoid sarcoma (Evans tumor): a clinicopathologic analysis of 19 cases with a unique observation in the pediatric population. Am J Surg Pathol 2005;29(2):204–10.

25. Reid R, de Silva MV, Paterson L, et al. Low-grade fibromyxoid sarcoma and hyalinizing spindle cell tumor with giant rosettes share a common t(7;16)(q34;p11) translocation. Am J Surg Pathol 2003;27(9):1229–36.

26. Mertens F, Fletcher CD, Antonescu CR, et al. Clinicopathologic and molecular genetic characterization of low-grade fibromyxoid sarcoma, and cloning of a novel FUS/CREB3L1 fusion gene. Lab Invest 2005;85(3):408–15.

27. Guillou L, Benhattar J, Gengler C, et al. Translocation-positive low-grade fibromyxoid sarcoma: clinicopathologic and molecular analysis of a series expanding the morphologic spectrum and suggesting potential relationship to sclerosing epithelioid fibrosarcoma: a study from the French Sarcoma Group. Am J Surg Pathol 2007;31(9):1387–402.

28. Doyle LA, Möller E, Dal Cin P, et al. MUC4 is a highly sensitive and specific marker for low-grade fibromyxoid sarcoma. Am J Surg Pathol 2011;35(5): 733–41.

29. Bhattacharya B, Dilworth HP, Iacobuzio-Donahue C, et al. Nuclear beta-catenin expression distinguishes deep fibromatosis from other benign and malignant fibroblastic and myofibroblastic lesions. Am J Surg Pathol 2005;29(5):653–9.

30. Montgomery EA, Devaney KO, Giordano TJ, et al. Inflammatory myxohyaline tumor of distal extremities with virocyte or Reed-Sternberg-like cells: a distinctive lesion with features simulating inflammatory

conditions, Hodgkin's disease, and various sarcomas. Mod Pathol 1998;11(4):384–91.

31. Meis-Kindblom JM, Kindblom LG. Acral myxoinflammatory fibroblastic sarcoma: a low-grade tumor of the hands and feet. Am J Surg Pathol 1998;22(8): 911–24.

32. Antonescu CR, Zhang L, Nielsen GP, et al. Consistent t(1;10) with rearrangements of TGFBR3 and MGEA5 in both myxoinflammatory fibroblastic sarcoma and hemosiderotic fibrolipomatous tumor. Genes Chromosomes Cancer 2011;50(10): 757–64.

EPITHELIOID LESIONS

Andrea T. Deyrup, MD, PhD[a,b,*]

KEYWORDS

• Epithelioid lesions • Mesenchymal tumors • Epithelioid vascular lesions

ABSTRACT

Epithelioid variants have been described for most mesenchymal tumors, including leiomyosarcoma, pleomorphic liposarcoma, epithelioid fibrous histiocytoma, and myxofibrosarcoma. Soft tissue tumors that commonly show epithelioid morphology include epithelioid vascular lesions, epithelioid sarcoma, sclerosing epithelioid fibrosarcoma, and epithelioid malignant peripheral nerve sheath tumor. Many of the entities described in this review were originally described as "simulating carcinoma" or "often mistaken for carcinoma" and this pitfall should be considered when evaluating epithelioid lesions in soft tissue. Many epithelioid soft tissue tumors express epithelial antigens to a varying degree and an immunohistochemical panel is essential for correct classification.

EPITHELIOID VASCULAR LESIONS

OVERVIEW

In 1979, Rosai and colleagues[1] proposed the term, *histiocytoid hemangioma*, to designate vascular lesions with distinctive epithelioid or histiocytoid appearance. Based on immunohistochemical and ultrastructural analysis, they suggested that the component cells were endothelial cells with histiocytic properties. The spectrum of lesions they included in this category included angiolymphoid hyperplasia with eosinophilia, inflammatory angiomatoses, "some reported cases of cutaneous angiosarcoma," and hemangioendothelioma of bone.

Since then, it has been recognized that epithelioid shape in endothelial cells does not reflect a unique line of differentiation but instead is a morphologic variant. The importance in recognizing endothelial differentiation in epithelioid vascular lesions resides primarily in avoiding misdiagnosis as carcinoma or a mesenchymal lesion. This pitfall is particularly hazardous because immunoreactivity for epithelial markers is well documented in epithelioid vascular neoplasms.[2–4]

Epithelioid vascular lesions span the spectrum from benign (epithelioid hemangioma [EH]) to malignant (epithelioid angiosarcoma); the clinical behavior of epithelioid hemangioendothelioma (EHE) is considered to fall between these two extremes, generally closer to the malignant end of the spectrum, and EHE is classified as malignant in the most recent edition of the World Health Organization (WHO) classification.[5]

EPITHELIOID HEMANGIOMA

OVERVIEW

EH is characterized microscopically by two dominant features, both of which may obscure the underlying vascular architecture: (1) epithelioid endothelial cells with abundant eosinophilic cytoplasm and (2) exuberant mixed inflammation.

The prominence of the inflammatory component is reflected in the terms used for this entity, including angiolymphoid hyperplasia with eosinophilia,[6] pseudopyogenic granuloma,[7] and inflammatory angiomatous nodule.[8]

EH affects individuals of all ages, with a female predominance, and arises most frequently in the head, primarily affecting the distribution of the superficial temporal artery, and in the distal extremities, usually the digits.[9,10] Involvement of the trunk, inguinal fold,[10] and penis[4] have also been reported.

Most EH are unifocal and arise in the subcutis where they may present with bleeding or irritational changes. Approximately 50% of patients develop multiple lesions, usually in the same anatomic site.

---

[a] Department of Orthopaedic Surgery, University of South Carolina School of Medicine, 701 Grove Road, Greenville, SC 29605, USA
[b] Pathology Consultants of Greenville, 8 Memorial Medical Court, Greenville, SC 29605-4449, USA
* Pathology Consultants of Greenville, 8 Memorial Medical Court, Greenville, SC 29605-4449.
E-mail address: atdeyrup@yahoo.com

Surgical Pathology 4 (2011) 865–885
doi:10.1016/j.path.2011.08.007

There has been some controversy regarding whether EH is a neoplastic or reactive condition.[9] Evidence supporting the latter includes

1. The observation that many of these tumors arise in the setting of a damaged blood vessel[9]
2. A common history of previous trauma
3. An associated inflammatory component
4. Tumor maturation.

Evidence supporting tumor malformation is primarily centered on the lesion's tendency to recur.

GROSS FEATURES OF EPITHELIOID HEMANGIOMA

The gross appearance is typically of a well-circumscribed nodule in the cutaneous or subcutaneous soft tissue. Although there may be focal hemorrhage, ectatic blood-filled spaces are not characteristic.

MICROSCOPIC FEATURES OF EPITHELIOID HEMANGIOMA

Epithelioid hemangiomas may arise in the dermis or in the subcutaneous tissue and are characterized by lobules of capillary-sized vessels lined by polygonal to cuboidal endothelial cells with abundant eosinophilic cytoplasm (Fig. 1). The cells protrude prominently into the vessel lumen, giving a hobnail or scalloped appearance to the vascular space, and may even seem to completely occlude the lumen (Fig. 2). Endothelial stratification or piling up is not seen.

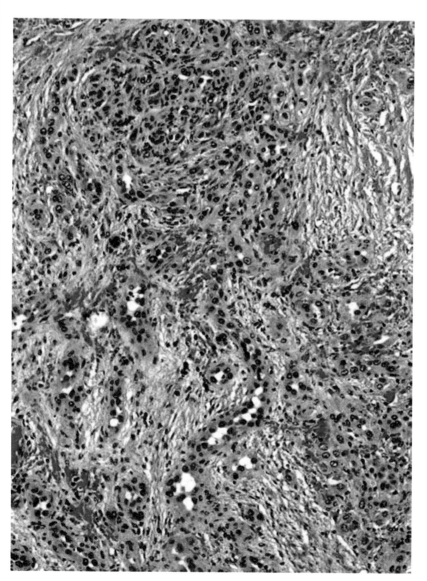

Fig. 1. Low-power view of EH showing lobular architecture.

Fig. 2. The polygonal endothelial cells have abundant eosinophilic cytoplasm and may partially occlude the vessel lumen. Nucleolii may be prominent; however, nuclear hyperchromasia and endothelial stratification are not seen.

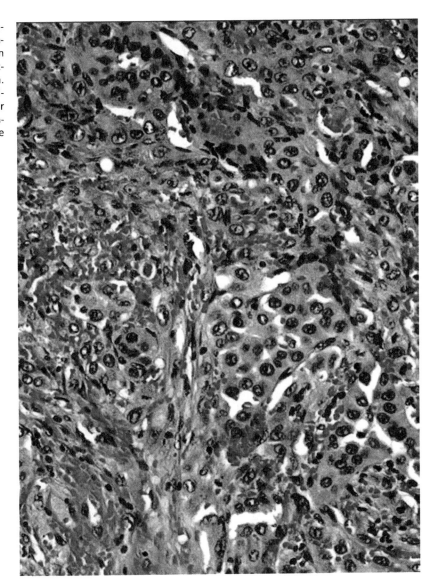

Key Features
EPITHELIOID HEMANGIOMA

- Polygonal to cuboidal endothelial cells that may obscure the vascular lumen

- Lobular architecture

- Mixed inflammatory infiltrate

- Bland cytology and absence of nuclear hyperchromasia

EHs are typically well marginated, although there may be focal infiltration of surrounding soft tissue, particularly in those lesions centered in the dermis. Peripherally, the vessels show increased maturation characterized by a well-formed smooth muscle wall, less-prominent epithelioid morphology, and more clearly defined vascular spaces.

The nuclei have fine chromatin with small, distinct nucleoli. Nuclear hyperchromasia, chromatin clumping, and variability in size and shape of the nuclei and nucleoli are not seen and should raise the possibility of an epithelioid angiosarcoma. Mitotic activity is typically low (0–2 mitotic figures/10 high-power fields [hpf]).

There is almost always an associated mixed inflammatory infiltrate that consists of eosinophils, plasma cells, and lymphocytes (**Fig. 3**). Lymphoid follicles can be seen and the low-power appearance may mimic a lymph node.

DIFFERENTIAL DIAGNOSIS OF EPITHELIOID HEMANGIOMA

Previously, the terms Kimura disease and epithelioid hemangioma were considered interchangeable. Now, however, it is recognized that these are two different disease processes.[11,12] Kimura disease is a chronic inflammatory disorder of unknown etiology that frequently presents as subcutaneous masses in the head and neck.

Histologically, the lesions consist of lymphoid nodules with distinct germinal centers, abundant eosinophils, and eosinophilic abscesses and minimal capillary proliferation. In contrast, the dominant finding in EHs is the vascular proliferation. In addition, EHs tend to be more superficial and lack germinal centers and eosinophilic abscesses.

Recently, a new epithelioid vascular lesion, cutaneous epithelioid angiomatous nodule (CEAN), has been described that shows histologic overlap with EH.[13] CEANs are typically solitary nodules or papules that are present for a short duration and that are confined to the dermis and predominantly affect the trunk and extremities. Unlike EH, mitotic activity is brisk in CEAN (up to 5 mitotic figures/10 hpf) and the polygonal endothelial cells are

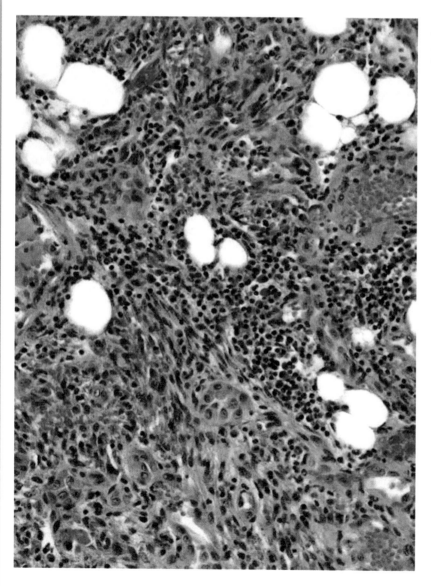

Fig. 3. Mixed inflammation with prominent eosinophilia is a common finding in EH.

Pitfalls
EPITHELIOID HEMANGIOMA

! Vascular differentiation may be obscured by enlarged, epithelioid endothelium, and extensive mixed inflammation.

! Unusual histologic features prompts diagnosis as hemangioendothelioma.

Key Features
EPITHELIOID HEMANGIOENDOTHELIOMA

• Myxohyaline stroma

• Cords of epithelioid cells without clear vessel formation

arranged in solid nests and sheets. Chronic inflammation, including eosinophils, is also typical. Other investigators have suggested that CEAN represents a variant of EH.[14]

Occasionally, pathologists consider the term, *epithelioid hemangioendothelioma*, in EHs with brisk mitotic activity or "worrisome" features in order to communicate a concern for more aggressive biologic behavior. It is critical to remember that EHE is a distinct entity that is rarely in the histologic differential diagnosis of EH due to the presence of myxohyaline stroma and the absence of prominent mixed inflammation and well-formed vessels.

The most important entity to exclude from the differential diagnosis of EH is epithelioid angiosarcoma. In a study of EHs of the penis, Fetsch and colleagues[4] noted that approximately 70% of their cases were interpreted as malignant by at least one contributing pathologist. Clues to the benign nature of the lesion include

1. Lobular architecture
2. Absence of diffuse infiltration into surrounding soft tissue, geographic tumor necrosis, and significant nuclear atypia
3. Peripheral maturation of vessels.

EPITHELIOID HEMANGIOENDOTHELIOMA

OVERVIEW

EHE of soft tissue was initially described by Weiss and Enzinger in 1982.[15] The term, *hemangioendothelioma*, was chosen by those investigators to indicate biological behavior that was intermediate between hemangioma and angiosarcoma because, in their initial study, approximately 10% of cases recurred and nearly 20% of tumors metastasized, usually to regional lymph nodes.

EHE of soft tissue affects both genders equally and, unlike EHE of bone and liver, is typically solitary. Tumors may arise in superficial or deep soft tissue in patients of any age, although pediatric cases are rare. The lesion presents as a mass

and may be painful possibly secondary to vascular occlusion because many EHE show angiocentric growth. In angiocentric lesions, veins are more commonly involved than arteries.

In 2001, an identical translocation was identified in two cases of EHE: t(1;3)(p36.3;q25).[16] Recently, Errani and colleagues[17] confirmed the presence of the t(1;3)(p36.3;q25) in EHE from multiple anatomic sites (bone, soft tissue, and liver) and described a unique fusion of the WWTR1-CAMTA1 genes.

GROSS FEATURES OF EPITHELIOID HEMANGIOENDOTHELIOMA

In contrast to other vascular tumors, EHE is generally not hemorrhagic and typically presents, instead, as an ill-defined tan to gray nodule. EHE arising in association with a blood vessel may appear as a fusiform expansion or as a mass encompassing the vessel.

MICROSCOPIC FEATURES OF EPITHELIOID HEMANGIOENDOTHELIOMA

EHE is characterized by cords and nests of bland epithelioid cells arranged in a myxohyaline stroma (Fig. 4). Blister cells, which are thought to represent rudimentary intracytoplasmic lumina in nascent blood vessels, may be seen. Typically, a well-formed vasculature, such as that seen in angiosarcoma or in hemangioma, is not present. EHEs may display areas with cytologic pleomorphism, increased mitotic activity (>1 mitotic figure/hpf), necrosis, and tumor cell spindling (Fig. 5).[18,19] Metaplastic bone has been described.[15,20] The interface with the adjacent soft tissue is typically infiltrative, although some cases are well circumscribed.

The endothelial markers, factor VIII–related antigen, CD31, CD34, and Fli-1, are usually positive in EHE.[15,20–23] Of the keratins, K18 and K7 are commonly expressed in EHE (100% and 50% of cases, respectively) and epithelial membrane antigen (EMA) may highlight the lining of primitive lumina.[2]

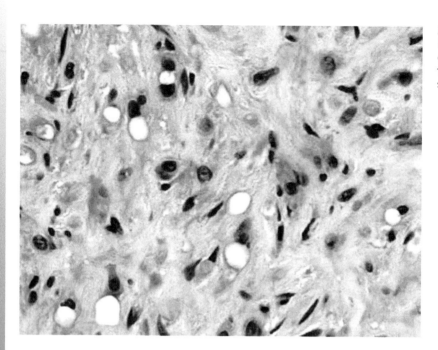

Fig. 4. EHE is characterized by nests and cords of epithelioid cells distributed in a myxohyaline stroma.

DIAGNOSIS AND DIFFERENTIAL DIAGNOSIS OF EPITHELIOID HEMANGIOENDOTHELIOMA

The diagnostic consideration with EHE is often metastatic carcinoma as opposed to other vascular or mesenchymal entities. Expression of epithelial antigens in EHE is a potential pitfall in excluding a carcinoma. Metastatic carcinomas, however, typically display greater cytologic atypia and more prominent mitotic activity than that seen in conventional EHE. Mucin stains confirm that the intracytoplasmic vacuoles are not epithelial mucin and endothelial markers, including CD31, CD34, and Fli-1, demonstrate endothelial differentiation.

EHE arising in the skin may mimic a mixed tumor due to the myxohyaline stroma and cord-like arrangement of the lesional cells. Absence of S-100 protein is a useful clue in excluding this entity.

Epithelioid angiosarcoma is not typically in the differential diagnosis of EHE. However, EHE-like areas may be seen in clearly malignant vascular tumors characterized by necrosis, brisk mitotic activity, and marked cytologic atypia. In such cases, a diagnosis of epithelioid angiosarcoma is warranted.

ES shares an immunophenotype with EHE (pancytokeratin and CD34 positive) and, therefore, may enter the differential diagnosis. Pancytokeratin is typically less diffuse in EHE and CD31 is almost always negative in epithelioid sarcoma (ES).[24]

PROGNOSIS OF EPITHELIOID HEMANGIOENDOTHELIOMA

The term, *hemangioendothelioma*, was selected to denote biologic behavior that was intermediate between hemangioma and angiosarcoma. Local recurrence is seen in approximately 12% of patients.[20,21] EHE metastasizes in 20% to 31% of cases, most often to regional lymph nodes and lung.[20,21,25] Three large series of EHE have shown death from disease in 13%[21] and 18%[20,25] of cases.

In their initial publication, Weiss and Enzinger suggested that cytologic atypia, cell spindling, and brisk mitotic activity were associated with more aggressive behavior.[15] In subsequent studies, these investigators and others have noted that although these features may correlate with more aggressive behavior; histologically bland EHE may also metastasize.[20,21]

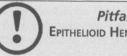

> **!** *Pitfalls*
> EPITHELIOID HEMANGIOENDOTHELIOMA
>
> ! Epithelial antigen expression and intracytoplasmic lumina mimic metastatic adenocarcinoma.
>
> ! Vascular differentiation may not be apparent.

Fig. 5. Marked nuclear pleomorphism, spindle morphology and brisk mitotic activity can be seen in epithelioid hemangioendotheliomas.

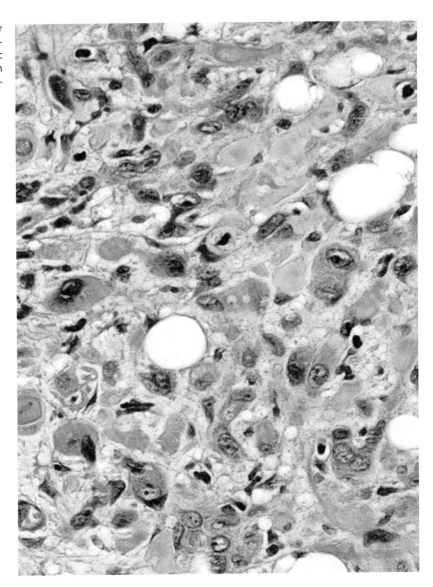

Additional studies have expanded the data on behavior: local recurrences occur in 10% to 15% of patients, metastatic rates range from 20% to 30%, and approximately 10% to 20% of patients die from disease.[15,20,21] Based on these data, EHE is classified by the WHO as a malignant tumor because the metastatic rate exceeds the limit of less than 2%.[5] Reliable criteria to predict aggressive behavior have been inconclusive.[25]

Recently, Deyrup and colleagues[25] identified two features that correlated with worse prognosis: size greater than 3.0 cm and mitotic count greater than 3 per 50 hpf. In patients with both features, the 5-year disease-specific survival was 59% whereas none of the patients whose tumors lacked both these features died.[25]

EPITHELIOID ANGIOSARCOMA

OVERVIEW

It is increasingly evident that angiosarcomas represent a heterogeneous group of tumors in which the clinical behavior is directly related to the site of disease and the clinical setting.[26] Epithelioid morphology can be seen in angiosarcomas arising in deep soft tissue and, less commonly, in those centered on the skin. Both sporadic cases and those associated with prior radiation therapy may have an epithelioid appearance.

Although Fletcher and colleagues[27] noted a male predominance in epithelioid angiosarcomas of deep soft tissue, cutaneous epithelioid angiosarcomas seem to be evenly distributed between the genders.[28] Two small series addressing epithelioid angiosarcomas of skin and deep soft tissue have suggested a predilection for the limbs (8 of 8 and 10 of 13 cases, respectively).[27,28] In a series of 69 sporadic cutaneous angiosarcomas; however, only 7% of the cases with epithelioid morphology arose in the extremities in contrast to 17% of those arising in the head and neck (Andrea T. Deyrup, MD, PhD, unpublished data, 2008).[18]

GROSS FEATURES OF EPITHELIOID ANGIOSARCOMA

Angiosarcomas tend to be extensively hemorrhagic, regardless of cell shape. They may have an infiltrative border with the surrounding tissue or a pseudocapsule may develop. Calcifications can be seen.

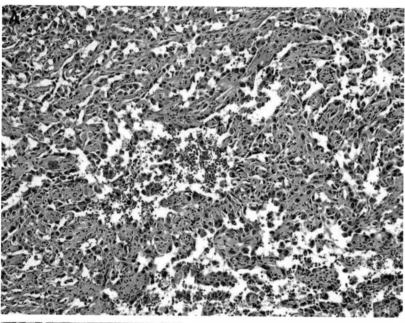
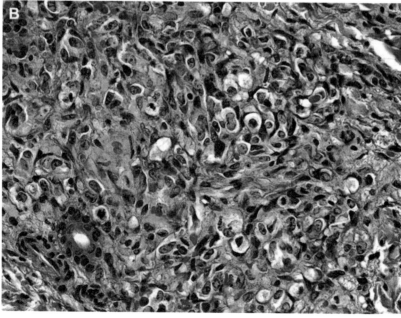

Fig. 6. Epithelioid angiosarcomas may show (A) anastomosing channels lined by markedly atypical polygonal endothelial cells or (B) solid sheets of epithelioid cells with minimal vasoformation.

Fig. 7. An immunohistochemical panel should be considered when the differential diagnosis includes epithelioid angiosarcoma and should include (*A*) CD31, (*B*) CD34, and (*C*) Fli-1.

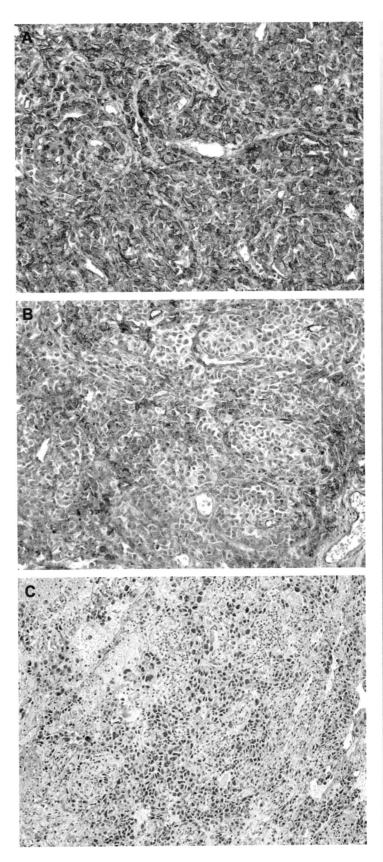

MICROSCOPIC FEATURES OF EPITHELIOID ANGIOSARCOMA

Epithelioid angiosarcomas may vary in appearance from relatively distinct vascular channels lined by atypical epithelioid cells (**Fig. 6**) to solid sheets of malignant cells that show only focal vasoformation (see **Fig. 6**). In the latter instance, clinical suspicion is critical in arriving at the correct diagnosis. The lesional cells show abundant eosinophilic cytoplasm and large nuclei with a prominent nucleolus. In addition to vasoformation, intracellular vacuoles encompassing red blood cells may also be seen.[27,28] Necrosis is a common feature, seen in more than half the reported cases, and mitotic activity is typically brisk, with scattered atypical mitotic figures.[27–29]

Markers of endothelial differentiation are typically positive in epithelioid angiosarcomas with CD31 showing a greater sensitivity than CD34 (97% vs 66%, respectively) (**Fig. 7**).[27–29] Fli-1 also shows great sensitivity in angiosarcomas and should be considered in a panel of immunohistochemical stains.

Epithelial antigens are frequently expressed in epithelioid angiosarcomas of deep soft tissue (**Fig. 8**).[27,30] In contrast, although Suchak and colleagues[28] found 66% of their cases of cutaneous epithelioid angiosarcomas to express EMA or pancytokeratin, none of the tumors evaluated by Bacchi and colleagues[29] or Marrogi and colleagues[31] was positive.

Key Features
EPITHELIOID ANGIOSARCOMA

- Pleomorphic, markedly atypical epithelioid cells with at least focal vasoformation
- Immunohistochemical expression of vascular markers CD34, CD31, and Fli-1

DIAGNOSIS AND DIFFERENTIAL DIAGNOSIS OF EPITHELIOID ANGIOSARCOMA

Epithelioid angiosarcomas with limited vasoformation may mimic poorly differentiated carcinoma, melanoma or lymphoma. The low incidence of angiosarcoma in the general population compared with the much higher incidence of carcinoma contributes to the diagnostic difficulty. This is complicated by the frequent expression of epithelial antigens in epithelioid angiosarcomas. Clues to the diagnosis include areas of hemorrhage or hemosiderin deposition, areas of dyshesion, and clinical features.

An extremely necrotic, cystic, or hemorrhagic angiosarcoma (regardless of cell shape) may mimic a resolving hematoma. A clinical history indicating a long duration should raise suspicion of a neoplastic process, particularly in the absence of coagulopathy.

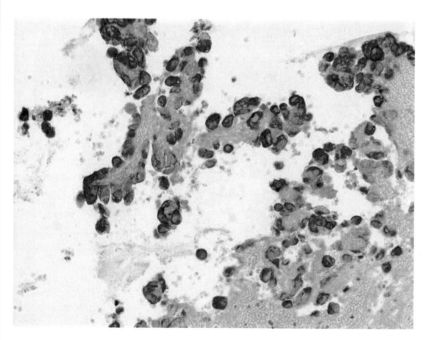

Fig. 8. Epithelial antigens may be positive in epithelioid angiosarcoma. Pancytokeratin highlights epithelioid endothelial cells in this image.

Key Features
EPITHELIOID SARCOMA

- Multiple nodules of brightly eosinophilic, monomorphic epithelioid cells with peripheral spindling embedded in a dense fibrous stroma and central necrosis (usual-type ES).

- Sheets of polygonal to rhabdoid epithelioid cells with enlarged, pleomorphic nuclei and prominent nucleoli.

- Co-expression of CD34 and pancytokeratin; absence of INI1.

Similar to epithelioid angiosarcoma, melanoma may have abundant cytoplasm and prominent nucleoli. Although S-100 protein expression has been evaluated in several angiosarcomas, only one case has shown positivity.[30,32] In addition, there is a reported case of epithelioid angiosarcoma with abundant S-100 protein–positive macrophages that mimicked melanoma.[33] Careful evaluation of the microscopic appearance combined with an immunohistochemical panel that includes HMB-45 and MART-1 help avoid this pitfall.

PROGNOSIS OF EPITHELIOID ANGIOSARCOMA

The prognosis for angiosarcomas of deep soft tissue, regardless of morphology, is dismal.[30] Sporadic cutaneous angiosarcomas with epithelioid morphology seem to behave more aggressively than cutaneous angiosarcomas that lack this feature[18]; however, the relationship between epithelioid morphology and clinical behavior is less well documented for angiosarcomas arising in other settings (ie, postradiation therapy and deep soft tissue).

EPITHELIOID SARCOMA

OVERVIEW

Epithelioid sarcoma (ES) is a sarcoma of undetermined lineage that shows epithelial differentiation. Two variants have been described; the entity originally described in 1970 by Enzinger is generally referred to as usual-type ES[34] whereas the tumor reported by Guillou and colleagues[35] in 1997 is designated as proximal-type ES.

Usual-type ES occurs primarily in young adult men and is most common in the distal upper extremities, in particular the fingers and hands.[36] The lesions may be solitary or multifocal and typically arise in the dermis/subcutaneous tissue. In the initial description, Enzinger emphasized the microscopic resemblance to necrotizing granulomas, chronic inflammation, and squamous cell carcinoma.[34]

Proximal-type ES is usually deep seated and most common in proximal anatomic sites, such as the pelvic and inguinal areas, axilla, and flank.[35,37] Patients are typically older than those affected by usual-type ES and the lesional cells show greater cytologic atypia and a more rhabdoid appearance. This variant is more aggressive than usual-type ES.[35,37]

GROSS FEATURES OF EPITHELIOID SARCOMA

Usual-type ES is characterized by small solitary or multiple dermal and/or subcutaneous nodules that may show surface ulceration. The cut surface is typically firm and white to gray with central necrosis and/or hemorrhagic discoloration. Proximal-type epithelioid sarcomas are generally larger but otherwise show similar features.

MICROSCOPIC FEATURES OF EPITHELIOID SARCOMA

Both usual-type and proximal-type ES are typically composed of multiple, ill-defined nodules with central necrosis (**Fig. 9**). Usual-type ES is characterized by relatively monomorphic, polygonal epithelioid cells that modulate to a more spindled shape peripherally (**Fig. 10**). Nucleoli are not typically prominent. The cells may be deceptively bland and inconspicuous, particularly in densely sclerotic soft tissue. Necrotic foci with a peripheral fringe of epithelioid cells can simulate granulomatous inflammation; mitotic activity is generally low (1–14 mitotic figures/10 hpf)[36] but more evident than that seen in inflammatory mimics of ES. Calcification and/or ossification may be present.[36] A variety of morphologic variants has been described, including myxoid,[38] angiomatoid,[39] and fibroma-like.[19,39]

In contrast to the histology of usual-type ES, proximal-type ES shows greater nuclear

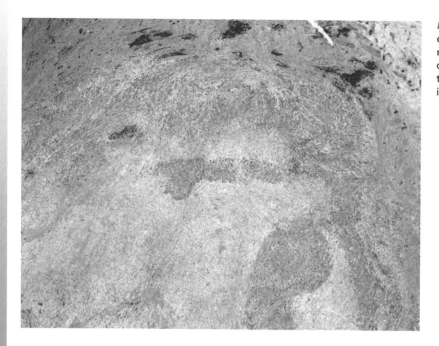

Fig. 9. A low-power view of ES shows the typical nodular architecture and central necrosis, suggestive of granulomatous inflammation.

pleomorphism and often has a rhabdoid appearance (**Fig. 11**). Nucleoli are prominent. Necrosis in proximal-type ES lacks the granulomatous appearance seen in usual-type ES.

The immunophenotype of ES is critical in correct diagnosis: pancytokeratin positive (more than 90% of cases) (**Fig. 12**), CD34 positive (more than 50% of cases) (see **Fig. 12**), and negative for INI1 (more than 85% of cases).[39,40] INI1 is a tumor suppressor that is expressed in normal tissue but negative in most tumor types, with some exceptions.[41–43] CD31 and Fli-1 are usually negative, excluding vascular neoplasia.[23,39] Subtyping of cytokeratin expression has shown most ES to be positive for keratin 8; keratin 5/6 shows focal expression in approximately 30% of cases.[44]

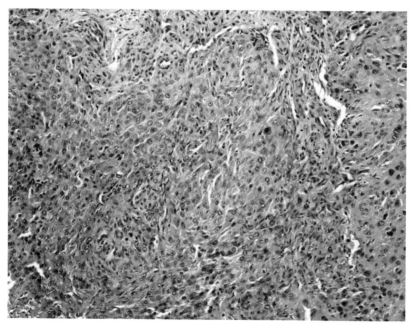

Fig. 10. Usual-type ES consists of eosinophilic epithelioid cells that blend peripherally into spindle cells.

Fig. 11. Proximal-type ES shows greater cytologic atypia than usual-type ES and may have a rhabdoid appearance.

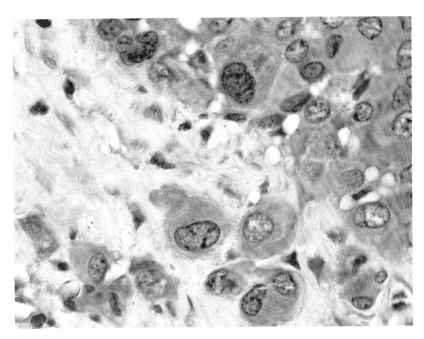

DIAGNOSIS AND DIFFERENTIAL DIAGNOSIS OF EPITHELIOID SARCOMA

Usual-type ES may have a deceptively bland appearance and, due to cellular palisading and central necrosis, may raise the possibility of granulomatous inflammation or deep granuloma annulare and necrobiotic granulomas; mitotic activity, although typically low in ES, usually exceeds that seen in such lesions. A benign neoplastic or reactive process may also enter the differential diagnosis. A high index of suspicion can help avoid misdiagnosis; even convincing cases of these entities may warrant a pancytokeratin immunohistochemical stain when arising in the distal extremity of a child.

ES-like hemangioendothelioma is a close mimic of usual-type ES due to its[45]

1. Multinodular growth pattern
2. Modulation of epithelioid to spindled shape
3. Strong cytokeratin expression.

The clinical presentation is also similar; patients tend to be young adults and tumors arise in the extremities. In contrast to usual-type ES, ES-like hemangioendothelioma is negative for CD34 but positive for CD31.

Squamous cell carcinoma is another potential mimic that can be distinguished from usual-type ES by absence of CD34 expression and presence of INI1 and cytokeratin 5/6.[44,46] Furthermore, squamous cell carcinoma is uncommon in the patient population affected by usual-type ES.

In considering a diagnosis of proximal-type ES, epithelioid angiosarcoma may enter the differential diagnosis. Both tumors display significant nuclear pleomorphism and prominent nucleoli and can co-express the vascular marker CD34 and pancytokeratin.[27,30] Vasoformation is a helpful clue; however, correct diagnosis is best supported by a panel of immunohistochemical stains, including CD31 and Fli-1, in addition to pancytokeratin and CD34.

PROGNOSIS OF EPITHELIOID SARCOMA

Recurrence is frequent in usual-type ES and metastases occur in 30% to 45% of cases. ES is unusual among sarcomas in that, in addition to frequent

Pitfalls
Epithelioid Sarcoma

! Usual-type ES may be deceptively bland and convincingly mimic a non-neoplastic process.

! Strong pancytokeratin expression raises the possibility of spindle squamous cell carcinoma (usual-type ES) or metastatic carcinoma (proximal-type ES).

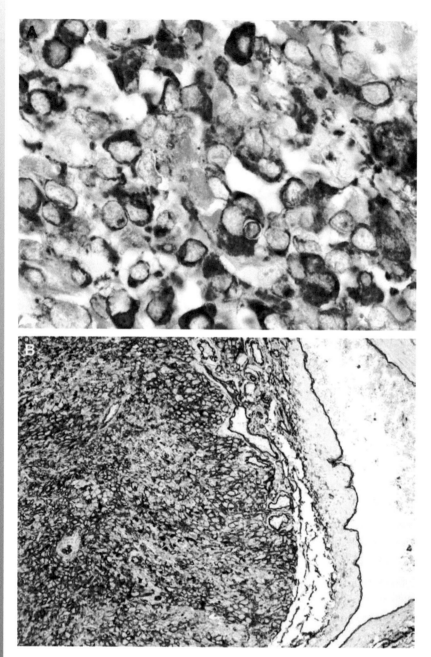

Fig. 12. ES is positive for pancytokeratin AE1/3 (*A*) and, in 50% of cases, CD34 (*B*).

pulmonary metastases, locoregional lymph nodes are also common sites of distant disease. ES is not graded by the WHO; increased mitotic activity, proximal location, and increasing tumor size correlate with a worse prognosis. ES is an indolent disease and a protracted clinical course can result in late metastases and patient death.

Proximal-type ES is more aggressive than usual-type ES; however, it is not clear if this is due to a tendency for larger size at diagnosis and the more proximal location. Forty-three to 75% of patients with proximal-type ES have metastatic disease, primarily to lymph node and lung, and 35% to 65% of patients die from disease.[35,36]

SCLEROSING EPITHELIOID FIBROSARCOMA

OVERVIEW

Sclerosing epithelioid fibrosarcoma (SEF) was initially described in 1995 by Meis-Kindblom and colleagues,[47] who noted its resemblance to infiltrating carcinoma. SEF typically presents as a painful enlarging mass in the deep soft tissues of the lower extremities and trunk and limb girdles. The genders are affected equally and patients are typically in their fourth decade.

Fibroblastic differentiation is supported by immunohistochemical as well as electron microscopic data.[47,48] Based on histologic and cytogenetic evidence, it has recently been suggested that SEF may be related to low-grade fibromyxoid sarcoma.[49] SEF, however, seems to pursue a more aggressive clinical course than low-grade fibromyxoid sarcoma, which may be due, in part, to difficulty and, therefore, delay in diagnosis.

GROSS FEATURES OF SCLEROSING EPITHELIOID FIBROSARCOMA

SEF is typically a large, well-circumscribed, lobulated/multinodular mass. The cut surfaces are gray to white and typically firm, although cystic change, necrosis, and myxoid/mucoid areas may be present. Calcification is rare.

Key Features
SCLEROSING EPITHELIOID FIBROSARCOMA

- Monomorphic clear epithelioid cells distributed in a variably hyalinized stroma with dense collagen bundles.
- Immunohistochemical stains essentially negative for hematopoietic, myoid, epithelial, and melanocytic antigens.

MICROSCOPIC FEATURES OF SCLEROSING EPITHELIOID FIBROSARCOMA

The classic appearance of SEF is epithelioid cells with moderate amounts of clear cytoplasm distributed in a variably hyalinized to sclerotic stroma. Typically, the cells are arranged in cords, linear arrays, or nests separated by densely eosinophilic collagen, similar to lobular breast carcinoma (Fig. 13). A pseudoalveolar appearance may result from central dyshesion of the tumor cells (Fig. 14). Broad paucicellular areas of dense fibrosis have been described in some cases and can result in misclassification as a benign mesenchymal tumor.[48]

Nuclear pleomorphism is uncommon and the lesional cells have a bland, monomorphic appearance with fine nuclear chromatin and small

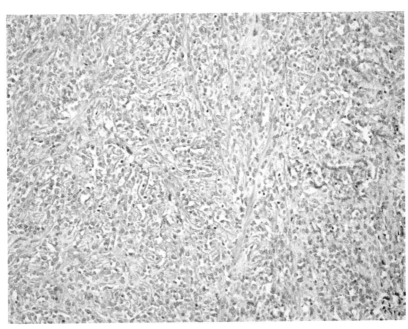

Fig. 13. Sclerosing epithelioid fibrosarcoma showing the characteristic bland clear cells distributed in a densely hyalinized stroma.

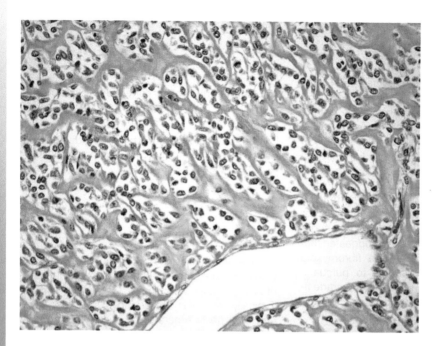

Fig. 14. Central dyshesion can give a pseudoalveolar appearance in sclerosing epithelioid fibrosarcoma.

nucleoli. Mitotic activity is variable but typically low. Larger tumors more frequently have at least focal necrosis.[48]

As is typical for fibrosarcomas as a group, the immunophenotype of SEF is not specific; vimentin expression is the only consistent finding.[47,48] Variable, focal EMA, S-100 protein, and cytokeratin expression have been described.[47]

DIAGNOSIS AND DIFFERENTIAL DIAGNOSIS OF SCLEROSING EPITHELIOID FIBROSARCOMA

The two primary diagnostic considerations for SEF are carcinoma and lymphoma, and the possibility of SEF may only be considered when epithelial or hematopoietic immunohistochemical stains are unexpectedly negative. The corollary to this is that a diagnosis of SEF should only be made after a broad immunohistochemical panel that excludes metastatic carcinoma, sclerosing lymphoma, and mesenchymal mimics, including sclerosing rhabdomyosarcoma, monophasic synovial sarcoma, and clear cell sarcoma of soft tissue.

Of the carcinomas, lobular breast carcinoma and renal cell carcinoma bear the greatest resemblance to SEF and can be excluded simply by a pancytokeratin immunohistochemical stain. Clear cell sarcoma of soft tissue expresses S-100 protein and other markers of melanocytic

differentiation. Sclerosing rhabdomyosarcoma and alveolar rhabdomyosarcoma express desmin and MyoD1, with the latter also typically expressing diffuse myogenin. Although EMA and pancytokeratin may be focal in synovial sarcoma, translocation analysis for the X:18 chromosomal translocation and evaluation of CD99 and bcl-2 expression clarify the matter.

PROGNOSIS OF SCLEROSING EPITHELIOID FIBROSARCOMA

Despite its bland histologic appearance, SEF is an aggressive sarcoma; a systematic review of the literature calculated metastatic rates of 44%, local recurrence in 37% of patients, and death from

Pitfalls
SCLEROSING EPITHELIOID FIBROSARCOMA

! No positive immunohistochemical stains necessitates a broad panel to exclude potential mimics.

! Bland appearance may result in a diagnosis as a benign or reactive lesion.

disease in 34% of patients after a mean duration of 46 months.[50] It is not clear if the poor prognosis is due, in part, to delay in diagnosis; 13% of patients had metastatic disease at the time of diagnosis and there was a mean duration of 33 months from first onset of symptoms to diagnosis. The most common sites of metastatic disease are the lung, bone, and pleura.[47,48,50] A high proportion (35%) of tumors metastasized to multiple sites.

EPITHELIOID MALIGNANT PERIPHERAL NERVE SHEATH TUMOR

OVERVIEW

Although typical epithelioid malignant peripheral nerve sheath tumor (MPNST) may show focal areas of epithelioid morphology, predominantly epithelioid MPNSTs are far less common, with a reported incidence of 5% of all MPNSTs.[51–53]

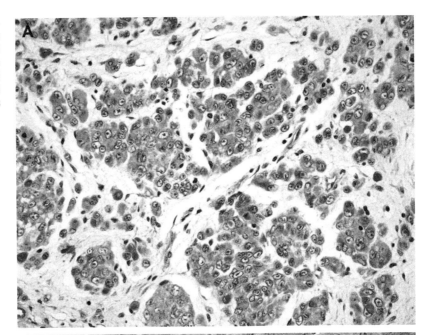
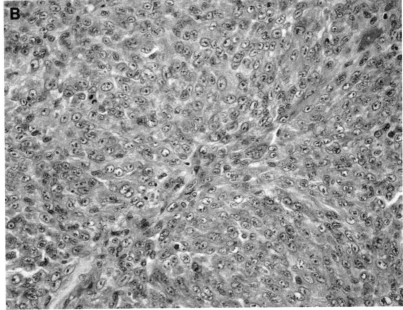

Fig. 15. Epithelioid malignant peripheral nerve sheath tumor composed of nodules of round to polygonal cells arranged in cords in a myxoid stroma (*A*) or solid sheets of cells (*B*).

Epithelioid MPNST was first described in a case report in 1954 by McCormack and colleagues as "malignant schwannoma"[54] with two subsequent cases of entirely epithelioid MPNST published in 1986.[51] A larger series by Laskin and colleagues[52] in 1991 further defined the entity.

Tumors typically present as an asymptomatic mass in superficial or deep soft tissue in patients in their fourth decade.[52,55] The genders are affected equally. Unlike typical MPNSTs, there is no definite association with neurofibromatosis 1.[51] Although it seems that epithelioid MPNSTs tend to arise in the setting of benign nerve sheath tumors (schwannoma or neurofibroma), this may be related to selection bias.[52,53]

GROSS FEATURES OF EPITHELIOID MALIGNANT PERIPHERAL NERVE SHEATH TUMOR

Epithelioid MPNSTs arising in the superficial soft tissue typically form a single nodule whereas those originating in deep soft tissue have a more lobulated, multinodular appearance and are frequently associated with a large nerve. The cut surface is tan-white and firm; however, there may be areas of necrosis and hemorrhage.

MICROSCOPIC FEATURES OF EPITHELIOID MALIGNANT PERIPHERAL NERVE SHEATH TUMOR

Epithelioid MPNST is composed of ill-defined nodules separated by fibrous septa. The epithelioid cells are round to polygonal and may be arranged in cords or syncytial nests distributed in a variably myxoid stroma (Fig. 15) or in solid sheets (see Fig. 15). The nuclei are large and vesicular with prominent, eosinophilic nucleoli, similar to those seen in melanoma. A population of malignant spindle cells is usually present, at least focally. Mitotic activity is variable. In tumors with prominent necrosis, viable tumor predominates adjacent to blood vessels.

In cases associated with a peripheral nerve, the malignant cells may infiltrate between nerve fibers, expanding the fascicles. A pre-existing benign nerve sheath tumor, either schwannoma or neurofibroma, can be present.[52,53]

In contrast to typical MPNST, S-100 protein expression is generally strong and diffuse with staining of both cytoplasm and nuclei (Fig. 16). Pancytokeratin and melanoma markers are usually negative.

DIAGNOSIS AND DIFFERENTIAL DIAGNOSIS OF EPITHELIOID MALIGNANT PERIPHERAL NERVE SHEATH TUMOR

The strong, diffuse expression of S-100 protein and prominent eosinophilic nucleoli can raise the possibility of amelanotic melanoma. More specific markers of melanin production (MART-1 and HMB-45) are typically negative. Clear cell sarcoma is another potential mimic; in this entity, in addition to evaluation of melanin-related

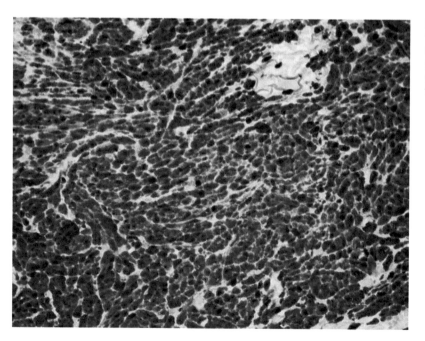

Fig. 16. Strong, diffuse S-100 protein expression in the cytoplasm and nuclei in epithelioid malignant peripheral nerve sheath tumor.

antigens, molecular studies can confirm the diagnosis by identifying EWS-gene rearrangements.

Epithelioid MPNST with prominent myxoid stroma may mimic extraskeletal myxoid chondrosarcoma which, although it may be focally S-100–protein positive, does not show the same diffuse expression seen in epithelioid MPNST.

PROGNOSIS OF EPITHELIOID MALIGNANT PERIPHERAL NERVE SHEATH TUMOR

MPNSTs are aggressive tumors with a high disease-related mortality. A recent series of MPNSTs found 5-year disease-specific survival of 35% and 50% for patients with neurofibromatosis 1 and sporadic cases, respectively.[56] Large studies of epithelioid MPNST have not been possible because of the few cases. There is no evidence to suggest, however, that these tumors have a better prognosis than typical MPNSTs.

As with most sarcomas, superficial epithelioid MPNSTs have a better prognosis than deeply situated tumors and tend to be somewhat smaller.[52] Lymph node metastases have been reported in epithelioid MPNSTs[55]; however, other series have not found a similar metastatic pattern.[52] Sites of metastasis are lung, pleura, and liver.

REFERENCES

1. Rosai J, Gold J, Landy R. The histiocytoid hemangiomas. A unifying concept embracing several previously described entities of skin, soft tissue, large vessels, bone, and heart. Hum Pathol 1979;10: 707–30.
2. Al-Abbadi MA, Almasri NM, Al-Quran S, et al. Cytokeratin and epithelial membrane antigen expression in angiosarcomas: an immunohistochemical study of 33 cases. Arch Pathol Lab Med 2007;131: 288–92.
3. Miettinen M, Fetsch JF. Distribution of keratins in normal endothelial cells and a spectrum of vascular tumors: implications in tumor diagnosis. Hum Pathol 2000;31:1062–7.
4. Fetsch JF, Sesterhenn IA, Miettinen M, et al. Epithelioid hemangioma of the penis: a clinicopathologic and immunohistochemical analysis of 19 cases, with special reference to exuberant examples often confused with epithelioid hemangioendothelioma and epithelioid angiosarcoma. Am J Surg Pathol 2004;28:523–33.
5. Fletcher CD, Unni KK, Mertens F. World Health Organization classification of tumours. Lyon (France): IARC Press; 2002.
6. Wells GC, Whimster IW. Subcutaneous angiolymphoid hyperplasia with eosinophilia. Br J Dermatol 1969;81:1–14.
7. Eady RA, Jones EW. Pseudopyogenic granuloma: enzyme histochemical and ultrastructural study. Hum Pathol 1977;8:653–68.
8. Jones EW, Bleehen SS. Inflammatory angiomatous nodules with abnormal blood vessels occurring about the ears and scalp (pseudo or atypical pyogenic granuloma). Br J Dermatol 1969;81:804–16.
9. Fetsch JF, Weiss SW. Observations concerning the pathogenesis of epithelioid hemangioma (angiolymphoid hyperplasia). Mod Pathol 1991;4:449–55.
10. Olsen TG, Helwig EB. Angiolymphoid hyperplasia with eosinophilia. A clinicopathologic study of 116 patients. J Am Acad Dermatol 1985;12:781–96.
11. Kuo TT, Shih LY, Chan HL. Kimura's disease. Involvement of regional lymph nodes and distinction from angiolymphoid hyperplasia with eosinophilia. Am J Surg Pathol 1988;12:843–54.
12. Googe PB, Harris NL, Mihm MC Jr. Kimura's disease and angiolymphoid hyperplasia with eosinophilia: two distinct histopathological entities. J Cutan Pathol 1987;14:263–71.
13. Brenn T, Fletcher CD. Cutaneous epithelioid angiomatous nodule: a distinct lesion in the morphologic spectrum of epithelioid vascular tumors. Am J Dermatopathol 2004;26:14–21.
14. Sangueza OP, Walsh SN, Sheehan DJ, et al. Cutaneous epithelioid angiomatous nodule: a case series and proposed classification. Am J Dermatopathol 2008;30:16–20.
15. Weiss SW, Enzinger FM. Epithelioid hemangioendothelioma: a vascular tumor often mistaken for a carcinoma. Cancer 1982;50:970–81.
16. Mendlick MR, Nelson M, Pickering D, et al. Translocation t(1;3)(p36.3;q25) is a nonrandom aberration in epithelioid hemangioendothelioma. Am J Surg Pathol 2001;25:684–7.
17. Errani C, Zhang L, Sung YS, et al. A novel WWTR1-CAMTA1 gene fusion is a consistent abnormality in epithelioid hemangioendothelioma of different anatomic sites. Genes Chromosomes Cancer 2011;50:644–53.
18. Deyrup AT, McKenney JK, Tighiouart M, et al. Sporadic cutaneous angiosarcomas: a proposal for risk stratification based on 69 cases. Am J Surg Pathol 2008;32:72–7.
19. Mirra JM, Kessler S, Bhuta S, et al. The fibroma-like variant of epithelioid sarcoma. A fibrohistiocytic/myoid cell lesion often confused with benign and malignant spindle cell tumors. Cancer 1992;69: 1382–95.
20. Mentzel T, Beham A, Calonje E, et al. Epithelioid hemangioendothelioma of skin and soft tissues: clinicopathologic and immunohistochemical study of 30 cases. Am J Surg Pathol 1997;21:363–74.
21. Weiss SW, Ishak KG, Dail DH, et al. Epithelioid hemangioendothelioma and related lesions. Semin Diagn Pathol 1986;3:259–87.

22. Rossi S, Orvieto E, Furlanetto A, et al. Utility of the immunohistochemical detection of FLI-1 expression in round cell and vascular neoplasm using a monoclonal antibody. Mod Pathol 2004;17:547–52.

23. Folpe AL, Chand EM, Goldblum JR, et al. Expression of Fli-1, a nuclear transcription factor, distinguishes vascular neoplasms from potential mimics. Am J Surg Pathol 2001;25:1061–6.

24. den Bakker MA, Flood SJ, Kliffen M. CD31 staining in epithelioid sarcoma. Virchows Arch 2003;443:93–7.

25. Deyrup AT, Tighiouart M, Montag AG, et al. Epithelioid hemangioendothelioma of soft tissue: a proposal for risk stratification based on 49 cases. Am J Surg Pathol 2008;32:924–7.

26. Fayette J, Martin E, Piperno-Neumann S, et al. Angiosarcomas, a heterogeneous group of sarcomas with specific behavior depending on primary site: a retrospective study of 161 cases. Ann Oncol 2007;18:2030–6.

27. Fletcher CD, Beham A, Bekir S, et al. Epithelioid angiosarcoma of deep soft tissue: a distinctive tumor readily mistaken for an epithelial neoplasm. Am J Surg Pathol 1991;15:915–24.

28. Suchak R, Thway K, Zelger B, et al. Primary cutaneous epithelioid angiosarcoma: a clinicopathologic study of 13 cases of a rare neoplasm occurring outside the setting of conventional angiosarcomas and with predilection for the limbs. Am J Surg Pathol 2011;35:60–9.

29. Bacchi CE, Silva TR, Zambrano E, et al. Epithelioid angiosarcoma of the skin: a study of 18 cases with emphasis on its clinicopathologic spectrum and unusual morphologic features. Am J Surg Pathol 2010;34:1334–43.

30. Meis-Kindblom JM, Kindblom LG. Angiosarcoma of soft tissue: a study of 80 cases. Am J Surg Pathol 1998;22:683–97.

31. Marrogi AJ, Hunt SJ, Cruz DJ. Cutaneous epithelioid angiosarcoma. Am J Dermatopathol 1990;12:350–6.

32. Prescott RJ, Banerjee SS, Eyden BP, et al. Cutaneous epithelioid angiosarcoma: a clinicopathological study of four cases. Histopathology 1994;25:421–9.

33. Brightman LA, Demierre MF, Byers HR. Macrophage-rich epithelioid angiosarcoma mimicking malignant melanoma. J Cutan Pathol 2006;33:38–42.

34. Enzinger FM. Epithelioid sarcoma: a sarcoma simulating a granuloma or a carcinoma. Cancer 1970;26:1029–41.

35. Guillou L, Wadden C, Coindre JM, et al. "Proximal-type" epithelioid sarcoma, a distinctive aggressive neoplasm showing rhabdoid features. Clinicopathologic, immunohistochemical, and ultrastructural study of a series. Am J Surg Pathol 1997;21:130–46.

36. Chase DR, Enzinger FM. Epithelioid sarcoma. Diagnosis, prognostic indicators, and treatment. Am J Surg Pathol 1985;9:241–63.

37. Hasegawa T, Matsuno Y, Shimoda T, et al. Proximal-type epithelioid sarcoma: a clinicopathologic study of 20 cases. Mod Pathol 2001;14:655–63.

38. Flucke U, Hulsebos TJ, van Krieken JH, et al. Myxoid epithelioid sarcoma: a diagnostic challenge. A report on six cases. Histopathology 2010;57:753–9.

39. Miettinen M, Fanburg-Smith JC, Virolainen M, et al. Epithelioid sarcoma: an immunohistochemical analysis of 112 classical and variant cases and a discussion of the differential diagnosis. Hum Pathol 1999;30:934–42.

40. Hornick JL, Dal Cin P, Fletcher CD. Loss of INI1 expression is characteristic of both conventional and proximal-type epithelioid sarcoma. Am J Surg Pathol 2009;33:542–50.

41. Kohashi K, Izumi T, Oda Y, et al. Infrequent SMARCB1/INI1 gene alteration in epithelioid sarcoma: a useful tool in distinguishing epithelioid sarcoma from malignant rhabdoid tumor. Hum Pathol 2009;40:349–55.

42. Cheng JX, Tretiakova M, Gong C, et al. Renal medullary carcinoma: rhabdoid features and the absence of INI1 expression as markers of aggressive behavior. Mod Pathol 2008;21:647–52.

43. Patil S, Perry A, Maccollin M, et al. Immunohistochemical analysis supports a role for INI1/SMARCB1 in hereditary forms of schwannomas, but not in solitary, sporadic schwannomas. Brain Pathol 2008;18:517–9.

44. Laskin WB, Miettinen M. Epithelioid sarcoma: new insights based on an extended immunohistochemical analysis. Arch Pathol Lab Med 2003;127:1161–8.

45. Billings SD, Folpe AL, Weiss SW. Epithelioid sarcoma-like hemangioendothelioma. Am J Surg Pathol 2003;27:48–57.

46. Orrock JM, Abbott JJ, Gibson LE, et al. INI1 and GLUT-1 expression in epithelioid sarcoma and its cutaneous neoplastic and nonneoplastic mimics. Am J Dermatopathol 2009;31:152–6.

47. Meis-Kindblom JM, Kindblom LG, Enzinger FM. Sclerosing epithelioid fibrosarcoma. A variant of fibrosarcoma simulating carcinoma. Am J Surg Pathol 1995;19:979–93.

48. Antonescu CR, Rosenblum MK, Pereira P, et al. Sclerosing epithelioid fibrosarcoma: a study of 16 cases and confirmation of a clinicopathologically distinct tumor. Am J Surg Pathol 2001;25:699–709.

49. Guillou L, Benhattar J, Gengler C, et al. Translocation-positive low-grade fibromyxoid sarcoma: clinicopathologic and molecular analysis of a series expanding the morphologic spectrum and suggesting potential relationship to sclerosing epithelioid fibrosarcoma: a study from the French Sarcoma Group. Am J Surg Pathol 2007;31:1387–402.

50. Ossendorf C, Studer GM, Bode B, et al. Sclerosing epithelioid fibrosarcoma: case presentation and a systematic review. Clin Orthop Relat Res 2008; 466:1485–91.

51. DiCarlo EF, Woodruff JM, Bansal M, et al. The purely epithelioid malignant peripheral nerve sheath tumor. Am J Surg Pathol 1986;10:478–90.

52. Laskin WB, Weiss SW, Bratthauer GL. Epithelioid variant of malignant peripheral nerve sheath tumor (malignant epithelioid schwannoma). Am J Surg Pathol 1991;15:1136–45.

53. McMenamin ME, Fletcher CD. Expanding the spectrum of malignant change in schwannomas: epithelioid malignant change, epithelioid malignant peripheral nerve sheath tumor, and epithelioid angiosarcoma: a study of 17 cases. Am J Surg Pathol 2001;25:13–25.

54. McCormack LJ, Hazard JB, Dickson JA. Malignant epithelioid neurilemoma (schwannoma). Cancer 1954;7:725–8.

55. Lodding P, Kindblom LG, Angervall L. Epithelioid malignant schwannoma. A study of 14 cases. Virchows Arch A Pathol Anat Histopathol 1986;409: 433–51.

56. Zou C, Smith KD, Liu J, et al. Clinical, pathological, and molecular variables predictive of malignant peripheral nerve sheath tumor outcome. Ann Surg 2009;249:1014–22.

SELECTED LESIONS FEATURING GIANT CELLS

Karokh H. Salih, MBChB, FICPath[a], Aatur D. Singhi, MD, PhD[b],
Elizabeth A. Montgomery, MD[b],*

KEYWORDS

- Tenosynovial giant cell tumor • Reticulohistiocytoma • Juvenile xanthogranuloma
- Giant cell fibroblastoma • Giant cell angiofibroma • Phosphaturic mesenchymal tumor

ABSTRACT

Many neoplasms of the soft tissues feature giant cells, but this article covers entities in which giant cells are a striking feature. Specifically, we consider tenosynovial giant cell tumor (localized and diffuse types; giant cell tumor of tendon sheath, and pigmented villonodular tenosynovitis), reticulohistiocytoma, juvenile xanthogranuloma, giant cell fibroblastoma (a variant form of dermatofibrosarcoma protuberans), giant cell angiofibroma (which is essentially a giant cell–rich form of solitary fibrous tumor), and phosphaturic mesenchymal tumor.

OVERVIEW

Many lesions can feature giant cells and these are discussed in other articles in this issue. For example, so-called giant cell malignant fibrous histiocytoma, classically reported in the retroperitoneum, is now known to be dedifferentiated liposarcoma,[1,2] which is addressed in "Liposarcomas" by Singhi and Montgomery elsewhere in this issue. Tumefactive extramedullary hematopoiesis contains megakaryocytes, and thus seemingly has giant cells.[3] When fibromatoses invade skeletal muscle, the injured skeletal myocytes form giant cells (**Fig. 1**), but this phenomenon is a pitfall rather than a tumor type.[4] Several types of tumors have giant cell patterns, including carcinomas and sarcomas, such as the leiomyosarcoma depicted

in **Fig. 2**, and these tumors can also contain osteoclastlike giant cells.[5,6] Certain soft tissue tumors, however, have giant cells as a key feature and some of these are addressed in this article.

TENOSYNOVIAL GIANT CELL TUMOR, LOCALIZED TYPE (GIANT CELL TUMOR OF TENDON SHEATH)

OVERVIEW

These tumors are typically encountered in middle-aged women but can arise at any age. They are

---

Key Features
LOCALIZED TYPE

- Arises at any age, women > men
- Most examples in digits (usually hands)
- Nodular circumscribed mass
- Sheets of histiocyte-like small cells and polygonal larger cells, background histiocytes, siderophages
- CD68+ in osteoclastlike cells and some of small round cells
- Desmin +
- Benign

---

[a] Department of Pathology, College of Medicine, University of Sulaimani, As-Sulaimaniyah, Iraq
[b] Department of Pathology, The Johns Hopkins Medical Institutions, 401 North Broadway, Weinberg 2242, Baltimore, MD 21231-2410, USA
* Corresponding author.
E-mail address: emontgom@jhmi.edu

Surgical Pathology 4 (2011) 887–913
doi:10.1016/j.path.2011.08.008
1875-9181/11/$ – see front matter © 2011 Elsevier Inc. All rights reserved.

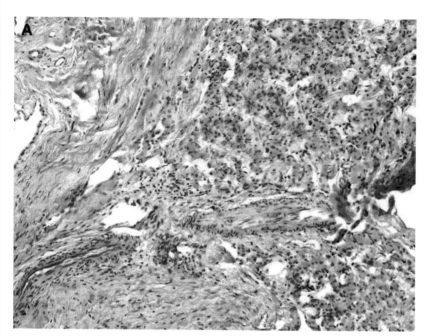

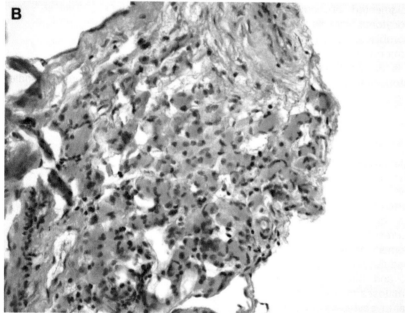

Fig. 1. (A) The interface of a fibromatosis (desmoid tumor, lower left) with skeletal muscle can produce giant cells as the skeletal myocytes round up (hematoxylin-eosin [H&E] stain, original magnification ×20). (B) Higher magnification of the damaged skeletal muscle giant cells (H&E stain, original magnification ×40).

classically encountered in the hand but other large joints can be affected.[7] Patients present with painless, slowly growing well-marginated masses closely related to synovial or tendon sheath or even the joint itself. Occasionally the tumors erode adjoining bone.[8] Local excision is generally curative but occasional tumors recur.

GROSS FEATURES

Localized tenosynovial giant cell tumors are small (<5 cm), lobulated extra-articular lesions with a solid white, gray, or brown cut surface depending on the amount of hemosiderin in any given lesion. They are often surrounded by a fibrous capsule.

Fig. 2. (*A*) A giant cell pattern in a leiomyosarcoma (H&E stain, original magnification ×40). The lesional cells contain brightly eosinophilic cytoplasm and atypical nuclei. (*B*) Desmin labeling in the leiomyosarcoma seen in *A* (immunohistochemical stain-Desmin, original magnification ×20).

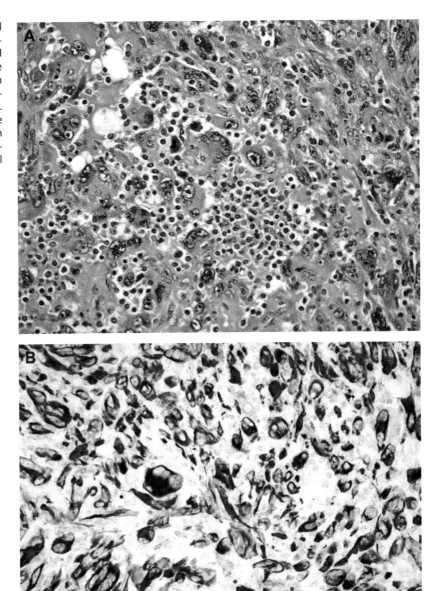

MICROSCOPIC FEATURES

Microscopically, the tumors have a focal fibrous capsule and a heterogeneous appearance from field to field (Fig. 3). The tumors consist of small, uniform histiocytelike cells with scant eosinophilic cytoplasm and various quantities of osteoclastlike giant cells, foamy macrophages, and hemosiderin-laden macrophages. Some tumors have few giant cells, whereas others have many. Larger mononuclear cells often accompany the small uniform ones. Mitotic figures can usually be identified and, when brisk, can indicate a propensity for recurrence. Some examples show stromal hyalinization, but necrosis is unusual (but not a feature predictive of malignant behavior).

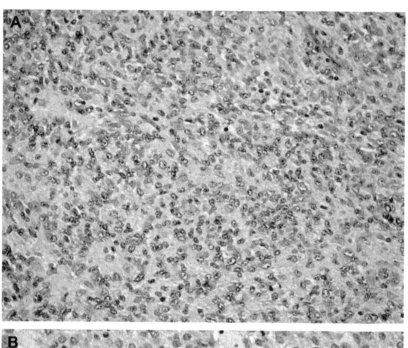

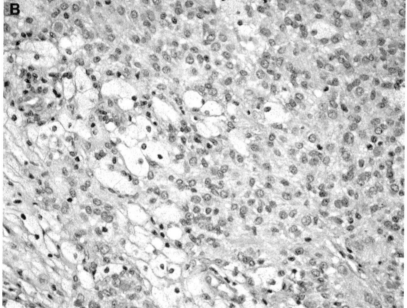

Fig. 3. (A) Tenosynovial giant cell tumor, localized type (giant cell tumor of tendon sheath). This field shows a monotonous population of rounded cells with modest amounts of pale pink cytoplasm (H&E stain, original magnification ×20). (B) Prominent foamy macrophages (H&E stain, original magnification ×20).

ANCILLARY STUDIES

Iron stains usually demonstrate iron even when it is not seen on routine staining. On immunolabeling, the mononuclear cells can show expression of CD45 and CD68, as well as actin. Clusterin staining is diffuse and strong in the large mononuclear cells and most cases show focal desmin expression in the larger cells. The large cells also express podoplanin but not CD163, CD21, CD35, and CXCL13. The smaller histiocytoid cells express CD163 but not the other markers.[9] The osteoclastlike cells express CD68. Translocations involving the short arm of chromosome 1 are often found (shared with the diffuse type) with fusions of CSF1 and COL6A3.[10]

Fig. 3. (*C*) Zone of plump larger cells in a tenosynovial giant cell tumor, localized type (H&E stain, original magnification ×20). (*D*) There is strong CD68 expression on the CD 68 stain (original magnification x10).

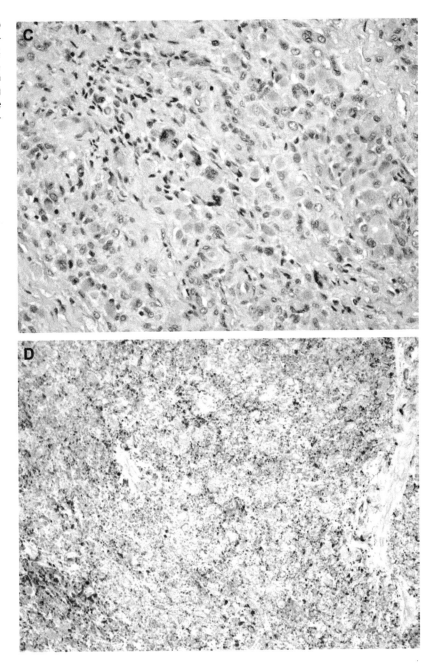

DIFFERENTIAL DIAGNOSIS

The differential diagnosis includes lesions of the distal extremities that can feature giant cells. The key malignant contenders are clear cell sarcoma (**Fig. 4**; see also "Clear Cell Tumors of Soft Tissue" by Auerbach and Cassarino elsewhere in this issue) and epithelioid sarcoma (see "Epithelioid Lesions" by Andrea T. Deyrup elsewhere in this issue). These can readily be separated from tenosynovial giant cell tumor with immunolabeling. Clear cell sarcoma consists of monotonous cells with prominent nucleoli and expresses S100 protein and melanoma markers, such as HMB45.

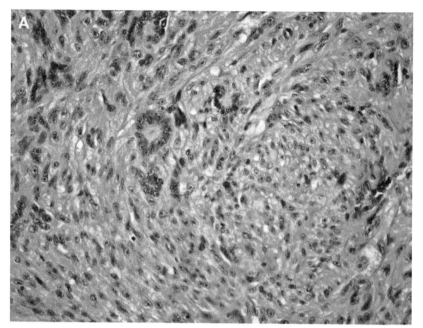

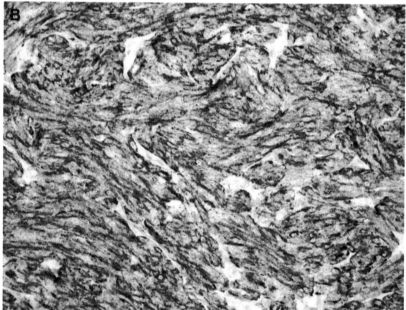

Fig. 4. (*A*) Clear cell sarcomas can contain prominent wreathlike giant cells with the same nuclear characteristics as the other lesional cells. Note that each nucleus contains a prominent nucleolus (H&E stain, original magnification ×20). (*B*) There is strong labeling with HMB45 in this clear cell sarcoma (immunohistochemical stain-HMB45, original magnification ×20).

△△ **Differential Diagnosis**
             LOCALIZED TYPE

- Clear cell sarcoma
- Epithelioid sarcoma
- Calcifying aponeurotic fibroma
- Fibrous histiocytoma
- Juvenile xanthogranuloma

The giant cells are tumor cells rather than osteoclastlike, such that the giant cells feature prominent nucleoli. Epithelioid sarcoma seldom has prominent giant cells but it classically arises in the distal upper extremity so when it does have giant cells, it can present a real pitfall. Epithelioid sarcomas typically express keratin and display loss of INI1. Calcifying aponeurotic fibromas (**Fig. 5**) also can contain giant cells but they are usually pediatric lesions rather than tumors of adult women, and their key features are calcification, chondroid change, and spindle cells.

Pitfall
LOCALIZED TYPE

! The most dangerous pitfall is with epithelioid sarcoma, a concern that is readily addressed with immunolabeling.

Osteoclastlike giant cells are not usually prominent in calcifying aponeurotic fibroma.

PROGNOSIS

Localized tenosynovial giant cell tumors are benign and only occasionally recur.

TENOSYNOVIAL GIANT CELL TUMOR, DIFFUSE TYPE (PIGMENTED VILLONODULAR TENOSYNOVITIS)

OVERVIEW

Pigmented villonodular tenosynovitis (PVNS) is the locally aggressive form of tenosynovial giant cell tumor. It is highly likely to recur and is difficult to completely resect without significant morbidity because it is highly infiltrative. It arises mostly in young adults with a female predominance. The lesions proliferate in intimate association with the synovium, producing papillary fronds. It can also

Key Features
DIFFUSE TYPE

- Arises in young adults, women > men
- Infiltrative, involves synovium, often of knee joint
- Infiltrative lesions composed of same components as the localized variant and have same immunolabeling pattern
- Locally aggressive with multiple recurrences, rare malignant behavior

be extra-articular.[11] Favored sites are the large joints, namely the knee, hip, and ankle.

GROSS FEATURES

These are large, shaggy tumors when they arise around the joint and infiltrative when not associated with a joint space. Occasionally they are associated with skin ulceration. The cut surface is rubbery with varying brown and yellow zones corresponding to fat and hemosiderin.

MICROSCOPIC FEATURES

The histologic features of PVNS overlap considerably with those of the localized type of tenosynovial giant cell tumor (Fig. 6). They consist of sheets of a mixed population of mononuclear cells

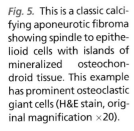

Fig. 5. This is a classic calcifying aponeurotic fibroma showing spindle to epithelioid cells with islands of mineralized osteochondroid tissue. This example has prominent osteoclastic giant cells (H&E stain, original magnification ×20).

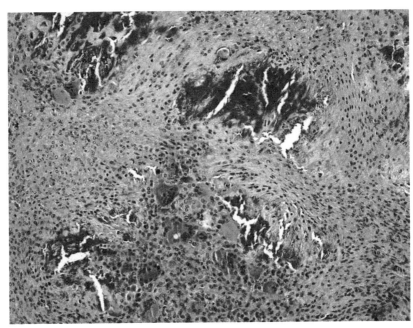

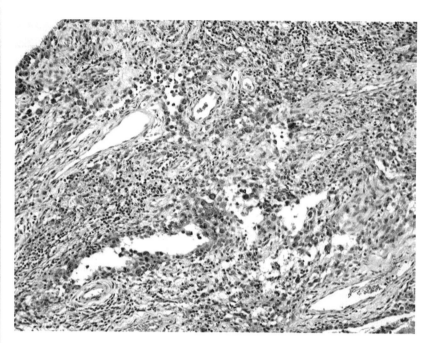

Fig. 6. Tenosynovial giant cell tumor, diffuse type (pigmented villonodular tenosynovitis/PVNS). This example undermines synovium and is rich in siderophages (H&E stain, original magnification ×20).

and osteoclastlike giant cells, siderophages, and other inflammatory cells, including eosinophils. There is variable stromal hyalinization and some cases have zones of necrosis. Mitotic activity is usually found. Rare examples are malignant, reported as either coexistence of classic lesion with malignant areas, occurrence of obvious sarcoma in an area of prior excision of PVNS, or malignant behavior in an otherwise unremarkable example of PVNS.[11–13] The lesion depicted in **Fig. 7** behaved in a malignant fashion and displayed more cytologic atypia than most examples of PVNS but arose in association with a classic example of PVNS.

ANCILLARY STUDIES

As for the localized type, in PVNS iron stains usually demonstrate iron even when it is inconspicuous on routine staining. Again, as per the localized type, clusterin staining is diffuse and strong in the large mononuclear cells and most

cases show focal desmin expression in the larger cells. The large cells also express podoplanin but not CD163, CD21, CD35, and CXCL13. The smaller histiocytoid cells express CD163 but not the other markers.[9] The osteoclastlike cells express CD68. Translocations involving the short arm of chromosome 1 are often found (shared with the diffuse type) with fusions of *CSF1* and *COL6A3*.[10]

DIFFERENTIAL DIAGNOSIS

As for the localized type, the differential diagnosis is with epithelioid sarcoma, and, in some cases, with lymphomas. Usually correlation with imaging findings is helpful, as most radiologists are adept at suggesting the diagnosis in the absence of biopsy information.

PROGNOSIS

PVNS is a destructive lesion prone to local recurrences. Rare examples, either with classic

Differential Diagnosis
DIFFUSE TYPE

- Epithelioid sarcoma
- Lymphoma

Pitfall
DIFFUSE TYPE

! The most dangerous pitfall is with epithelioid sarcoma, a concern that is readily addressed with immunolabeling.

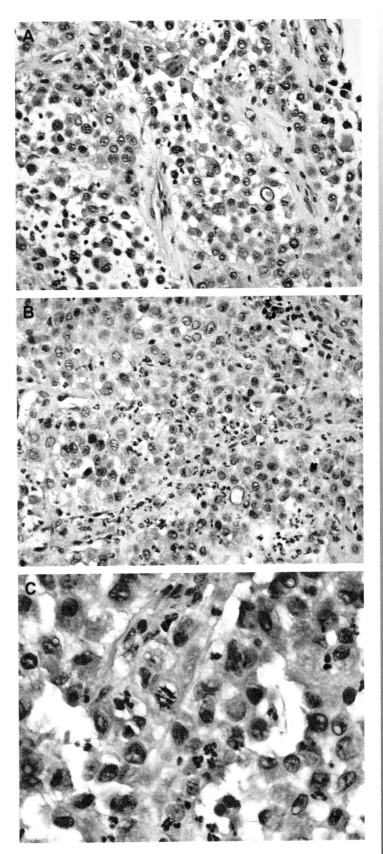

Fig. 7. Malignant PVNS. (*A*) This field shows larger nuclei than typically encountered (H&E stain, original magnification ×20). (*B*) Note the epithelioid appearance (H&E stain, original magnification ×20). (*C*) Malignant PVNS showing mitotic activity and hemosiderin deposition (H&E stain, original magnification ×40).

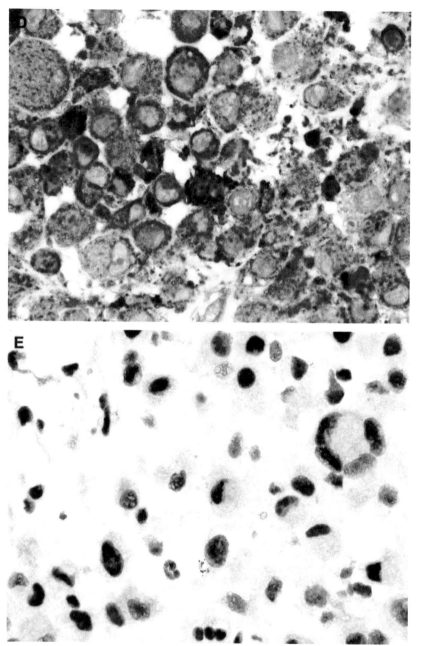

Fig. 7. (*D*) Prominent CD68 labeling in an example of malignant PVNS (immunohistochemical stain-CD68, original magnification ×40). (*E*) Intact INI1 nuclear expression argues against epithelioid sarcoma (immunohistochemical stain-INI1, original magnification ×40).

histology or with overtly sarcomatous changes, have metastasized and deaths are recorded.[11–13]

JUVENILE XANTHOGRANULOMA

OVERVIEW

Juvenile xanthogranuloma (JXG) is classically a lesion of infants, arising in the cutaneous tissue of the head and neck, trunk, and proximal limbs. This tumor belongs to the family of non-Langerhans cell histiocytoses (histiocytoses of mononuclear phagocytes other than Langerhans cells) and is distinct but related to other macrophage-related proliferations, such as Rosai-Dorfman disease. It results from proliferation of dendrocytes, usually dermal dendrocytes, and there is some ambiguity related to its pathogenesis (reactive vs neoplastic).[14] Lesions appear as brownish plaques or nodules and are usually solitary. JXG is a tumor of first 2 decades of life; 10% may be present at birth and only 10% occur in adults. It usually presents as a solitary cutaneous lesion of the head and neck region; this is usually referred to as superficial JXG. When it occurs as a subcutaneous or intramuscular lesion, it is called deep JXG. Systemic JXG refers to a rare disorder featuring multiple cutaneous, subcutaneous, and visceral lesions of JXG.[15] Association with juvenile myelomonocytic leukemia and increased incidence in neurofibromatosis type 1 is reported.[16] This tumor has been reported in virtually every organ of the body, but usually it presents as a superficial cutaneous nodule, or deeper subcutaneous lesion, in the eyes, viscera, and central nervous system. Deep lesions usually occur as solitary intramuscular lesions in infants and young children.

GROSS FEATURES

Skin lesions are well marginated with a yellow cut surface, whereas deep lesions are more poorly demarcated with a yellow to whitish surface.

MICROSCOPIC FEATURES

Skin lesions are covered by a thin layer of epidermis stretched over the lesion (**Fig. 8**). There is a dense infiltrate composed of polygonal to spindled cells with delicately vacuolated sparse cytoplasm. There are various numbers of eosinophils and lymphocytes. Toutonlike giant cells are characteristic but occasionally absent. The deep lesions have fewer giant cells and other inflammatory cells. The giant cells in JXG are usually located at the periphery of the lesion. Touton-type giant cells with wreathlike nuclei are characteristic of this lesion but are not always present in early lesions. Early lesions show only a monotonous infiltrate of macrophages with abundant eosinophilic cytoplasm, which accumulates lipid with time and becomes foamy, a change that is usually accompanied by lesional fibrosis. Such lesions in which the mononuclear cells are devoid of lipid are sometimes called nonlipidized JXG or the mitotic form of JXG, as mitoses are usually numerous in such cases.

ANCILLARY STUDIES

Both superficial and deep types express CD68, CD-163, HAM56, Factor-XIIIa, HHF35, CD4, LCA, and vimentin[17] but not S100 protein and CD1a.

DIFFERENTIAL DIAGNOSIS

The differential diagnosis is with other histiocytoses and with Rosai-Dorfman disease. The key histiocytosis to consider is Langerhans cell histiocytosis, which has overlapping morphology in that it expresses CD68 and has eosinophils but the histiocytes in Langerhans histiocytosis are more reniform and enlarged and feature

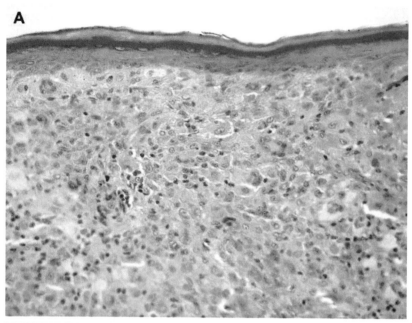

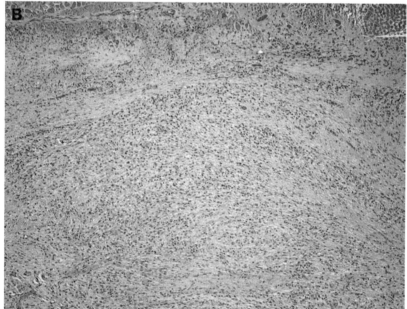

Fig. 8. Juvenile xanthogranuloma. (A) Note the thinned overlying epidermis and scattered giant cells (H&E stain, original magnification ×40). (B) In this deep example of JXG, skeletal muscle can be seen at the top of the field. The lesion consists of sheets of histiocytoid cells (H&E stain, original magnification ×10).

nuclear grooves. Further, they express CD1a and S100 protein, whereas the cells of JXG do not. Rosai-Dorfman disease is characterized by S100 protein reactive histiocytes that exhibit emperipolesis of lymphocytes and other cells (Fig. 9). The differential diagnosis of superficial JXG also includes multicentric reticulohistiocytosis, melanoma, and xanthomatized dermatofibroma.

Melanoma can be considered in some cases of JXG that have few foamy histiocytes and lack Touton giant cells, especially when presenting with epidermal ulceration. The clue to diagnosis is negativity for melanocytic markers (Melan-A, HMB45, and tyrosinase).

Dermatofibroma (DF) with a prominent xanthomatous component may be difficult to differentiate from superficial JXG, or when JXG is not lipidized. Both Touton giant cells and eosinophils may be found in dermatofibroma, which makes them unreliable in distinguishing these 2 lesions;

Fig. 8. (*C*) The lesional cells are round with frothy eosinophilic cytoplasm. There is an eosinophil in the center of the field (H&E stain, original magnification ×40). (*D*) Strong CD68 labeling in many cells in JXG (immunohistochemical stain-CD68, original magnification ×20).

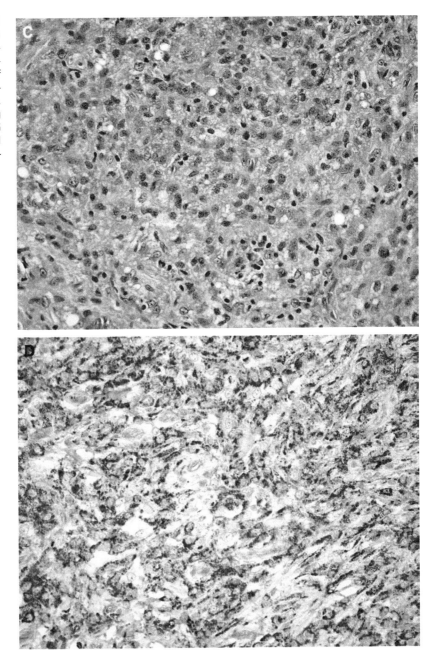

however, peripheral entrapments of keloidlike collagen in DF is a very useful feature in this situation. Immunohistochemical studies can be helpful, as CD4 positivity tilts the balance in favor of JXG.[18]

Deep JXGs needed to be differentiated mainly from deep malignant fibrous histiocytoma/undifferentiated pleomorphic sarcoma, and from diffuse-type tenosynovial giant cell tumor, as well as from epithelioid leiomyosarcoma with osteoclastlike giant cells.

Malignant fibrous histiocytoma can be differentiated from JXG by the presence of frank cytologic atypia, areas of necrosis, and lack of Touton giant cells.

Atypical diffuse tenosynovial giant cell tumor contains mononucleated and multinucleated cells with a histiocytic appearance and numerous mitoses that are similar to those of JXG; however, atypical diffuse tenosynovial giant cell tumor is usually located closely to large joints, and it shows

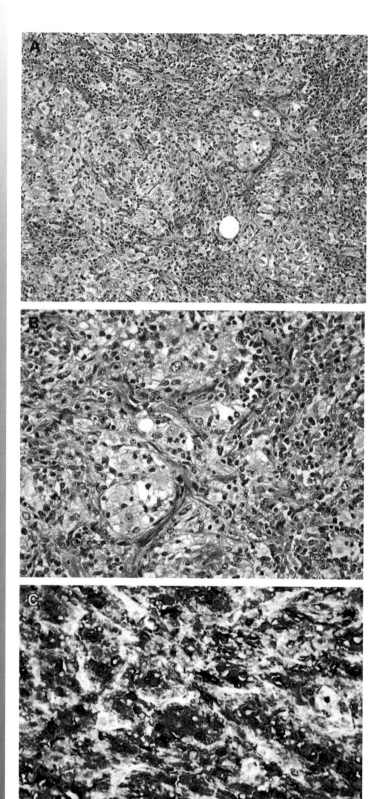

Fig. 9. Rosai-Dorfman disease. (*A*) Large histiocytes are the eye-catching feature in this area (H&E stain, original magnification ×20). (*B*) The cells have engulfed lymphocytes and eosinophils that remain intact in their cytoplasm (emperipolesis) (H&E stain, original magnification ×40). (*C*) On S100 protein labeling, the histiocytes of Rosai-Dorfman disease show both nuclear and cytoplasmic expression, whereas the emperipolesed cells are negative (immunohistochemical stain-S-100, original magnification ×40).

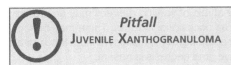

an infiltrative growth pattern. Additionally, the lack of the typical larger dendritic cells in tenosynovial giant cell tumor is a very helpful feature. These cells show broad eosinophilic cytoplasm, large vesicular nuclei, and occasional intranuclear pseudoinclusions. JXG also differs from giant cell tumor of soft tissue (GCTST) by displaying Touton-type giant cell morphology (the giant cells in GCTST are predominantly of osteoclast-type) and by the absence of hemosiderin, which can be confirmed by negativity of stain for iron.

Leiomyosarcoma with osteoclastlike giant cells differs from deep JXG by the presence of, at least focally, a distinctive fascicular growth pattern of spindle-shaped cells with eosinophilic cytoplasm and with typical cigar-shaped nuclei. Nuclear atypia is usually more striking and some mitotic figures can by atypical.

PROGNOSIS

Pediatric lesions tend to regress, whereas adult lesions, although less common, do not.

Large lesions can produce morbidity, owing to the size and location, but these are predominantly benign tumors. Infants with large retroperitoneal masses or liver, bone marrow, or central nervous system involvement usually survive with chemotherapy treatment. Death despite chemotherapy has been reported in rare cases of multisystem JXG.[19]

RETICULOHISTIOCYTOMA

OVERVIEW

Reticulohistiocytoma is classified as one of the diseases belonging to class II of histiocytic proliferations (non-Langerhans histiocytosis, non-X-histiocytosis) in the World Health Organization classification of histiocytic disorders, and can be solitary or multicentric (reticulohistiocytosis).

Solitary reticulohistiocytoma (also known as isolated reticulohistiocytoma, reticulohistiocytoma cutis, solitary epithelioid reticulohistiocytoma, or

giant cell reticulohistiocytosis) occurs in adults, with men affected more than women, usually arising in skin of the head or hands. Multiple lesions can occur in absence of systemic disease in about 20% of patients.[20]

The typical lesion forms a red or yellow papule unassociated with systemic manifestations. These tumors are benign and resolve spontaneously, and hence are believed to be an immune-related tumefaction rather than a neoplastic proliferation.

Multicentric reticulohistiocytosis (also previously called lipoid dermo-arthritis) is a systemic disease with a spectrum of symptoms, including symmetric erosive seronegative arthritis, hyperlipidemia, fever, and weight loss. The disease is typically found in middle-aged white women, and sometimes it is associated with autoimmune diseases, such as vasculitis (polyarteritis nodosa) or connective tissue diseases (rheumatoid arthritis, systemic lupus erythematosus, and others). It is also reported as a paraneoplastic disorder in about 15% to 28% of patients.[21]

GROSS FEATURES

Solitary reticulohistiocytoma (SRE) is usually a superficial, circumscribed, mildly elevated, solitary lesion of skin (mostly of the head) with a yellow-tan color cut surface located in the dermis with an average diameter of 5 mm, and more than one lesion can be seen in a subset of patients in absence of systemic disease.

Multicentric reticulohistiocytoma (MRE) is characterized by multiple lesions with a similar gross morphology in skin and mucous membranes and sometimes in synovium.

MICROSCOPIC FEATURES

Reticulohistioctyomas are dermal nodules and consist of sheets of mononuclear and frequent multinucleated histiocytes (Fig. 10).

All lesions show a mixture of mononuclear and multinucleated histiocytes, fibroblasts, xanthoma cells, and inflammatory cells.[22]

The histiocytes are plump with abundant granular eosinophilic cytoplasm (hence the designation "epithelioid"), darker in the center and lighter staining at the periphery of the cells, reminiscent of oncocytic cells of the thyroid. The granules are PAS positive and diastase resistant. Multinucleate cells are frequent. These are often several times larger than the mononuclear histiocytes and have cytoplasm with a ground glass appearance, with a random arrangement of nuclei. The giant cells in the multicentric variant tend to be smaller with fewer nuclei than those in solitary reticulohistiocytoma.

Key Features
RETICULOHISTIOCYTOMA

- Non-Langerhans histiocytosis, non-X-histiocytosis, usually seen in adults.

- Solitary and multicentric variants.

- Solitary reticulohistioctyoma is seen as red or yellow cutaneous papules.

- Multicentric reticulohistiocytoma is a systemic disease associated with systemic seronegative arthritis, hyperlipidemia, weight loss, and fever.

- May be seen with autoimmune diseases or malignancy as a paraneoplastic syndrome.

- Small lesion (5 mm) present as dermal nodules with a yellow-tan color. Lesions of multicentric type are similar and also involve mucous membranes and synovium.

- In both solitary and multicentric reticulohistiocytoma there is a mixture of mononuclear and multinucleated histiocytes, fibroblasts, xanthoma cells, and inflammatory cells. The mononuclear cells have abundant eosinophilic cytoplasm with a ground glass cytoplasm.

- Express histiocytic immunohistochemical markers (CD68, HAM56, and lysozyme) but are negative for MAC387 and CD13. Other markers include CD-163 and microphthalmia-associated transcription factor.

Nuclear atypia of varying degrees may be present, as well as occasional mitoses. There may be focal nuclear spindling of the histiocytes, but this is rarely extensive, and necrosis is absent.

Typical lesions in early stages contain mixed inflammatory cell infiltrate with lymphocytes, plasma cells, eosinophils, mast cells, histiocytes, and neutrophils, whereas later lesions show larger numbers of giant cells and fewer lymphocytes. Older lesions tend to have fewer inflammatory components and giant cells and more stromal fibrosis.[23]

ANCILLARY STUDIES

The immunohistochemical profile of SRE and MRE is consistent with their histiocytic nature, thus both mononuclear and multinucleate forms are positive for CD68, HAM56, and lysozyme but are negative for MAC387 and CD13.[22] The plump epithelioid cells express CD163 and in some cases there is focal nuclear immunoreactivity for microphthalmia-associated transcription factor. Desmin, smooth muscle actin (SMA), S100 protein, and CD34 are negative.[24]

DIFFERENTIAL DIAGNOSIS

Reticulohistiocytoma should be differentiated from juvenile xanthogranuloma, granulomatous conditions (like lepromatous leprosy and acute cutaneous leishmaniasis), skin lesions of Rosai-Dorfman

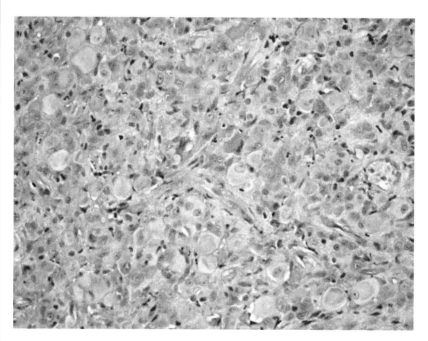

Fig. 10. Reticulohistiocytoma. The cells are epithelioid (H&E stain, original magnification ×40).

disease, Spitz nevus, melanoma, epithelioid sarcoma, malignant fibrous histiocytoma, and histiocytic sarcoma.

JXG is distinguished from reticulohistiocytoma by the presence of Touton giant cells, which are usually at the periphery of the lesion. The giant cell component in juvenile xanthogranuloma is not a prominent feature. Additionally, it is likely to be a pediatric lesion, whereas reticulohistiocytomas are lesions of adults.

Differentiating reticulohistiocytoma from lepromatous leprosy is through demonstration of acid-fast bacilli. In acute cutaneous leishmaniasis, the histiocytes contain round to oval Leishman-Donovan bodies, which can be demonstrated by Giemsa and Wright stains.

Skin lesions of Rosai-Dorfman disease feature a dense dermal histiocytic infiltrate; however, there are multiple lymphoid aggregates with germinal centers at the periphery of the nodular histiocytic aggregates and numerous blood vessels surrounded by plasma cells. Engulfment of lymphocytes, plasma cells, and neutrophils without destroying them (emperipolesis) by the histiocytes is a characteristic feature. Dilated lymphatic with intraluminal histiocytes are sometimes seen in the centers of the nodules.

Melanomas are usually composed of large pleomorphic cells with large nuclei and prominent nucleoli, with expression of S-100 protein and pan-melanocytic markers. The same set of markers can be used for differentiating Spitz nevus from reticulohistiocytoma.

Malignant fibrous histiocytoma/high-grade pleomorphic undifferentiated sarcoma is usually more deeply seated than reticulohistiocytoma,

and the cytologic features are frankly malignant with high mitotic rate and frequent abnormal mitotic figures. Areas of necrosis and hemorrhage are common.

The same can be said of epithelioid sarcoma and histiocytic sarcoma, which display a frankly malignant cytologic profile, quite unlike the benign cytologic features of cells in solitary and multicentric reticulohistiocytoma.

The multisystemic presentation of MRE sometimes results in a clinical misdiagnosis as rheumatoid arthritis, which usually fails to respond to standard treatments. Some cases of MRE may be associated with connective tissue diseases, autoimmune diseases, and malignancy, thus its recognition may alert the pathologist to the possibility of the associated diseases.

PROGNOSIS

Solitary reticulohistiocytoma has an excellent prognosis and is treated by simple surgical excision.

The outlook for patients with MRE is less satisfactory. Treatment consists of corticosteroid therapy or chemotherapy with methotrexate, which may lead to complete remission or stabilization of the disease.[24]

GIANT CELL FIBROBLASTOMA

OVERVIEW

Giant cell fibroblastoma can be regarded as the childhood variant of dermatofibrosarcoma protuberans (DFSP). It mostly arises in the first decade of life but adult examples are known. It generally presents as a slow-growing, painless subcutaneous mass.[25] Like DFSP, it arises in the truck/shoulder girdle area and proximal lower limb.

GROSS FEATURES

The tumors are irregularly shaped with ill-defined, infiltrative borders. They display a firm to somewhat

Key Features
GIANT CELL FIBROBLASTOMA

- Children in first decade

- Dermis and subcutis

- Loose fascicles of spindle cells in collagenous to myxoid stroma with variable numbers of giant cells often surrounding pseudovascular cystic spaces

- CD34+

rubbery consistency with a gray-white to tan-yellow cut surface.

MICROSCOPIC FEATURES

Giant cell fibroblastoma is poorly marginated and infiltrates the skin and subcutis (**Fig. 11**). It infiltrates directly under the squamous epithelium often without a Grenz zone. It has a broad spectrum of histologic patterns, including cellular foci, more densely collagenized paucicellular areas, and sinusoidlike spaces. The neoplasm involves both the mid and lower dermis, encircling but not obliterating cutaneous adnexal structures. The overlying skin shows slight hyperkeratosis, acanthosis, and papillomatosis. Some tumors show extensions into subjacent skeletal muscle. The cellular areas contain parallel, slender to plump, elongated, sometimes wavy spindle cells closely associated with wiry collagen fibers. The spindle cells have a bland uniform appearance with rare normal mitotic figures. Tumors show irregular sinusoidlike spaces rimmed by either a continuous or discontinuous layer of pleomorphic or giant cells. Occasionally, these cells aggregate along the perimeter of the sinusoidal spaces. Exfoliated multinucleated cells, clumped erythrocytes, and, less commonly, lymphocytes can be found in the spaces. Giant cell fibroblastoma occasionally has displayed a focal storiform pattern. The borders of the lesion infiltrate as tentaclelike cellular projections into the adjacent adipose tissue.

ANCILLARY STUDIES

On immunolabeling, like DFSP, giant cell fibroblastoma classically expresses CD34 and can also express CD99, but not SMA, desmin, epithelial membrane antigen, and cytokeratins.[26–28] It is

genetically identical to DFSP and transition of giant cell fibroblastoma to DFSP is known. Like DFSP, it has a characteristic translocation (t[17;22]) that results in a fusion of COL1A to PDGFB1.[29–31]

DIFFERENTIAL DIAGNOSIS

Surprisingly, the differential diagnosis of giant cell fibroblastoma revolves around lesions other than DFSP. DFSP is cellular with a tight storiform pattern, whereas giant cell fibroblastoma has a loose myxoid pattern that might be confused with cutaneous myxoma/angiomyxoma or neurofibroma. These tumors lack all giant cells and neurofibromas express S100 protein; however, in cases with transition to DFSP, other cellular lesions would be considered, including juvenile xanthogranuloma, Rosai-Dorfman disease, and Langerhans cell histiocytosis. These lesions all lack CD34 expression.

Fibromatosis is a consideration, although it is usually a deep lesion that when superficial does not encircle skin appendages but rather replaces them. It lacks giant cells (other than where they are formed by damaged entrapped skeletal muscle) and lacks cystic spaces. Is seldom expresses CD34.

Fibrous hamartoma of infancy, like giant cell fibroblastoma, is a pediatric lesion. It consists of fat, spindle cells, and small round cells in various mixtures but it lacks cystic spaces and giant cells.

Lymphangioma is also frequently a pediatric lesion but, in lymphangiomas, the cystic spaces are lined by endothelial cells.

Differential Diagnosis
GIANT CELL FIBROBLASTOMA

- Cutaneous myxoma/angiomyxoma

- Neurofibroma

- Juvenile xanthogranuloma

- Rosai-Dorfman disease

- Langerhans cell histiocytosis

- Fibrous histiocytoma

- Fibromatosis

- Fibrous hamartoma of infancy

- Lymphangioma

Fig. 11. Giant cell fibroblastoma. (*A*) The lesion proliferates directly under the epidermis and is moderately cellular. Note the cystic space in the lower part of the field (H&E stain, original magnification ×10). (*B*) Giant cells in giant cell fibroblastoma (H&E stain, original magnification ×40).

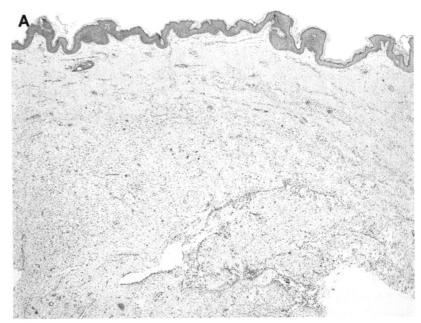

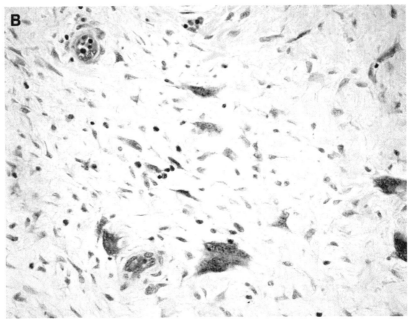

PROGNOSIS

Giant cell fibroblastoma is prone to local recurrences (up to 50%) but metastases have not been reported. Because it may evolve to DFSP, complete excision is suggested.

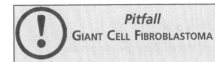

Pitfall
GIANT CELL FIBROBLASTOMA

! The pseudovascular spaces are presumably a degenerative feature and these are not vascular lesions.

GIANT CELL ANGIOFIBROMA (GIANT CELL–RICH SOLITARY FIBROUS TUMOR)

OVERVIEW

Solitary fibrous tumors are tumors of adults that have been reported all over the body. Those that are giant cell rich form a subset that seems to arise in the upper half of the body, most typically the orbit, where they were first reported as "giant cell angiofibroma."[32] Most lesions diagnosed as hemangiopericytoma in the past would be subsumed under solitary fibrous tumor by current criteria,[33] including orbital lesions.[34] In contrast, we know now that the rare true hemangiopericytomas are in the family of myopericytoma (discussed in "Myofibroma, Myopericytoma, Myoepithelioma, and Myofibroblastoma of Skin and Soft Tissue" by LeBlanc and Taube elsewhere in this issue).[33]

GROSS FEATURES

Solitary fibrous tumors with or without giant cells are typically well-marginated tumors up to 10 cm. They have a firm, white cut surface.

MICROSCOPIC FEATURES

Solitary fibrous tumors (with and without giant cells) have variable cellularity, focal myxoid change, wiry collagen, and angulated cells. Some zones are densely sclerotic. They have a characteristic vascular pattern consisting of staghorn-shaped vessels (hemangiopericytomatous vessels). Most cases have few mitoses but criteria for malignancy that have been offered include greater than 4 mitoses per high-power field (HPF), nuclear crowding and pleomorphism, and necrosis. Examples with prominent giant cells have the same background features as other examples (Fig. 12).

Key Features
Giant Cell–Rich Solitary Fibrous Tumor/Giant Cell Angiofibroma
• Adults
• Classic site is orbit
• Well-marginated slow-growing mass
• Staghorn vessels, wiry collagen, "patternless pattern," giant cells
• CD34+

⚠⚠ *Differential Diagnosis*
Giant Cell–Rich Solitary Fibrous Tumor/Giant Cell Angiofibroma
• Synovial sarcoma
• Nerve sheath tumors
• Adult type fibrosarcoma
• Giant cell fibroblastoma

ANCILLARY STUDIES

These lesions express CD34, CD99, and BCL2, but not S100 protein.

DIFFERENTIAL DIAGNOSIS

The differential diagnosis is the differential diagnosis of solitary fibrous tumor, which is principally with synovial sarcoma (covered in detail in "Spindle Cell Sarcomas" by Cyril Fisher, elsewhere in this issue), nerve sheath tumors, adult type fibrosarcoma, and giant cell fibroblastoma. Giant cell fibroblastoma is likely to arise in children in a superficial location. Synovial sarcoma shares a vascular pattern consisting of vessels with a staghorn configuration but is always CD34 negative. Adult type fibrosarcomas (which often arise in association with DFSP) can be CD34 reactive but are more cellular and lack the typical staghorn vascular pattern. Benign nerve sheath tumors express S100 protein, and malignant peripheral nerve sheath tumors usually appear more overtly sarcomatous than solitary fibrous tumor.

PROGNOSIS

These tumors are generally benign. It is not clear from the literature whether malignant behavior has been reported specifically in giant cell–rich lesions.

Pitfall
Giant Cell–Rich Solitary Fibrous Tumor/Giant Cell Angiofibroma
! Easily mistaken for nerve sheath tumors

PHOSPHATURIC MESENCHYMAL TUMOR

OVERVIEW

Phosphaturic mesenchymal tumor (PMT; mixed connective tissue variant [PMTMCT]) is a rare but unique distinct lesion that is classically associated with oncogenic osteomalacia (OO), a syndrome that results from phosphate wasting.[35] The renal phosphate wasting is mediated by metabolic substances released by the neoplasm, and may be curable by removal of the tumor; however, PMTs without OO have been reported.[35]

This tumor may arise in soft tissue (about 50% of reported cases) or bone. The most likely sites are extremities; a minority of cases arise in the sinonasal region and only rarely in the axial skeleton. No particular association with age or sex has been noted.[36]

Occasionally, other types of tumors are associated with oncogenic osteomalacia but most examples of oncogenic osteomalacia are associated with tumors of the type noted here.

GROSS FEATURES

Most PMTs range in size from 2 to 10 cm; however, some can be extremely small and difficult to localize, necessitating a thorough clinical and radiological evaluation for their detection.[36] Because these lesions are partly calcified in many cases, they may display a gritty cut surface.

MICROSCOPIC FEATURES

PMT has a range of appearances (**Fig. 13**). Overall, lesions are composed of spindle to stellate cells with moderate amounts of cytoplasm in a matrix that is focally calcified, irregular, stippled and amorphous, or myxochondroid. The appearance has been called "grungy" by Folpe and colleagues.[36] The prototypical PMTMCT is characterized by a low to moderately cellular proliferation with low mitotic activity (<1/10 HPF) featuring ill-defined sheets of bland-appearing spindle cells with round normochromatic nuclei and indistinct nucleoli, within a myxochondroid and osteoidlike "smudgy" matrix containing foci of flocculent dystrophic calcification. The cells may be rounded rather than spindle shaped, and thus reminiscent of glomus cells. Scattered clusters of osteoclastlike giant cells are frequently noted, often associated with hemorrhage. Other complementary features include microcystic change imparting a sievelike appearance to the stroma, prominent vasculature

with a hemangiopericytomalike pattern, blood-filled lakes, foci of mature adipose tissue, and formation of a partial shell of metaplastic bone.[35]

The extremely rare malignant PMT is reminiscent of an undifferentiated spindle cell sarcoma, featuring areas of high cellularity, high nuclear grade (markedly enlarged nuclei with irregular coarse chromatin and bizarre nuclear morphology), and a mitotic index greater than 5/10 HPF.

ANCILLARY STUDIES

These tumors have variable expression of smooth muscle–specific actin and do not express CD34, S-100 protein, desmin, or cytokeratin.[36] Immunolabeling against fibroblast growth factor 23 (FGF23) yields a granular cytoplasmic reaction in most cases.[36] This is the protein that is produced by the tumor and interferes with transepithelial transport of phosphate in renal tubules leading to phosphaturia. Alterations in the *FGF23* gene can also be detected by reverse transcriptase polymerase chain reaction in these lesions.[37]

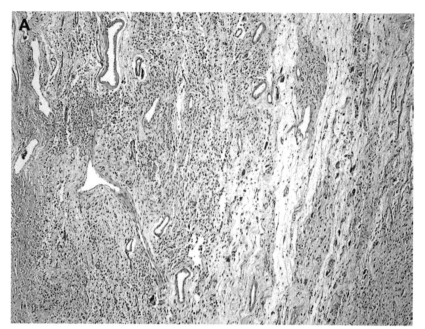

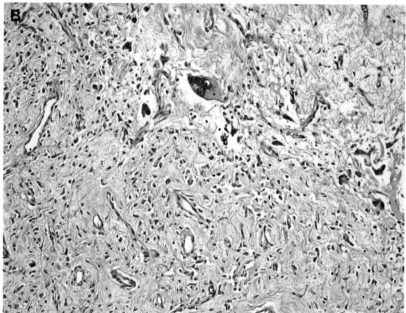

Fig. 12. Giant cell–rich solitary fibrous tumor/giant cell angiofibroma. (A) This lesion shows spindle cells and large ectatic vessels. Most examples have been reported in the orbit, but this tumor arose in the wall of the esophagus (H&E stain, original magnification ×10). (B) Higher magnification showing giant cells (H&E stain, original magnification ×20).

DIFFERENTIAL DIAGNOSIS

The differential diagnosis of PMT is essentially with lesions displaying a hemangiopericytomatous-type vascular pattern and with tumoral calcinosis (Fig. 14). In contrast to most of the tumors with a hemangiopericytoma vascular pattern, however, PMT has zones with other features rather than the relatively monotonous appearance of solitary fibrous tumor or synovial sarcoma. Tumoral

△△ Differential Diagnosis
PHOSPHATURIC MESENCHYMAL TUMOR

1. Diffuse-type tenosynovial giant cell tumor
2. Giant cell tumor of soft tissue
3. Hemangiopericytoma
4. Malignant fibrous histiocytoma
5. Sclerosing hemangioma

Fig. 13. Phosphaturic mesenchymal tumor. (*A*) Low
magnification shows a mineralized tumor with zones
of amorphous debris (H&E
stain, original magnification ×10). (*B*) Higher magnification of the image
shown in *A* (H&E stain,
original magnification ×20).

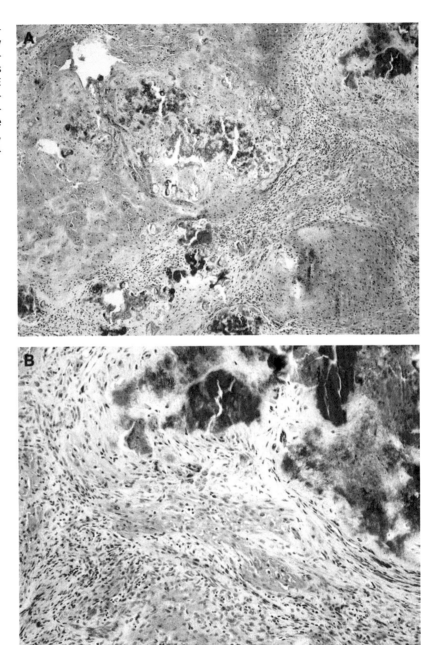

which patients manifest extraskeletal deposits of
hydroxyapatite crystals that invoke a granulomatous response and ossification—the tumors
behave in a benign fashion. These tumors appear
similar to the "grungy" component of PMT but
lack the spindle cells and vascular pattern.
Patients with syndromic lesions have mutations

of *GALNT3*, *FGF23*, and *KL* genes but not
osteomalacia.

In the years preceding the standardized recognition of this tumor, various types of tumors have been
mistaken for PMTMCT. For soft tissue tumors,
these include tenosynovial giant cell tumor—diffuse
type, GCTST, hemangiopericytoma, malignant

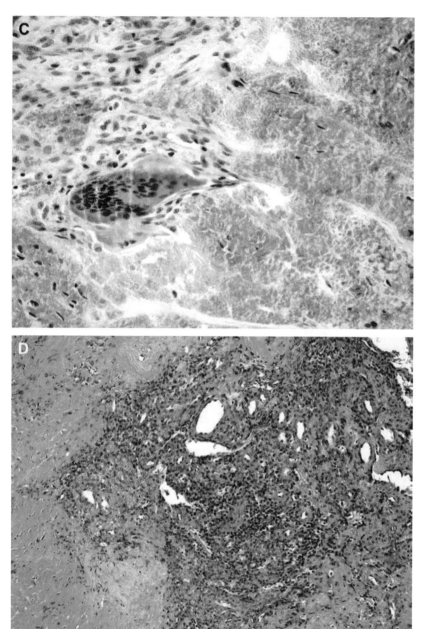

Fig. 13. (*C*) An osteoclastic-type giant cell adjacent to "grungy" material (H&E stain, original magnification ×100). (*D*) This area shows a hemangiopericytomalike vascular pattern (H&E stain, original magnification ×20).

fibrous histiocytoma, and sclerosing hemangioma (a variant of dermatofibroma).

Tenosynovial giant cell tumor—diffuse type lacks the typical matrix of PMT and the distinctive highly vascular bland spindle-cell proliferation; the polymorphous cellular composition of siderophages, foam cells, and inflammatory cells of GCTST is not seen in PMT and the tumor is FGF23 negative.

GCTST (of low malignant potential) has some features that overlap with those of PMTMCT,

such as osteoclastlike giant cells, partial fibrohistiocytic differentiation, and an occasional shell of woven bone; but it lacks the typical myxochondroid matrix of PMTMCT and highly vascular spindle-cell morphology.

GCTST is a rare soft tissue tumor with features similar to giant cell tumor of bone, hence it is sometimes known as osteoclastoma of soft tissue. It is most frequent in middle-aged adults, although there is a wide age distribution, including pediatric

Fig. 14. Tumoral calcinosis. (*A*) Amorphous material with a giant cell reaction (H&E stain, original magnification ×20). (*B*) Higher magnification of the same tumor (H&E stain, original magnification ×40).

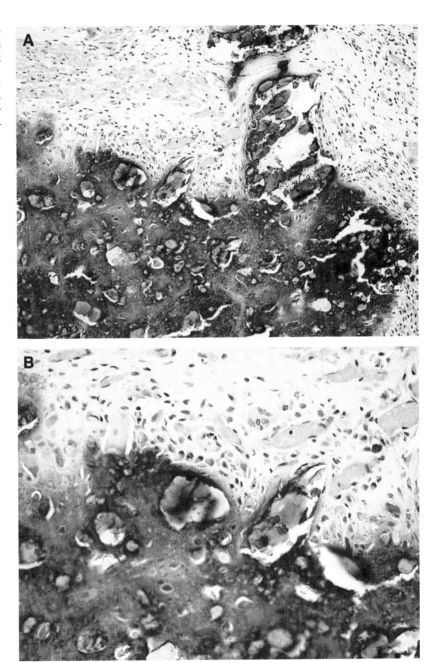

examples. There is no particular gender or racial predilection. The tumor is typically a solid, well-defined nodular lesion, usually arising from subcutaneous and dermal connective tissue in two-thirds of cases, and the other third arises from tissues below the plane of superficial fascia. The most common sites are the extremities, followed by trunk, abdomen and pelvis, and head and neck.[38,39] The size ranges from 0.5 to 10.0 cm, and tumors display a fleshy brown to gray cut surface with hemorrhage and cystic change, and an occasional focal gritty texture, as some of the tumors may develop a shell of reactive bone in their periphery.

GCTST is generally considered the microscopic counterpart of giant cell tumor of bone. At low-power magnification, a lobulated or multinodular architecture is noted, with cellular nodules separated by septa of fibrous connective tissue. These septa contain a variable number of hemosiderin-laden macrophages, whereas the nodules are composed of numerous multinucleated osteoclastlike giant cells distributed uniformly among round to spindle-shaped mononuclear cells. About a third of tumors contain foci of vascular invasion, which may lead to misdiagnosis of malignancy, but this is a feature seen in otherwise benign tumors and does not indicate malignancy. The stroma is often vascular and there may be stromal hemorrhage, hemosiderin deposition, blood-filled cysts, or aneurysmal bone cystlike areas. The stroma can also show variable fibrosis and collections of foamy macrophages, but necrosis is rare. Metaplastic bone of lamellar or woven type may be seen at the margin of the tumor. SMA can be demonstrated in the mononuclear cells, and occasional tumors may show focal cytokeratin or S100 protein expression. CD68 expression is characteristically diffuse and strong in the osteoclastlike giant cells, but only focal in the mononuclear cells.

PMT differs from hemangiopericytoma by displaying its typical matrix and lacking walled hyalinized "staghorn" vascular channels, as well as by positivity for FGF23 and negativity for CD34.

PROGNOSIS

The vast majority of PMTMCTs are benign and curable by local surgical resection, which leads to dramatic reversal of the biochemical abnormalities related to phosphate, remineralization of bone, and disappearance of symptoms.

Records of very few malignant cases of PMTMCT show metastatic spread to skeleton and lungs; however, the tumors are generally amenable to control via use of chemotherapy.[36]

Pitfall
PHOSPHATURIC MESENCHYMAL TUMOR

! Misdiagnosis of PMT should be avoided through recognition of the typical grungy matrix and clinical association with osteomalacia.

REFERENCES

1. Coindre JM, Hostein I, Maire G, et al. Inflammatory malignant fibrous histiocytomas and dedifferentiated liposarcomas: histological review, genomic profile, and MDM2 and CDK4 status favour a single entity. J Pathol 2004;203(3):822–30.
2. Coindre JM, Mariani O, Chibon F, et al. Most malignant fibrous histiocytomas developed in the retroperitoneum are dedifferentiated liposarcomas: a review of 25 cases initially diagnosed as malignant fibrous histiocytoma. Mod Pathol 2003;16(3):256–62.
3. Remstein ED, Kurtin PJ, Nascimento AG. Sclerosing extramedullary hematopoietic tumor in chronic myeloproliferative disorders. Am J Surg Pathol 2000;24(1):51–5.
4. Guillou L, Coquet M, Chaubert P, et al. Skeletal muscle regeneration mimicking rhabdomyosarcoma: a potential diagnostic pitfall. Histopathology 1998;33(2):136–44.
5. Fletcher CD. Leiomyosarcoma with osteoclast-like giant cells. Histopathology 1993;22(1):94–5.
6. Mentzel T, Calonje E, Fletcher CD. Leiomyosarcoma with prominent osteoclast-like giant cells. Analysis of eight cases closely mimicking the so-called giant cell variant of malignant fibrous histiocytoma. Am J Surg Pathol 1994;18(3):258–65.
7. Ushijima M, Hashimoto H, Tsuneyoshi M, et al. Giant cell tumor of the tendon sheath (nodular tenosynovitis). A study of 207 cases to compare the large joint group with the common digit group. Cancer 1986;57(4):875–84.
8. Uriburu IJ, Levy VD. Intraosseous growth of giant cell tumors of the tendon sheath (localized nodular tenosynovitis) of the digits: report of 15 cases. J Hand Surg Am 1998;23(4):732–6.
9. Boland JM, Folpe AL, Hornick JL, et al. Clusterin is expressed in normal synoviocytes and in tenosynovial giant cell tumors of localized and diffuse types: diagnostic and histogenetic implications. Am J Surg Pathol 2009;33(8):1225–9.
10. Moller E, Mandahl N, Mertens F, et al. Molecular identification of COL6A3-CSF1 fusion transcripts in tenosynovial giant cell tumors. Genes Chromosomes Cancer 2008;47(1):21–5.
11. Somerhausen NS, Fletcher CD. Diffuse-type giant cell tumor: clinicopathologic and immunohistochemical analysis of 50 cases with extraarticular disease. Am J Surg Pathol 2000;24(4):479–92.
12. Bertoni F, Unni KK, Beabout JW, et al. Malignant giant cell tumor of the tendon sheaths and joints (malignant pigmented villonodular synovitis). Am J Surg Pathol 1997;21(2):153–63.
13. Li CF, Wang JW, Tzeng CC, et al. Clinicopathologic, immunohistochemical, and biogenetic analyses of

benign versus malignant diffuse-type tenosynovial giant cell tumors. Mod Pathol 2007;20:18a.

14. Hernandez-Martin A, Baselga E, Drolet BA, et al. Juvenile xanthogranuloma. J Am Acad Dermatol 1997;36(3 Pt 1):355–67 [quiz: 368–9].

15. Dehner LP. Juvenile xanthogranulomas in the first two decades of life: a clinicopathologic study of 174 cases with cutaneous and extracutaneous manifestations. Am J Surg Pathol 2003;27(5): 579–93.

16. Zvulunov A, Barak Y, Metzker A. Juvenile xanthogranuloma, neurofibromatosis, and juvenile chronic myelogenous leukemia. World statistical analysis. Arch Dermatol 1995;131(8):904–8.

17. Zelger B, Cerio R, Orchard G, et al. Juvenile and adult xanthogranuloma. A histological and immunohistochemical comparison. Am J Surg Pathol 1994; 18(2):126–35.

18. Nascimento AG. A clinicopathologic and immunohistochemical comparative study of cutaneous and intramuscular forms of juvenile xanthogranuloma. Am J Surg Pathol 1997;21(6):645–52.

19. Sonoda T, Hashimoto H, Enjoji M. Juvenile xanthogranuloma. Clinicopathologic analysis and immunohistochemical study of 57 patients. Cancer 1985; 56(9):2280–6.

20. Purvis WE 3rd, Helwig EB. Reticulohistiocytic granuloma (reticulohistiocytoma) of the skin. Am J Clin Pathol 1954;24(9):1005–15.

21. Campbell DA, Edwards NL. Multicentric reticulohistiocytosis: systemic macrophage disorder. Baillieres Clin Rheumatol 1991;5(2):301–19.

22. Zelger B, Cerio R, Soyer HP, et al. Reticulohistiocytoma and multicentric reticulohistiocytosis. Histopathologic and immunophenotypic distinct entities. Am J Dermatopathol 1994;16(6):577–84.

23. Tajirian AL, Malik MK, Robinson-Bostom L, et al. Multicentric reticulohistiocytosis. Clin Dermatol 2006; 24(6):486–92.

24. Miettinen M, Fetsch JF. Reticulohistiocytoma (solitary epithelioid histiocytoma): a clinicopathologic and immunohistochemical study of 44 cases. Am J Surg Pathol 2006;30(4):521–8.

25. Shmookler BM, Enzinger FM, Weiss SW. Giant cell fibroblastoma. A juvenile form of dermatofibrosarcoma protuberans. Cancer 1989;64(10):2154–61.

26. Diwan AH, Skelton HG 3rd, Horenstein MG, et al. Dermatofibrosarcoma protuberans and giant cell fibroblastoma exhibit CD99 positivity. J Cutan Pathol 2008;35(7):647–50.

27. Terrier-Lacombe MJ, Guillou L, Maire G, et al. Dermatofibrosarcoma protuberans, giant cell fibroblastoma, and hybrid lesions in children: clinicopathologic comparative analysis of 28 cases with molecular data—a study from the French Federation of Cancer Centers Sarcoma Group. Am J Surg Pathol 2003; 27(1):27–39.

28. Dal Cin P, Sciot R, de Wever I, et al. Cytogenetic and immunohistochemical evidence that giant cell fibroblastoma is related to dermatofibrosarcoma protuberans. Genes Chromosomes Cancer 1996;15(1):73–5.

29. Macarenco RS, Zamolyi R, Franco MF, et al. Genomic gains of COL1A1-PDFGB occur in the histologic evolution of giant cell fibroblastoma into dermatofibrosarcoma protuberans. Genes Chromosomes Cancer 2008;47(3):260–5.

30. Kashima A, Yamashita A, Moriguchi S, et al. Detection of COL1A1-PDGFB fusion transcripts and platelet-derived growth factor alpha and beta receptors in giant cell fibroblastoma of the postsacrococcygeal region. Br J Dermatol 2006;154(5):983–7.

31. Maire G, Martin L, Michalak-Provost S, et al. Fusion of COL1A1 exon 29 with PDGFB exon 2 in a der(22)t(17;22) in a pediatric giant cell fibroblastoma with a pigmented Bednar tumor component. Evidence for age-related chromosomal pattern in dermatofibrosarcoma protuberans and related tumors. Cancer Genet Cytogenet 2002;134(2): 156–61.

32. Dei Tos AP, Seregard S, Calonje E, et al. Giant cell angiofibroma. A distinctive orbital tumor in adults. Am J Surg Pathol 1995;19(11):1286–93.

33. Guillou L, Gengler C. Solitary fibrous tumour and haemangiopericytoma: evolution of a concept. Histopathology 2006;48(1):63–74.

34. Furusato E, Valenzuela IA, Fanburg-Smith JC, et al. Orbital solitary fibrous tumor: encompassing terminology for hemangiopericytoma, giant cell angiofibroma, and fibrous histiocytoma of the orbit: reappraisal of 41 cases. Hum Pathol 2011;42(1):120–8.

35. Weidner N, Santa Cruz D. Phosphaturic mesenchymal tumors. A polymorphous group causing osteomalacia or rickets. Cancer 1987;59(8):1442–54.

36. Folpe AL, Fanburg-Smith JC, Billings SD, et al. Most osteomalacia-associated mesenchymal tumors are a single histopathologic entity: an analysis of 32 cases and a comprehensive review of the literature. Am J Surg Pathol 2004;28(1):1–30.

37. Bahrami A, Weiss SW, Montgomery E, et al. RT-PCR analysis for FGF23 using paraffin sections in the diagnosis of phosphaturic mesenchymal tumors with and without known tumor induced osteomalacia. Am J Surg Pathol 2009;33(9):1348–54.

38. Folpe AL, Morris RJ, Weiss SW. Soft tissue giant cell tumor of low malignant potential: a proposal for the reclassification of malignant giant cell tumor of soft parts. Mod Pathol 1999;12(9):894–902.

39. Oliveira AM, Dei Tos AP, Fletcher CD, et al. Primary giant cell tumor of soft tissues: a study of 22 cases. Am J Surg Pathol 2000;24(2):248–56.

GASTROINTESTINAL TRACT MESENCHYMAL LESIONS

Dora Lam-Himlin, MD

KEYWORDS

• Mesenchymal lesions • Gastrointestinal tract • Intra-abdominal • Pattern based

ABSTRACT

This article reviews the most common and characteristic mesenchymal lesions found in the gastrointestinal tract and intra-abdominal location in a pattern-based approach: spindle and epithelioid tumors (gastrointestinal stromal tumor, schwannoma, glomus tumor, leiomyoma and leiomyosarcoma, inflammatory fibroid polyp, perineurioma, melanoma, calcifying fibrous tumor, sclerosing mesenteritis, mesenteric fibromatosis, and inflammatory myofibroblastic tumor), and clear and granular tumors (clear cell sarcoma, granular cell tumor, gangliocytic paraganglioma, and ganglioneuroma). Information includes gross and histologic features, diagnosis and differential diagnosis, and histologic and other diagnostic techniques, including immunohistochemistry related to projected patient outcome, along with prognosis, staging, and treatment.

schwannoma, glomus tumor, leiomyoma and leiomyosarcoma, inflammatory fibroid polyp [IPF], perineurioma, melanoma, calcifying fibrous tumor, sclerosing mesenteritis, mesenteric fibromatosis, and inflammatory myofibroblastic tumor [IMT]) and tumors with clear or granular cytoplasm (clear cell sarcoma [CCS], granular cell tumor [GCT], gangliocytic paraganglioma, and ganglioneuroma). Although the differential diagnosis of mesenchymal lesions can be challenging, the histologic pattern, location of the lesion's epicenter and immunohistochemistry aid in diagnosis (**Table 1**).

OVERVIEW

Mesenchymal lesions are rare in the gastrointestinal tract. Although most soft tissue neoplasms can occur in an intra-abdominal location, there are several lesions that are distinctive to this site. Some lesions may develop in a variety of sites but have a unique clinical and prognostic profile within the abdomen. This article reviews the most common and characteristic mesenchymal lesions found in the gastrointestinal tract and intra-abdominal location in a pattern-based approach; these include spindle and epithelioid tumors (gastrointestinal stromal tumor [GIST],

SPINDLED AND EPITHELIOID LESIONS CENTERED ON THE MUSCULARIS PROPRIA

GASTROINTESTINAL STROMAL TUMOR

Gross Features

GISTs may be found anywhere along the tubal gastrointestinal tract. They are generally well-circumscribed, firm white masses, which can be multinodular and have variable cyst formation, hemorrhage, necrosis, and mucosal ulceration. Tumors vary in diameter from less than 1 cm to 35 cm, but most are between 5 cm and 10 cm. Typically, they arise from the wall of the gut (muscularis propria) and extend inward toward the mucosa, outward toward the serosa, or in both directions; some examples are serosal or centered on the muscularis mucosa. Infrequently, lesions invade through the muscularis mucosae to involve the mucosa, a poor prognostic indicator.

The author has nothing to disclose.
Mayo Clinic Arizona, 13400 East Shea Boulevard, Scottsdale, AZ 85259, USA
E-mail address: Lamhimlin.Dora@mayo.edu

Surgical Pathology 4 (2011) 915–962
doi:10.1016/j.path.2011.08.010

Table 1
Mesenchymal lesions of the gastrointestinal tract organized by pattern and compartment

		Spindled and Epithelioid Lesions of the Gastrointestinal Tract	
Tumor	Major Compartment	Microscopic Features	Ancillary Studies
Gastrointestinal Stromal Tumor	Muscularis propria	Epithelioid or spindle cell variants. Fascicles of spindle cells with blunt or tapered nuclei. Paranuclear vacuoles. Organoid and palisading patterns	CD117+, DOG1+, CD34+, h-caldesmon+, variable SMA+, rare desmin+, rare S-100+, rare cytokeratin+ *KIT* or *PDGFRA* mutation
Schwannoma	Muscularis propria	Prominent lymphoid cuff with lymphoid aggregates. Fascicles of spindle cells with wavy nuclei. Intralesional chronic inflammation. Less palisading than extra-gastrointestinal lesions	S-100+, variable CD34+, variable GFAP+, calretinin–
Glomus Tumor	Muscularis propria	Solid sheets of uniformly round cells with prominent cell borders and clear cytoplasm. Intimately associated with vessels	SMA+, calponin+, h-caldesmon+, desmin–
Leiomyoma	Muscularis mucosae	Perpendicularly intersecting fascicles of spindle cells with blunt-ended nuclei and eosinophilic cytoplasm	SMA+, desmin+, h-caldesmon+, calponin+
Leiomyosarcoma	Muscularis mucosae; muscularis propria	Perpendicularly intersecting fascicles of spindle cells with blunt-ended nuclei and eosinophilic cytoplasm. Nuclear atypia, mitotic activity, focal necrosis	SMA+, desmin+, h-caldesmon+
Inflammatory Fibroid Polyp	Submucosa; extension into mucosa	Storiform bland spindle or stellate cells with whorling around vessels (onion skin). Prominent backdrop of eosinophils. Multinucleated giant cells	CD34+, *PDGFRA* mutation
Perineurioma (Benign Fibroblastic Polyp)	Mucosa; lamina propria	Bland ovoid spindle cells expand the lamina propria without crypt destruction. Adjacent crypts may show serrated changes	EMA+, Glut1+, Claudin1+
Primary Melanoma of Gastrointestinal Tract	Mucosa	Spindle or epithelioid cells with nuclear pleomorphism, prominent macronucleoli, mitoses. Pigment may be seen in 50%	S-100+, HMB-45+, Melan-A+, MART-1+, MITF+

Tumor	Major Compartment	Microscopic Features	Ancillary Studies
Calcifying Fibrous (Pseudo) Tumor	Serosa (gastric)	Circumscribed, unencapsulated lesion. Paucicellular dense collagen, lymphoid aggregates, psammomatous or dystrophic calcification, scant fibroblasts	Variable CD34+ or SMA+
Sclerosing Mesenteritis	Mesentery	Fascicles of fibrous tissue entrapping fat. Fat necrosis, inflammation, sparse spindle cells	SMA+, IgG4+ plasma cells
Mesenteric (Intra-Abdominal) Fibromatosis	Mesentery	Long, sweeping intersecting fascicles of myofibroblasts. Conspicuous small collapsed or gaping vessels running in parallel with fascicles	SMA+, nuclear β-catenin+, CD34−, spurious CD117+ depending on manufacturer
Inflammatory Myofibroblastic Tumor (Inflammatory Fibrosarcoma)	Mesentery	Bland myofibroblasts arranged in fascicular or storiform pattern. Prominent backdrop of chronic inflammatory cells, predominantly plasma cells	SMA+, ALK1+ (55%)

Clear and Granular Lesions of the Gastrointestinal Tract

Tumor	Major Compartment	Microscopic Features	Ancillary Studies
Clear Cell Sarcoma	Muscularis propria	Packets or nests of uniform round cells with prominent central macronucleoli. Clear or granular cytoplasm. Touton giant cells	S-100+, HMB-45+, Melan-A+, MITF+ t(12;22)(q13;q12); EWS-ATF1 or EWS-CREB1
Granular Cell Tumor	Submucosa	Sheets of large polygonal cells with abundant granular cytoplasm. Overlying squamous mucosa may show pseudoepitheliomatous hyperplasia	S-100+, CD68+, CEA+
Gangliocytic Paraganglioma	Submucosa with extension into mucosa	Triad of Schwannian spindle cells, ganglion cells, and nested epithelioid cells in varying proportions	Spindle cells: S-100+ Ganglion cells: NSE+, CD56+, synaptophysin+, chromogranin+ Epithelioid cells: keratin+
Ganglioneuroma	Mucosa (sporadic ganglioneuroma; ganglioneuromatous polyposis) Muscularis propria (diffuse ganglioneuromatosis)	Sheets or fascicles of spindled Schwann cells with variable proportions of interspersed ganglion cells	Spindle cells: S-100+ Ganglion cells: NSE+, CD56+, synaptophysin+, chromogranin+

Key Features
GASTROINTESTINAL STROMAL TUMOR

1. Tumors are usually found centered on the muscularis propria but may be centered on the serosa or muscularis mucosae.

2. Lesions are composed of spindle or epithelioid cells, or a mixture of the two, arranged in fascicles or whorls.

3. Skeinoid fibers may be present in the stroma, especially in small intestinal tumors.

4. Lesions are reactive with CD117, DOG1, and CD34; variable reactivity is seen with smooth muscle actin (SMA), S-100, and *platelet-derived growth factor receptor α (PDGFRA)*.

5. Location, size, and mitotic count are important prognostic indicators.

Light Microscopic Features

The lesions are composed of uniform spindled or epithelioid cells, sometimes mixed in varying proportions.[1] The spindle cells are elongated with blunt-ended or tapered nuclei, paranuclear vacuoles, and a moderate amount of eosinophilic, slightly fibrillary cytoplasm (**Figs. 1** and **2**). The cells form cellular sheets and fascicles with whorled or storiform patterns (**Fig. 3**), sometimes with nuclear palisading similar to that seen in nerve sheath tumors. Epithelioid cells show more abundant cytoplasm with prominent vacuolation, perinuclear halos, and well-defined cell borders, sometimes arranged as organoid nests (**Fig. 4**). Variations include clear cell, signet ring, oncocytic, rhabdoid, and plasmacytoid change. True pleomorphic tumors are rare, although degenerative nuclear features may be observed. The stroma is scanty and may be myxoid or hyalinized (**Fig. 5**) with giant cells and a variable lymphoplasmacytic infiltrate. Skeinoid fibers (eosinophilic globules of dense collagen) are sometimes seen, especially in small intestinal GISTs (**Figs. 6** and **7**). Lesions that have been treated with imatinib or related tyrosine kinase inhibitors may show hypocellularity, necrosis, myxoid change, and clusters of foamy cells with variable amounts of residual tumor (**Fig. 8**).

Other Diagnostic Techniques for GIST

GISTs show differentiation toward the interstitial cells of Cajal. Approximately 95% of GISTs show diffuse membranous and cytoplasmic reactivity for CD117 (c-kit) (**Fig. 9**), sometimes with a paranuclear dot pattern.[2] Depending on location, 60% to 70% are immunoreactive for CD34, 30% to 40% for SMA, 5% for S-100 protein, and 1% to 2% for cytokeratin.[3,4] Desmin is positive in only approximately 1% of cases, but h-caldesmon is often positive in GIST, which can cause misdiagnosis as leiomyosarcoma; smooth muscle tumors, however, are negative for CD117. Approximately 5% of GISTs are *KIT* negative, and deleted on

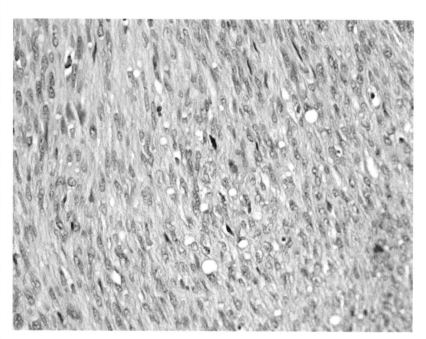

Fig. 1. This example of a GIST shows uniform spindle cells with tapered or blunt-ended nuclei and abundant paranuclear vacuoles (hematoxylin-eosin [H&E], original magnification ×400).

Fig. 2. This epithelioid GIST has markedly uniform cells arranged in a vaguely organoid pattern (H&E, original magnification ×400).

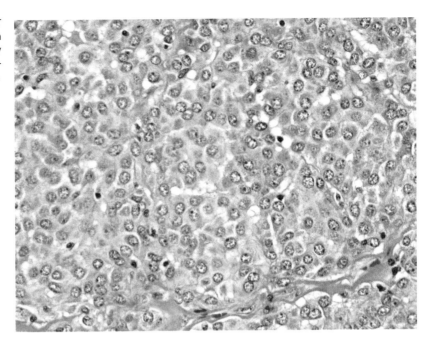

GIST 1 (DOG1) is useful for diagnosis of KIT-negative GIST.[5] More than 75% of these also show diffuse positivity for protein kinase C theta.[6,7]

Regarding genetics, 90% of GISTs contain mutations in either the gene for the receptor tyrosine kinases *KIT* or *PDGFRA*, which leads to constitutional (ligand-independent) activation of the receptors.[5,8–10] *KIT* mutations mostly involve exon 11 and less commonly exons 9, 8, 13, and 17. *PDGFRA* mutations are identifiable in up to 8% of tumors, in exons 12, 14, or 18, and are usually found in epithelioid gastric tumors that tend to be less aggressive; however, GISTs with a common Asp842Val substitution in exon 18 are

Fig. 3. A low-power view of a spindle cell GIST shows a storiform or whorling pattern (H&E, original magnification ×100).

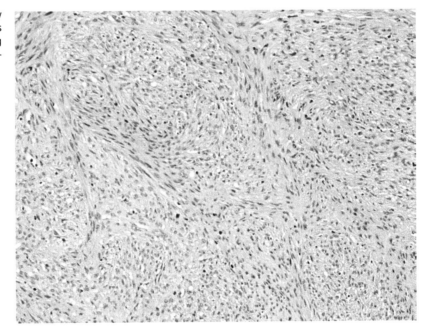

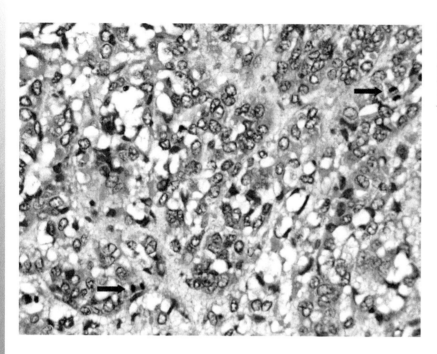

Fig. 4. This malignant epithelioid GIST shows nuclear atypia, prominent vacuolation, and abundant mitoses (*arrows*) (H&E, original magnification ×400).

resistant to imatinib.[11] GISTs associated with neurofibromatosis type 1 (NF-1) and a subset of those in pediatric age groups lack mutations of both *KIT* and *PDGFRA*. Similar germline mutations are found in patients with familial GISTs, with 100% penetrance.[6]

Assessment of management and patient outcome is increasingly reliant on mutational analysis. For example, the best responses to imatinib (approximately 65% of cases) are seen in tumors with exon 11 mutations. Those with *KIT* exon 9 Ala502_Tyr503dup mutants occur predominantly

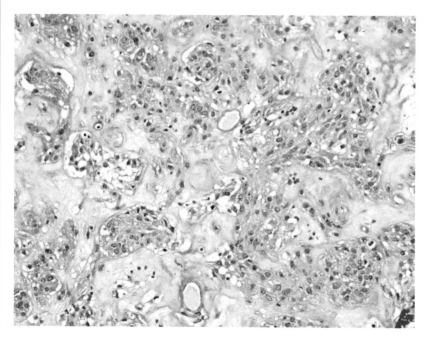

Fig. 5. A hyalinized background may be a prominent finding in some GISTs (H&E, original magnification ×200).

Fig. 6. Brightly eosinophilic skeinoid fibers punctuate this example of GIST. These are most commonly seen in small intestinal tumors (H&E, original magnification ×200).

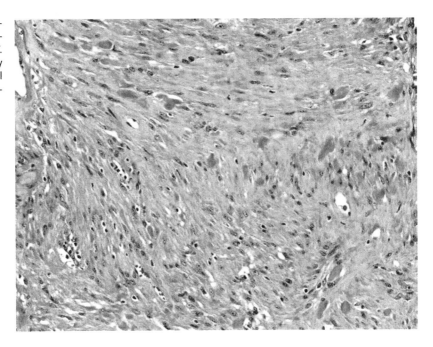

in small intestinal and colonic GISTs and are more aggressive and less responsive to imatinib (34%–40%).[5] The most recent National Comprehensive Cancer Network Task Force on GIST strongly recommends mutational analysis for *KIT* and *PDGFRA* be performed if imatinib therapy is begun for unresectable or metastatic disease. They also recommend consideration of mutational analysis in patients with primary disease, especially those with high-risk lesions. Additional mutations can arise in the course of therapy and impart secondary resistance to imatinib.[12] Sunitinib, another kinase inhibitor, is currently advocated as second-line therapy in this situation.

Fig. 7. Higher magnification of a skeinoid fiber, so named as they look like a skein of yarn (H&E, original magnification ×1000 oil immersion).

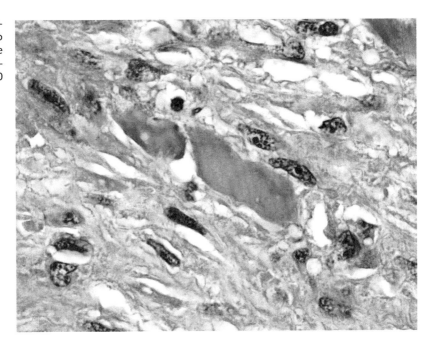

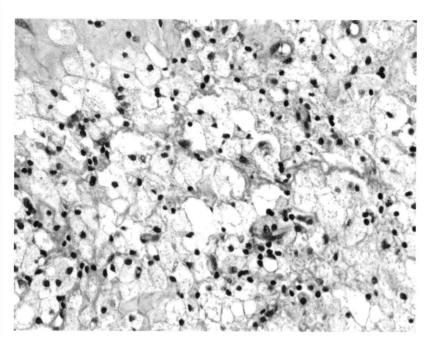

Fig. 8. This GIST has been treated with imatinib and exhibits characteristic post-treatment changes including prominent foamy cell change. Other areas were markedly paucicellular and showed myxoid change (H&E, original magnification ×400).

Differential Diagnosis

Because GISTs may be effectively treated with small molecule kinase inhibitor therapy (imatinib or sunitinib), it is essential to differentiate these tumors from mimics. The main differential diagnoses include smooth muscle tumors, such as leiomyomas and leiomyosarcomas; neural tumors, such as schwannomas; and occasionally fibroblastic and myofibroblastic lesions, such as fibromatosis and solitary fibrous tumors.[13,14] Most diagnostic difficulties can be resolved by the use of immunohistochemistry. For example, smooth muscle tumors should be reactive for actin and nonreactive for CD117, whereas neural tumors should be reactive for S-100 and nonreactive for CD117.

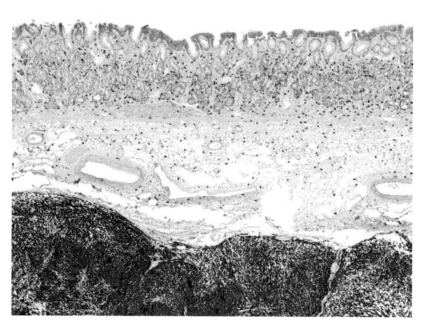

Fig. 9. A CD117 immunohistochemical stain strongly and diffusely highlights this gastric GIST centered on the muscularis propria (original magnification ×20).

In the cases of fibroblastic and myofibroblastic tumors, such as fibromatosis and solitary fibrous tumor, these tumors may show variable CD117 reactivity. The rabbit polyclonal antibody, A4502, manufactured by Dako (Carpinteria, CA, USA) has been reported to stain the cytoplasm of lesional fibroblasts and myofibroblasts. These false-positive tumors lack *KIT* mutations and respond only minimally to imatinib treatment. Despite the reactivity to CD117 antibody, morphology should aid in diagnosis. Fibromatosis demonstrates conspicuous vessels running in parallel with long, sweeping fascicles of spindle cells. Solitary fibrous tumor shows prominent staghorn vessels in a background of dense, hyalinized collagen and spindle cells arranged in a patternless pattern (imagine a group of shoaling fish).

Melanoma can be another diagnostic pitfall because metastases tend to spread to the small bowel or may present as anal or esophageal primaries. In addition, many melanomas are reactive for CD117, and spindle cell melanomas often lack the more specific melanocytic immunohistochemical markers, such as Melan-A and HMB-45. Melanomas typically demonstrate pleomorphism, however, a finding that is exceptionally rare in GISTs. Immunohistochemistry for S-100 is particularly helpful, because melanomas show strong and diffuse S-100 reactivity, whereas GISTs are nonreactive.

Prognosis, Staging, and Therapy

GISTs may recur many years after treatment and have the potential to metastasize. Histologic grading, staging, and prognostication of these tumors rely on mitotic count, size, and anatomic location.

Histologic grading of GISTs is determined by mitotic activity. Low-grade tumors (G1) have a mitotic rate of 5 or fewer mitoses per 5 mm^2, and high-grade tumors (G2) have a mitotic rate of greater than 5 mitoses per 5 mm^2. Most staging manuals express this as a mitotic count per 50 high-power fields (hpf); however, modern wide-field objectives may cover 5 mm^2 in as few as 20 hpf. Although most soft tissue sarcomas are staged according to histologic grade, this system is not appropriate for GISTs because most have mitotic rates below the thresholds used for soft tissue sarcomas. In addition, GISTs often manifest aggressive features with mitotic rates below the thresholds used for soft tissue tumor grading (the lowest tier of mitotic rates for soft tissue sarcomas being 10 mitoses per 10 hpf).

The Union for International Cancer Control (UICC) TNM staging criteria for GISTs defines the pT category by size, with cutoffs at 2 cm or smaller (T1), more than 2 to 5 cm (T2), more than 5 to 10 cm (T3), and more than 10 cm (T4). Because the main prognostic indicators for staging (size and mitotic count) are continuous variables, prognosis of GISTs exists along a spectrum and complete separation of benign and malignant GISTs cannot be achieved.

In addition to size and mitotic count, the anatomic location of the tumor affects prognosis and is taken into account during staging. For example, gastric GISTs have a more favorable outcome than tumors arising in other locations.[15] Guidelines using combinations of location, maximum dimension, and mitotic count for stratifying risk have been proposed, as in **Table 2**. The UICC divides staging of GISTs into two groups according to anatomic location, with different cutoffs defined by size and mitotic rate (**Table 3**). The first group includes gastric GISTs and primary omental GISTs. The second group includes GISTs arising in the small intestine, esophagus, colon, rectum, and mesentery.

Regional lymph node involvement is rare for GISTs, and N0 represents no regional lymph node metastasis, whereas N1 represents any regional lymph node metastasis. Lymphadenectomy is unnecessary except in rare instances when suspicious or enlarged lymph nodes are encountered. Similarly, M0 is no distant metastasis, and M1 is any distant metastasis. These tumors generally metastasize to a limited subset of anatomic sites[16]; they predominantly involve the liver or peritoneal surfaces where there can be disseminated intra-abdominal disease presenting as innumerable metastatic nodules. Rarely,

Table 2
Risk assessment in gastointestinal stromal tumors

Tumor Parameters		Risk of Progressive Disease			
Mitotic Index	Size	Stomach	Duodenum	Jejunum/Ileum	Rectum
≤5/50 hpf	≤2 cm	None	None	None	None
	>2–≤5 cm	Very low	Low	Low	Low
	>5–≤10 cm	Low	Insufficient data	Low	Insufficient data
	>10 cm	Moderate	High	High	High
>5/50 hpf	≤2 cm	None	Insufficient data	High	High
	>2–≤5 cm	Moderate	High	High	High
	>5–≤10 cm	High	Insufficient data	High	Insufficient data
	>10 cm	High	High	High	High

Data from Miettinen M, Lasota J. Gastrointestinal stromal tumors: pathology and prognosis at different sites. Semin Diagn Pathol 2006;23(2):70–83.

GISTs metastasize to the lungs, which is associated with a rectal primary or very advanced disease.[17]

Diagnostic Algorithm

Recognition of a spindled or epithelioid lesion that is centered on the muscularis propria yields a differential diagnosis that includes smooth muscle tumors, such as leiomyoma and leiomyosarcoma, as well as neural lesions, such as schwannoma. Other lesions that may be centered on the mesentery and extend to the muscularis propria include mesenteric fibromatosis and sclerosing mesenteritis. Given the limited differential diagnosis, confirmation of a diagnosis of GIST is straightforward with the aid of a limited panel of immunohistochemical stains. Most GISTs are reactive for CD117, DOG1, and CD34 and have variable reactivity for SMA, S-100, and *PDGFRA*.

SCHWANNOMA

Gross Features

Gastrointestinal schwannomas occur most commonly in the stomach and involve the muscularis propria with occasional involvement of the submucosa (**Fig. 10**). They may be found anywhere along the tubal gastrointestinal tract. The lesions are generally well-circumscribed, unencapsulated, firm white masses, ranging from 0.5 to 1.2 cm.

Light Microscopic Features

Schwannomas in the gastrointestinal tract share histologic similarities with their peripheral nervous system counterparts but differ in their lack of a capsule. The lesions are composed of wavy spindle cells arranged in interlacing fascicles and

---

⚠ **Pitfalls**
GASTROINTESTINAL STROMAL TUMOR

! The rabbit polyclonal antibody, A4502, manufactured by Dako has been reported to stain the cytoplasm of lesional fibroblasts and myofibroblasts, including some examples of fibromatosis and solitary fibrous tumor. These false-positive tumors lack *KIT* mutations and respond only minimally to imatinib treatment.

! Two percent to 10% of GISTs lack CD117 reactivity. These are predominantly epithelioid in cell morphology. DOG1 anitbody labels GISTs that lack CD117 expression.

! Melanomas may show reactivity for CD117. These lesions typically show, however, more pleomorphism than GISTs and are reactive for S-100.

 Key Features
SCHWANNOMA

1. Gastrointestinal schwannomas are centered on the muscularis propria.

2. They differ from their somatic counterparts in being unencapsulated, less palisaded, and nonreactive for calretinin immunohistochemistry.

3. A lymphoid cuff is a prominent and useful diagnostic feature.

4. Schwannomas are benign and resection is curative.

Table 3
Stage grouping by anatomic location for gastrointestinal stromal tumor

	Gastric GIST				Small Intestinal GIST			
				Mitotic Rate				Mitotic Rate
Stage IA	T1, T2	N0	M0	Low	T1, T2	N0	M0	Low
Stage IB	T3	N0	M0	Low				
Stage II	T1, T2	N0	M0	High	T3	N0	M0	Low
	T4	M0	M0	Low				
Stage IIIA	T3	N0	M0	High	T1	N0	M0	High
					T4	N0	M0	Low
Stage IIIB	T4	N0	M0	High	T2, T3, T4	N0	M0	High
Stage IV	Any T	N1	M0	Any rate	Any T	N1	M0	Any rate
	Any T	Any N	M1	Any rate	Any T	Any N	M1	Any rate

Data from Sobin LH, Gospodarowicz MK, Wittekind C, editors. UICC International Union Against Cancer. TNM classification of malignant tumours. 7th edition. Chichester (United Kingdom): Wiley-Blackwell, John Wiley & Sons Inc; 2010.

demonstrate only loose palisading (**Fig. 11**). The tumor has a prominent lymphoid cuff with germinal center formation and contains scattered lymphoid cells throughout.

Other Diagnostic Techniques

Schwannomas strongly label with S-100 protein and low-affinity nerve growth factor receptor. They can show labeling with CD34, glial fibrillary acidic protein (GFAP), and collagen type IV with a pericellular pattern.[18] Calretinin is negative in the gastrointestinal tract schwannoma compared with its peripheral nervous system counterpart, which characteristically labels with calretinin. These tumors are nonreactive for smooth muscle markers and CD117.

Differential Diagnosis

The primary differential diagnoses include spindle cell lesions that arise in the gastrointestinal tract and involve the muscularis propria, including GIST, mesenteric fibromatosis, and smooth muscle tumors, such as leiomyoma and leiomyosarcoma. Although GIST shares an important key

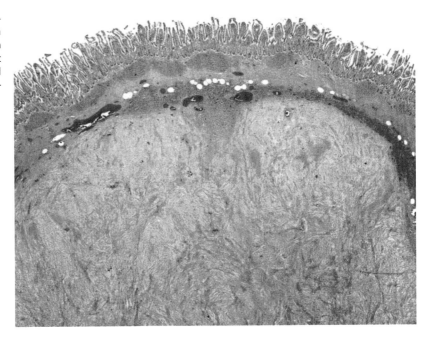

Fig. 10. This jejunal schwannoma is centered on the muscularis propria and exhibits a prominent lymphoid cuff with germinal center formation (H&E, original magnification ×20).

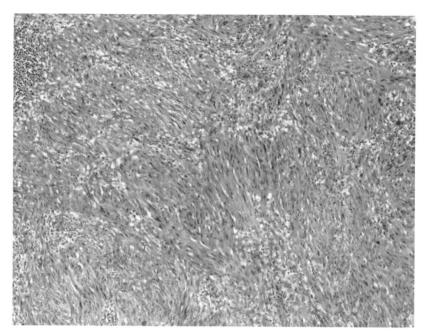

Fig. 11. The spindle cells in a gastrointestinal schwannoma show loose, subtle palisading compared with their peripheral nervous system counterparts; pleomorphism, hyalinization, mitoses, and ancient change are rare. Note the sprinkling of lymphocytes in the background (H&E, original magnification × 100).

feature of residing in the muscularis propria, GIST lacks the prominent lymphoid cuff and intralesional inflammatory cells. In addition, GIST shows immunolabeling with CD117 and lacks S-100 reactivity. Mesenteric fibromatosis is centered on the mesentery but may involve the muscularis propria by direct extension. This lesion is infiltrative and poorly demarcated compared with the well-circumscribed schwannoma. Mesenteric fibromatosis also lacks a lymphoid cuff and S-100 reactivity but does express nuclear β-catenin. Finally, smooth muscle tumors may arise from the muscularis propria but more commonly arise from the muscularis mucosae. Histologically, the spindle cells of smooth muscle tumors are arranged in perpendicularly aligned fascicles and have a more brightly eosinophilic cytoplasm with blunt-ended nuclei. These tumors also lack a lymphoid cuff or inflammatory backdrop. Immunohistochemistry shows expression of smooth muscle markers actin, desmin, calponin, and caldesmon.

Prognosis and Therapy

Schwannomas are benign lesions and excision is curative.

Diagnostic Algorithm

Recognizing that the spindle cell lesion is centered on the muscularis propria limits the differential diagnosis to GIST, mesenteric fibromatosis, and smooth muscle tumors. Histologically, the presence of a lymphoid cuff should aid in the diagnosis. A panel of immunohistochemical stains (S-100+, CD117–, actin–, desmin–, β-catenin–) confirms the diagnosis.

⚠️ Differential Diagnosis
Schwannoma

1. GIST: this lesion is also centered on the muscularis mucosae but has markedly uniform spindled or epithelioid cells and lacks a lymphoid cuff. In addition, this tumor labels with CD117 and is generally nonreactive for S-100.

2. Mesenteric fibromatosis: this lesion arises in the mesentery and has infiltrative margins. It lacks a lymphoid cuff and S-100 reactivity. A β-catenin immunostain is reactive in mesenteric fibromatosis.

3. Smooth muscle tumors: these typically arise in the muscularis mucosae but may arise in the muscularis propria. These lesions have perpendicularly intersecting fascicles of spindle cells that are immunoreactive for smooth muscle markers and nonreactive for S-100.

Pitfalls
SCHWANNOMA

! GISTs may exhibit prominent palisading of the spindle cells, mimicking a typical somatic schwannoma. It is helpful to remember that gastrointestinal schwannomas do not have strong palisading but do have a prominent lymphoid cuff; immunohistochemical stains (S-100 and CD117) may be useful in diagnosis.

Key Features
GLOMUS TUMOR

1. Glomus tumors are multinodular lesions centered on the muscularis propria.

2. They are composed of sheets of exquisitely uniform round cells with prominent cell borders.

3. The cells are intimately associated with small gaping hemangiopericytoma-like vessels.

4. The cells are derived from modified smooth muscle and immunolabel with actin, calponin, and h-caldesmon but not with desmin, keratin, or CD117.

GLOMUS TUMOR

Gross Features

Glomus tumors may be found anywhere along the gastrointestinal tract, but the majority are gastric. They are well-marginated, oval, intramural masses with a median diameter of 2.5 cm and may reach sizes larger than 5 cm.[19,20] Grossly, they bulge into the mucosa or outward toward the serosa. The cut surface is white to pink and often shows hemorrhage.

Light Microscopic Features

At low power, glomus tumors have multiple cellular nodules with intervening strands of residual muscularis propria and areas of hemorrhage and calcification. The overlying mucosa may be ulcerated.

The tumor is composed of solid sheets of uniformly round cells with prominent cell borders and clear cytoplasm (**Fig. 12**). The nuclei have delicate chromatin and inconspicuous nucleoli. These cells are intimately associated with gaping hemangiopericytoma-like vessels.

Other Diagnostic Techniques

Glomus tumors are composed of modified smooth muscle cells and these tumors express smooth muscle actin, calponin, and h-caldesmon on immunohistochemistry (**Fig. 13**). They are nonreactive for desmin, keratin, and chromogranin.

Fig. 12. Glomus tumors are composed of sheets of uniformly round cells that have sharply defined cell membranes and are intimately associated with gaping hemangiopericytoma-like vessels (H&E, original magnification ×200).

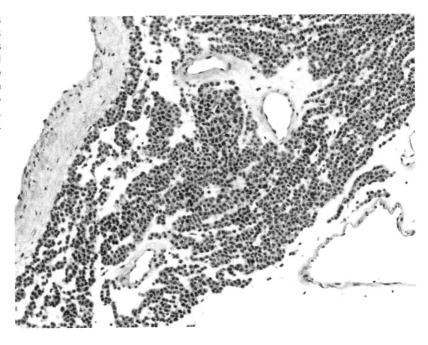

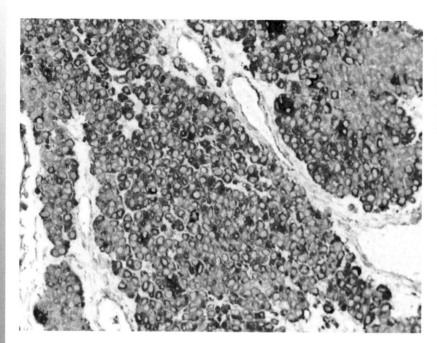

Fig. 13. Glomus tumors are composed of modified smooth muscle cells and express smooth muscle markers. This example labels with smooth muscle actin (immunohistochemistry, original magnification ×400).

Some examples have focal synaptophysin and CD34. These tumors are negative for CD117 and lack *KIT* mutations.[20]

Differential Diagnosis

Because of the exquisitely uniform and round cells, the main differential diagnoses include GIST and endocrine tumors (carcinoids). A negative immunohistochemical stain for CD117 excludes GIST. Immunohistochemical stains for endocrine markers may be mixed, because glomus tumors sometimes express synaptophysin. Negative reactivity for chromogranin and keratin, however, as well as labeling for smooth muscle markers, such as actin, calponin, or h-caldesmon, confirms the diagnosis of glomus tumor.

Prognosis and Therapy

The majority of glomus tumors are benign. Due to their vascular nature, the lesions may cause melena and rarely significant hemorrhage. Excision of these lesions is curative. Rare cases may metastasize, but there are no histologic features that can predict behavior.[20]

Diagnostic Pitfalls

As discussed previously, glomus tumors may express synaptophysin. This stain, in conjunction with the uniformly round cells, may lead to misdiagnosis as an endocrine neoplasm (carcinoid). Additional immunostains show the lesion is nonreactive for chromogranin and keratin, and labels with smooth muscle markers actin, calponin, and h-caldesmon.

△△ **Differential Diagnosis**
GLOMUS TUMOR

1. GIST: both lesions are centered on the muscularis propria and may exhibit epithelioid morphology, but only GIST expresses CD117.

2. Well-differentiated endocrine neoplasm (carcinoid): carcinoid tumors express chromogranin and keratin, whereas glomus tumors do not. In addition, glomus tumors express smooth muscle markers such as actin.

 Pitfalls
GLOMUS TUMOR

! Glomus tumors may express synaptophysin, leading to misdiagnosis of carcinoid tumor. Additional immunohistochemical stains (chromogranin, keratin, and actin) aid in correct diagnosis.

SPINDLED AND EPITHELIOID LESIONS CENTERED ON THE MUSCULARIS MUCOSAE

SMOOTH MUSCLE TUMORS: LEIOMYOMA AND LEIOMYOSARCOMA

Gross Features

Leiomyoma and its malignant counterpart, leiomyosarcoma, may arise in either the muscularis mucosae or muscularis propria throughout the gastrointestinal tract. Benign leiomyomas tend to arise in the muscularis mucosae (**Fig. 14**), whereas leiomyosarcomas may be centered on the muscularis propria. Most benign and malignant lesions in the gastrointestinal tract produce a polypoid luminal mass. The gross features are similar to those seen in uterine smooth muscle tumors and include a well-circumscribed, tan-white, whorled cut surface with rubbery texture. As with their gynecologic counterparts, the presence of necrosis indicates malignancy.

Light Microscopic Features

Both benign and malignant lesions are composed of spindle cells with brightly eosinophilic cytoplasm and blunt-ended nuclei arranged in perpendicularly oriented fascicles (**Fig. 15**). Benign leiomyomas have bland nuclear features and lack necrosis and mitoses. The presence of any nuclear atypia, necrosis, or mitoses is indication of

> **Key Features**
> **LEIOMYOMA AND LEIOMYOSARCOMA**
>
> 1. Leiomyomas tend to arise from the muscularis mucosae, whereas leiomyosarcomas may arise from the muscularis propria.
>
> 2. Both tumors are composed of perpendicularly intersecting fascicles of spindle cells with brightly eosinophilic cytoplasm and blunt-ended nuclei.
>
> 3. Both tumors express smooth muscle markers actin, desmin, and calponin.
>
> 4. The presence of any nuclear atypia, necrosis, or mitoses meets the criteria for leiomyosarcoma.

malignancy (**Fig. 16**).[21–24] Leiomyosarcomas may also take on an epithelioid pattern.

Other Diagnostic Techniques

Immunohistochemistry for smooth muscle markers actin, desmin, h-caldesmon, and calponin are reactive in both leiomyomas and leiomyosarcomas (**Fig. 17**).[25,26] Leiomyomas are typically reactive for h-caldesmon, whereas leiomyosarcomas are nonreactive. Both lesions are nonreactive

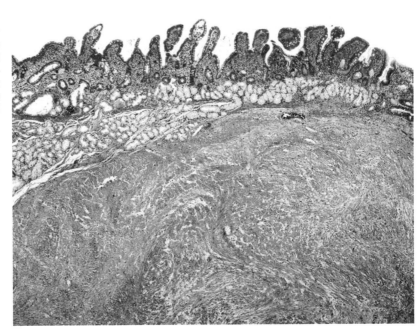

Fig. 14. Leiomyomas tend to arise from the muscularis mucosae anywhere along the gastrointestinal tract and may form polypoid luminal masses; this example is from the duodenum (H&E, original magnification ×40).

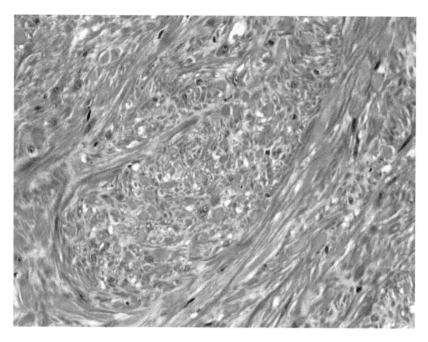

Fig. 15. Leiomyomas of the gastrointestinal tract histologically resemble their uterine and soft tissue counterparts, with perpendicularly intersecting fascicles of spindle cells demonstrating brightly eosinophilic cytoplasm and blunt-ended nuclei (H&E, original magnification ×400).

for CD117 and CD34.[26,27] Keratin labeling has been reported in leiomyosarcomas.

Differential Diagnosis

As with other spindle cell lesions in the gastrointestinal tract, recognition of the epicenter location is helpful in diagnosis. The differential diagnosis for spindle cell lesions involving the muscular layers includes GIST, schwannoma, mesenteric fibromatosis, and IMT. GISTs are perhaps the most important differential diagnosis, because they may be treated with targeted therapy and are much more common than smooth muscle tumors. GISTs

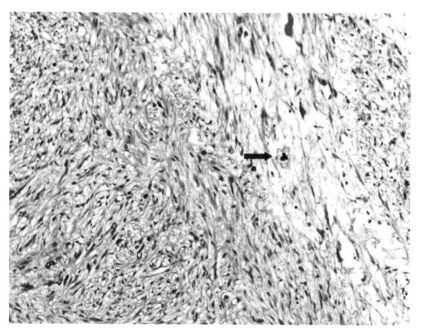

Fig. 16. This smooth muscle tumor in the muscularis propria of the colon shows nuclear atypia and mitotic activity with a tripolar mitosis (*arrow*); either of these features qualifies it as a leiomyosarcoma (H&E, original magnification ×200).

Differential Diagnosis
LEIOMYOMA AND LEIOMYOSARCOMA

1. GIST: this lesion is centered on the muscularis mucosae but has markedly uniform spindled or epithelioid cells and lacks the distinctive perpendicularly intersecting fascicles seen in smooth muscle tumors. In addition, this tumor labels with CD117 and has only scant reactivity for smooth muscle markers.

2. Schwannoma: this lesion is centered on the muscularis mucosae but has a prominent lymphoid cuff and a sprinkling of inflammatory cells throughout the lesion. It is immunoreactive for S-100 and nonreactive for smooth muscle markers.

3. Mesenteric fibromatosis: this lesion arises in the mesentery and has infiltrative margins. A β-catenin immunostain shows nuclear reactivity.

4. Inflammatory myofibroblastic tumor: these arise in the mesentery, have a storiform pattern of spindle cells with a prominent inflammatory backdrop, and are reactive for ALK.

typically reside in the muscularis propria, not the muscularis mucosae. Their spindle cells tend to demonstrate whorling and lack the perpendicularly intersecting fascicles seen in smooth muscle

tumors. In addition, GISTs show immunolabeling with CD117 and CD34, and show scant labeling for actin and desmin. Schwannomas also reside in the muscularis propria but have a prominent lymphoid cuff, a feature not seen in smooth muscle tumors. Schwannomas also express S-100 reactivity and are nonreactive for actin and desmin. Mesenteric fibromatosis is centered on the mesentery but may involve the muscularis propria by direct extension. This lesion is infiltrative and poorly demarcated compared with the well-demarcated leiomyoma. Mesenteric fibromatosis also lacks the pleomorphism seen in leiomyosarcoma and expresses nuclear β-catenin. IMTs arise in the mesentery but may extend into the muscularis propria. These lesions tend to have a strong inflammatory backdrop and express activin receptor-like kinase (ALK), both features that are not seen in smooth muscle tumors.

Prognosis and Therapy

Leiomyomas are benign lesions and resection is curative. Leiomyosarcomas, alternatively, are malignant smooth muscle tumors. The prognosis is generally poor and dependent on staging, with approximately 75% of patients dying of disease. Polypoid exophytic lesions of the rectum are reported to have a better prognosis. Targeted therapy, such as in GIST, is not available for leiomyosarcomas.

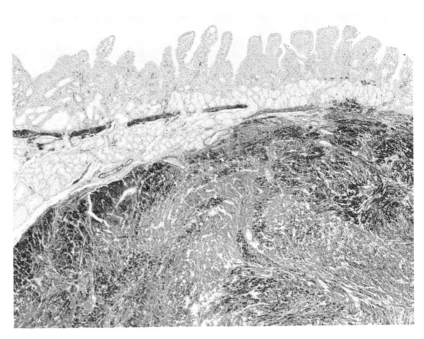

Fig. 17. An immunohistochemical stain for smooth muscle actin shows diffuse reactivity in this leiomyoma and highlights its origin from the muscularis mucosae (immunohistochemistry, original magnification ×40).

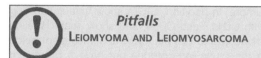

Pitfalls
LEIOMYOMA AND LEIOMYOSARCOMA

! In the small intestine, GISTs are far more common than smooth muscle tumors. Exclusion of GIST by immunohistochemistry in this location may be prudent.

! Leiomyosarcomas may take on an epithelioid morphology, making histologic diagnosis challenging. In addition, as these malignant lesions become poorly differentiated, they may lose some smooth muscle markers; some examples have been reported as keratin reactive.

Diagnostic Algorithm

In a resection specimen, recognition that a spindle cell or epithelioid lesion is arising from the muscular layers of the gastrointestinal tract is the first step to diagnosis. In difficult cases, immunohistochemistry may be helpful to confirm smooth muscle differentiation (actin+, desmin+, h-caldesmon+, and calponin+) and to exclude GIST (CD117), schwannoma (S-100), mesenteric fibromatosis (β-catenin), and IMT (ALK). A careful search for areas of nuclear atypia, necrosis, or mitotic figures should be performed for all smooth muscle tumors to exclude the possibility of malignancy.

SPINDLED AND EPITHELIOID LESIONS CENTERED IN THE SUBMUCOSA

INFLAMMATORY FIBROID POLYP

Gross Features

IFPs can arise anywhere in the gastrointestinal tract, with the stomach the most common site (70%).[28] These submucosal-based lesions are sessile or polypoid and the overlying mucosa may be ulcerated. Most lesions are single and well demarcated, ranging in size from less than 1 cm to 12 cm, with an average size of 1.5 cm. The cut surface is tan-gray and firm.

Light Microscopic Features

IFPs are centered in the submucosa and may have erosion, ulceration, or prominent reactive epithelial changes in the overlying mucosa (Fig. 18). The lesions are not encapsulated but are well marginated. They are composed of bland spindle cells arranged in whorls, often centered around prominent vessels, imparting an onion-skin appearance (Fig. 19). The cells have open nuclear chromatin and inconspicuous nucleoli. Some cases have marked stromal edema and multinucleated giant cells. Nearly all examples have numerous background eosinophils and scattered lymphoplasmacytic cells with occasional lymphoid aggregates.

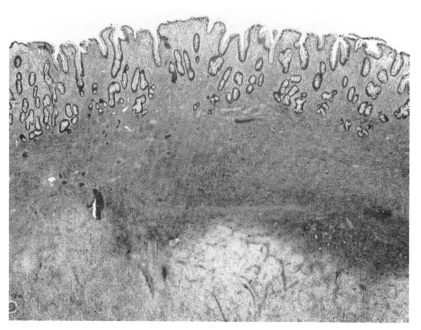

Fig. 18. Centered in the submucosa, this IFP splays the fibers of the muscularis mucosae and involves the lamina propria. The deeper portion of the lesion shows edema (H&E, original magnification ×20).

Key Features
INFLAMMATORY FIBROID POLYP

1. IFPs are centered in the submucosa.

2. The lesions are composed of bland spindle cells with a predilection for whorling around prominent vessels (onion-skin vessels) and have a backdrop of numerous eosinophils and lymphoid aggregates.

3. Some examples have scattered multinucleated giant cells.

4. The spindle cells are reactive for CD34 immunohistochemistry and the lesions harbor *PDGFRA* gene mutations.

5. IFPs are benign.

Other Diagnostic Techniques

The spindle cells in most examples of IFPs are reactive for CD34 immunohistochemistry, a helpful diagnostic tool (**Fig. 20**).[29] IFPs were previously believed reactive lesions, but molecular studies have shown that they harbor *PDGFRA* gene mutations with PDGFRA protein expression. In the gastric location, the mutation is found in exon 18, and in the small bowel location, the mutation is found in exon 12.[30,31] No *KIT* mutations have been reported in these lesions, and they are nonreactive for CD117 immunohistochemistry.[28]

Differential Diagnosis

The differential diagnosis includes many of the other lesions discussed previously; however, the submucosal epicenter of this lesion is a helpful clue to diagnosis. Although GIST and schwannoma are in the differential diagnosis, these lesions are usually centered on the muscularis propria, not the submucosa. In addition, GIST is reactive for CD117, and schwannoma is reactive for S-100, whereas IFP is nonreactive for both of these immunohistochemical markers. Other lesions in the differential diagnosis include mesenteric fibromatosis and IMT; these lesions are not centered in the submucosa but are located in the mesentery. Both of these lesions are nonreactive for CD34, whereas IFPs almost uniformly show reactivity. In addition, mesenteric fibromatosis has nuclear reactivity for β-catenin and IMT expresses ALK, findings which are not seen in IFP.

Endoscopic biopsies may capture only a superficial portion of the lesion, demonstrating lamina propria involvement by a spindle cell lesion and not revealing its submucosal epicenter (**Fig. 21**). In these cases, it may be difficult to distinguish IFP from perineuroma (benign fibroblastic polyp) or eosinophilic granuloma, lesions that are both usually found in the lamina propria. In these cases, immunohistochemistry can be especially useful; perineuriomas express epithelial membrane antigen (EMA), Glut1, and Claudin1, and eosinophilic granulomas express Langerhans cell markers CD68, S-100, and CD1a, whereas IFPs do not express any of these markers.

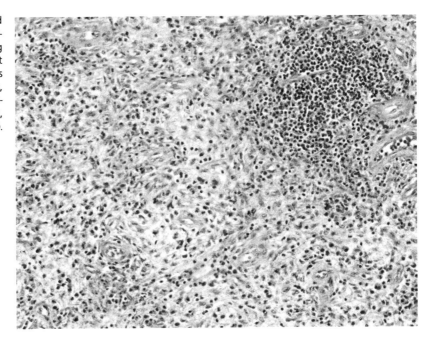

Fig. 19. IFPs are composed of bland spindle cells arranged in a whorling pattern with prominent small vessels, aggregates of lymphoplasmacytic cells, and a conspicuous backdrop of eosinophils (H&E, original magnification ×200).

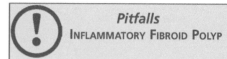

Differential Diagnosis
INFLAMMATORY FIBROID POLYP

1. GIST: this lesion is centered on the muscularis propria and expresses CD117 immunoreactivity. In comparison, IFP is centered in the submucosa and is nonreactive for CD117.

2. Schwannoma: this lesion is centered on the muscularis propria and expresses S-100 immunoreactivity. In comparison, the IFP is centered in the submucosa and is nonreactive for S-100.

3. Inflammatory myofibroblastic tumor: this lesion is centered on the mesentery and expresses ALK. In comparison, the IFP is centered in the submucosa and is nonreactive for ALK.

4. Mesenteric fibromatosis: this lesion is centered on the mesentery and expresses nuclear β-catenin. In comparison, the IFP is centered in the submucosa and is nonreactive for β-catenin.

5. Perineurioma: this lesion is centered in the lamina propria and expresses EMA, Glut1, and Claudin1. In comparison, the IFP is centered in the submucosa and is nonreactive for EMA, Glut1, and Claudin1.

6. Eosinophilic granuloma: this lesion is centered in the lamina propria and expresses CD68, S-100, and CD1a. In comparison, the IFP is centered in the submucosa and is nonreactive for CD68, S-100, and CD1a.

Pitfalls
INFLAMMATORY FIBROID POLYP

! These lesions were once viewed as reactive proliferations or "submucosal granuloma with eosinophilic infiltration" and sometimes confused with eosinophilic granulomas, neurofibromas, and hemangiopericytomas. They are now recognized as distinct neoplasms with *PDGFRA* gene mutations.

Prognosis and Therapy

IFPs are benign lesions but may cause local injury. Gastric outlet obstruction and/or hemorrhage may occur with gastric lesions, and intussesception is common with small bowel lesions. Colonic lesions are frequently found as an incidental polyp, but some examples have been associated with obstruction. Endoscopic or surgical excision is curative.

Diagnostic Algorithm

As discussed previously, recognition of the lesion's submucosal location is perhaps the most important key to diagnosis because it limits the number of differential diagnoses. Difficult cases may need the aid of immunohistochemistry to exclude perineurioma (EMA+, Glut1+, Claudin1+, and CD34–) and eosinophilic granuloma (CD68+, S-100+, CD1a+, and CD34–).

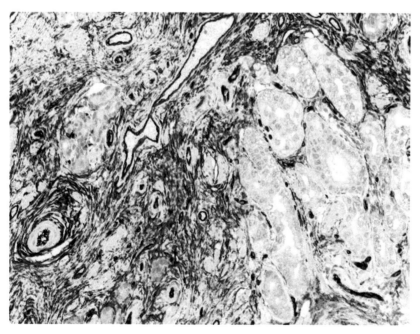

Fig. 20. A CD34 immunohistochemical stain highlights the spindle cells in this IFP. Note the predilection for the spindle cells to whorl around vessels, producing an onion-skin appearance (immunohistochemistry, original magnification ×200).

Fig. 21. A superficial biopsy of an IFP obtained endoscopically may demonstrate a spindle cell lesion in the lamina propria with rich eosinophilia, but the submucosal epicenter is not appreciated. Cases such as this may need immunohistochemistry to aid in diagnosis (H&E, original magnification ×200).

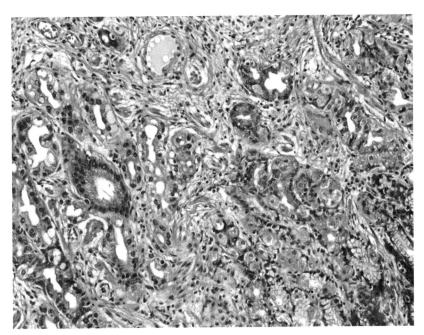

SPINDLED AND EPITHELIOID LESIONS CENTERED IN THE MUCOSA

PERINEURIOMA (BENIGN FIBROBLASTIC POLYP)

Gross Features

Perineuriomas (originally termed benign fibroblastic polyp) are essentially limited to the colonic lamina propria and are seen endoscopically as small mucosal polyps with a median size of 3 mm (2–6 mm range).

Light Microscopic Features

The lesion consists of bland spindle cells expanding the lamina propria and separating and distorting colonic crypts but not causing crypt destruction (**Fig. 22**). The cells have oval to elongated nuclei and pale eosinophilic to amphophilic cytoplasm (**Fig. 23**). Adjacent crypts and overlying epithelium frequently show serrated changes (**Fig. 24**).[32,33]

Other Diagnostic Techniques

More than half of perineuriomas and their associated serrated epithelial changes have recently been shown to harbor BRAF and KRAS mutations, suggesting that the lesions are mixed stromal/epithelial polyps rather than purely spindle cell proliferations.[33] Immunohistochemistry labels perineuriomas with epithelial membrane antigen (EMA) (**Fig. 25**) and Glut1, with variable expression of Claudin1 and CD34.[33,34] These lesions are nonreactive for S-100, GFAP, SMA, CD117, and keratin.

Differential Diagnosis

The main differential diagnoses include other lesions that similarly expand the lamina propria with spindle cells, including IFP, mucosal nerve sheath tumors, and ganglioneuromas. IFPs are

Key Features
PERINEURIOMA

1. Perineuriomas are identified on colonoscopy as small colonic polyps, most often in the distal colon and rectum.

2. The lesion is centered in the mucosa with bland spindle cells expanding the lamina propria and separating but not damaging adjacent crypts.

3. The spindle cells are frequently associated with serrated changes in the epithelium and more than half of the lesions harbor BRAF or KRAS mutations.

4. The lesion is benign and recurrences have not been reported.

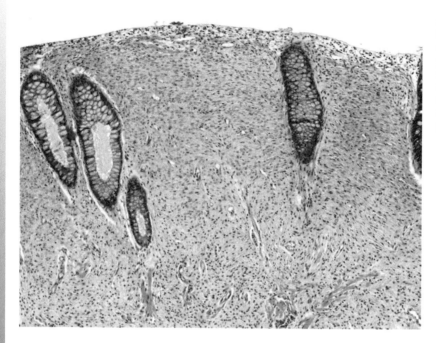

Fig. 22. This example of a perineurioma shows expansion of the lamina propria by a sheet of uniform, bland spindle cells that separate the colonic crypts without destruction (H&E, original magnification ×100).

centered in the submucosa, and, although they may extend upward to involve the lamina propria, these lesions have a prominent backdrop of eosinophils and are reactive for CD34 whereas perineuriomas lack inflammatory cells and only occasionally show variable expression of CD34. Mucosal nerve sheath tumors are histologically similar to perineuriomas, with an epicenter in the lamina propria and bland spindle cells. The most helpful tool in differentiating these lesions is the use of immunohistochemistry; mucosal nerve sheath tumors are S-100 positive whereas perineuriomas are nonreactive. Ganglioneuromas also contain abundant spindle cells that involve the lamina propria, but the presence of ganglion cells should be a clue to the correct diagnosis.

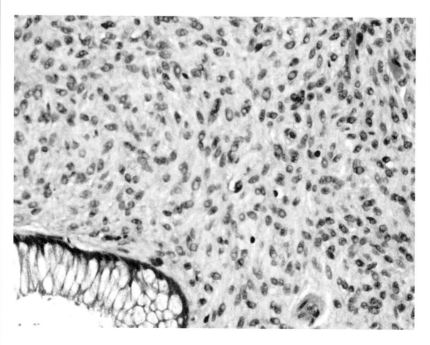

Fig. 23. On higher power, the spindle cells in a perineurioma appear uniform and bland with small nuclei (H&E, original magnification ×400).

Differential Diagnosis
PERINEURIOMA

1. Inflammatory fbroid polyp: the spindle cells in this lesion may extend into the lamina propria, but the main portion of the lesion is centered in the submucosa. In addition, a prominent backdrop of eosinophils and reactivity for CD34 immunohistochemistry is characteristic.

2. Mucosal nerve sheath tumor: these lesions are also centered in the lamina propria and histologically look similar to perineuriomas but express S-100 immunoreactivity.

3. Ganglioneuromas: abundant spindle cells in the lamina propria are present, but careful examination shows the presence of ganglion cells.

Prognosis and Therapy

Perineuriomas are benign mixed epithelial and stromal polyps usually found incidentally on colonoscopy. Excision by endoscopic polypectomy is curative and no recurrences have been reported.

Diagnostic Algorithm

As with other lesions, identifying the location of the lesion's epicenter is the first step in diagnosis. The presence of a spindle cell lesion that is expanding the lamina propria in a colonic polyp should yield

Pitfalls
PERINEURIOMA

! Fibrosis of the lamina propria may mimic this lesion. Lamina propria fibrosis, however, may be crypt destructive and does not typically produce an exophytic polyp.

a limited differential diagnosis. If the diagnosis cannot be made on routine histology, immunohistochemistry may be useful. A panel to confirm perineurial differentiation (EMA, Glut1, and Claudin1) and to exclude peripheral nerve sheath differentiation (S-100) is adequate.

PRIMARY MELANOMA OF THE GASTROINTESTINAL TRACT

Gross Features

Primary melanomas of the gastrointestinal tract are exceptionally rare, comprising less than 1% of all gastrointestinal malignancies. They are most commonly found at the anus, with esophagus the second most common location. Small tumors may appear flat or sessile, whereas larger tumors are bulky and may be polypoid. Less than one-half of these tumors are pigmented.

Light Microscopic Features

Melanoma is known to have variable morphologic appearances. The characteristic lesion shows

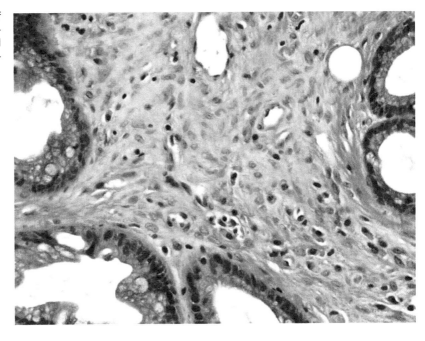

Fig. 24. This example of a perineurioma shows adjacent glands with serrated changes (H&E, original magnification ×400).

Key Features
MELANOMA

1. Primary melanoma of the gastrointestinal tract is most common in the anus, followed by the esophagus.

2. Less than 50% of tumors are pigmented.

3. An in situ component in the overlying epithelium is sometimes present.

4. The lesion resembles melanoma in other sites and is composed of sheets of epithelioid or spindled cells that have pleomorphism, prominent central nucleoli, and frequent mitoses.

5. Immunohistochemistry for S-100 is the most sensitive marker, whereas HMB-45, Melan-A, MART-1, and tyrosinase are more specific. CD117 is positive in many cases.

sheets or nests of epithelioid cells, but spindle cell variants are also common. The cells may be pigmented and are pleomorphic with prominent central nucleoli, intranuclear pseudoinclusions, and frequent mitoses. The overlying epithelium may demonstrate an in situ component, but this feature may be absent (**Figs. 26** and **27**). Pagetoid spread of melanoma cells into the overlying epithelium is characteristic.

Other Diagnostic Techniques

As with melanomas in any site, immunohistochemistry may be vital in making the diagnosis, especially in tumors lacking an in situ component. HMB-45, Melan-A, and tyrosinase are useful specific markers of melanocytic differentiation. Although S-100 is a nonspecific marker, it is the most sensitive, making it a mainstay in the workup of melanoma. CD117 has been shown to be reactive in up to 86% of anal melanomas.[35]

Differential Diagnosis

The morphologic patterns of melanoma are so varied that numerous neoplasms might be considered in the differential diagnosis, including poorly differentiated carcinoma, lymphoma, small cell neoplasms, epithelioid and spindle cell mesenchymal neoplasms, and pleomorphic sarcomas. The top differential diagnosis for the gastrointestinal melanoma is mostly limited to poorly differentiated carcinoma, GIST, perianal Paget disease, and lymphoma. Separation of these entities relies heavily on immunohistochemistry. Poorly differentiated carcinoma may lose some of the keratin markers, but performing multiple keratin markers (high molecular weight and low molecular weight) is recommended, because most demonstrate reactivity to at least one; melanomas are keratin negative. Distinguishing GIST from a spindle cell melanoma requires use of CD34, which is positive in up to 70% of GISTs and negative in melanomas, and S-100, which is strongly and diffusely positive

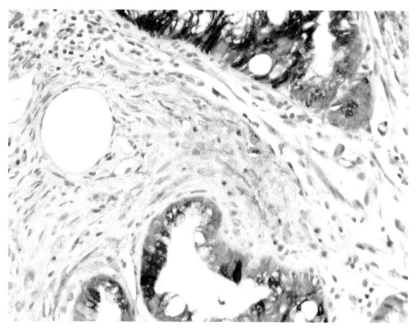

Fig. 25. The spindle cells in this perineurioma show weak reactivity with EMA immunohistochemistry (immunohistochemistry, original magnification ×400).

Fig. 26. This primary anal melanoma is undermining the squamous mucosa; an in situ component is not evident (H&E, original magnification ×200).

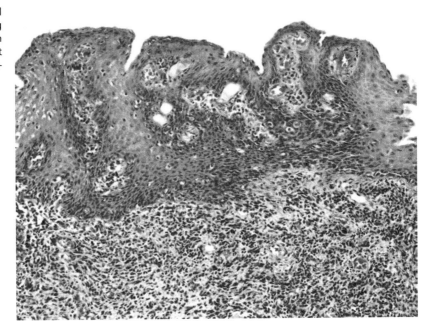

in melanomas and negative in GISTs.[35] Use of CD117 is of limited utility as both tumors may express this marker. Perianal Paget disease enters the differential diagnosis because of melanoma's tendency toward pagetoid spread of single cells into the overlying mucosa. In the perianal location, immunohistochemistry is indispensable for distinguishing melanoma from Paget disease, which is reactive for cytokeratin and demonstrates mucin positivity but is nonreactive for S-100. Lymphomas may involve the gastrointestinal mucosa but demonstrates CD45 (leukocyte common antigen) reactivity.

Prognosis and Therapy

Prognosis is poor and 5-year survival rates range from 6% to 22%; esophageal rates are less than 5%. Tumors are often high stage at the time of diagnosis with 26% of patients having metastatic disease at the time of presentation; the mean survival after diagnosis of metastatic disease is approximately 6 months. Wide local excision is the treatment of choice to decrease morbidity from radical surgery, especially because no survival benefit has been demonstrated for abdominoperitoneal resection. In patients who had *KIT* mutations, tyrosine kinase inhibitors have been successful.

△△ **Differential Diagnosis**
MELANOMA

1. Poorly differentiated carcinoma: performing at least two keratins (high molecular weight and low molecular weight) helps identify poorly differentiated carcinoma, because melanoma is typically negative for keratin.

2. GIST: both GIST and melanoma may label with CD117, so additional immunostains are necessary. CD34 highlights most GISTs whereas S-100 is negative.

3. Perianal Paget disease: this lesion is reactive for cytokeratin and demonstrates mucin on histochemical staining, features not seen in melanoma.

4. Lymphoma: CD45 immunoreactivity identifies cells as lymphoid in nature.

 Pitfalls
MELANOMA

! Melanomas may exhibit spindled morphology in combination with CD117 reactivity. In the gastrointestinal tract, care should be taken not to mistake this lesion for GIST. A high index of suspicion for melanoma and additional immunohistochemical markers, such as S-100, CD34, and more-specific melanocytic markers, are recommended.

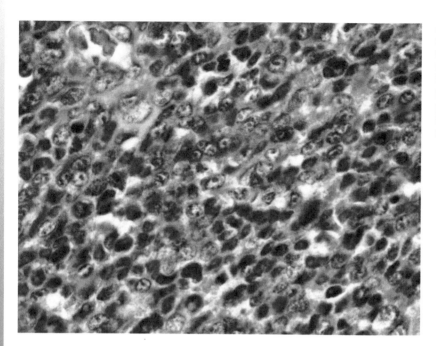

Fig. 27. Less than half of melanomas show pigment, as seen in this example. Note the prominent centrally located nucleoli and the nuclear pleomorphism (H&E, original magnification ×1000 oil immersion).

Diagnostic Algorithm

Diagnosis of melanoma in the gastrointestinal tract requires a high index of suspicion and melanoma should always be considered among the differential diagnosis of gastrointestinal tumors. Immunohistochemistry is almost always necessary to confirm the diagnosis. A panel of at least two keratins, CD117, CD34, S-100, CD45, HMB-45, and Melan-A/MART-1 is recommended to help exclude histologic mimics.

SPINDLED AND EPITHELIOID LESIONS CENTERED ON THE SEROSA

CALCIFYING FIBROUS (PSEUDO) TUMOR

Gross Features

This lesion is described in a variety of locations in the soft tissues as well as the pleura, peritoneum, mediastinum, paratesticular area, adrenal, heart, and lung. In the gastrointestinal tract, calcifying fibrous tumor has been described involving only the stomach or mesentery. The lesion is found primarily at the gastric body serosa, and the majority involve, at least in part, the muscularis propria.[36] These tumors are small (mean 1.9 cm), well-marginated, unencapsulated, firm, tan-yellow to white masses with a gritty cut surface.

Light Microscopic Features

Tumors show a characteristic hypocellular hyalinized sclerotic background with wavy, vaguely

Key Features
CALCIFYING FIBROUS TUMOR

1. Gastric calcifying fibrous (pseudo) tumors are unencapsulated, well-demarcated lesions limited to the serosa and mesentery with common involvement of the muscularis propria.

2. The lesions are markedly paucicellular with a background of hyalinized sclerotic tissue with bland fibroblasts, lymphoid aggregates, and psammomatous or dystrophic calcifications.

3. The tumors are benign and resection is curative.

storiform coarse collagen and scattered or patchy mononuclear inflammatory infiltrates composed predominantly of plasma cells and lymphocytes (**Fig. 28**). Small lymphoid aggregates are a common, and occasionally prominent, finding (**Fig. 29**). Both psammomatous and dystrophic calcifications may be found scattered within the lesion (**Fig. 30**).

Other Diagnostic Techniques

Calcifying fibrous tumors are variably reactive for CD34 and SMA and are nonreactive for CD117, S-100, desmin, ALK, h-caldesmon, and *PDGFRA*.

Fig. 28. This calcifying fibrous (pseudo) tumor is centered on the serosa of the gastric body and is composed of a hypocellular bland spindle cell population in a background of hyalinized sclerotic tissue with focal calcification (*arrow*) (H&E, original magnification ×20).

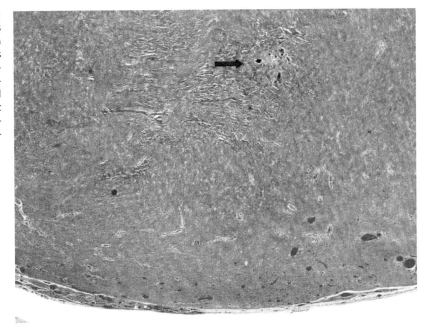

Tumors have not been shown to harbor genetic mutations in *KIT* or *PDGFRA*.[36]

Differential Diagnosis

The differential diagnosis primarily includes sclerotic or burnt-out variations of other mesenchymal lesions that involve the muscularis propria or mesentery, such as a sclerosing and calcified GIST or IMT; calcifying fibrous tumor was originally believed to be a burnt-out IMT. Gastric GISTs may be hyalinized with dystrophic calcifications in approximately 50% of cases.[37] Psammomatous calcifications and lymphoplasmacytic infiltrates, however, are not features of regressing GIST and sclerosing GISTs contain residual spindle cells

Fig. 29. Higher magnification of a calcifying fibrous tumor shows low cellularity, lymphoid aggregates, and a lymphoplasmacytic background (H&E, original magnification ×100).

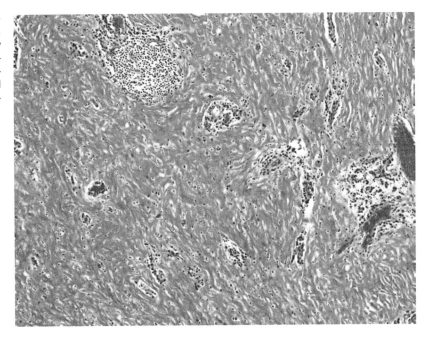

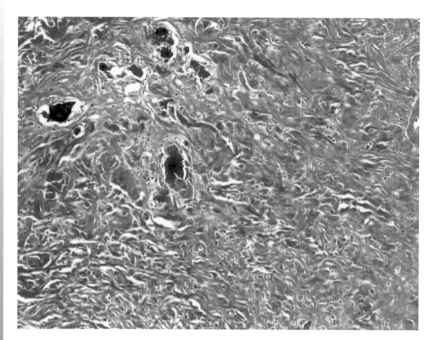

Fig. 30. Calcifications in a calcifying fibrous tumor may be psammomatous or dystrophic. Note the paucicellular densely collagenized background (H&E, original magnification ×100).

that coexpress CD117 and CD34.[37] Although IMTs have a prominent lymphoplasmactyic infiltrate, they express ALK, a finding not seen in calcifying fibrous tumors.[38]

Lower on the differential list are IFP, schwannoma, and sclerosing leiomyoma. Owing to focal CD34 reactivity in abdominoperitoneal calcifying fibrous tumors, IFP might be considered. Unlike IFP, however, calcifying fibrous tumors commonly involve the muscularis propria and the subserosa, lack the cellularity and the onion-skin pattern of IFP, and are wild-type for *PDGFRA*. The presence of focal peritumoral lymphoid cuffs in some cases may be reminiscent of gastric schwannoma but this can be excluded by the complete lack of S-100 reactivity. Similarly, sclerosing leiomyoma is a possibility that can also be excluded by absence of smooth muscle tumor cells on histologic and immunohistochemical assessment.

Prognosis and Therapy

These lesions are benign and prognosis is excellent. Excision is curative and recurrences have not been reported.

Diagnostic Algorithm

Most cases of calcifying fibrous tumor may be made on routine histology based on the gastric location and characteristic histologic features. Difficult cases, however, may benefit from immunohistochemistry to exclude other mesenchymal neoplasms of the stomach, such as GIST (CD117), IMT (ALK), schwannoma (S-100), and leiomyoma (actin).

SPINDLED AND EPITHELIOID LESIONS CENTERED ON THE MESENTERY

SCLEROSING MESENTERITIS

Gross Features

Sclerosing mesenteritis commonly affects the small bowel mesentery, presenting as a large, isolated mass, although up to 20% of patients have multiple lesions. The lesions are firm, white masses that extend into and encase surrounding tissue.

Light Microscopic Features

Sclerosing mesenteritis is composed of long sclerotic bands of fibrous tissue infiltrating fat and separating it into vague lobules (**Fig. 31**). There is an associated background of lymphoplasmacytic inflammatory cells and areas of fat necrosis (**Fig. 32**). Lymphocytic phlebitis or venulitis is often seen, a finding shared with IgG4-related sclerosing disorders (**Fig. 33**).

Other Diagnostic Techniques

There is no specific immunohistochemical profile for sclerosing mesenteritis, and diagnosis relies heavily on routine histology. The proliferating cells often express myofibroblastic markers actin and calponin but lack reactivity for desmin or caldesmon. Some cases show numerous IgG4 staining

Key Features
SCLEROSING MESENTERITIS

1. Most examples of sclerosing mesenteritis are solitary lesions centered on the mesentery and infiltrating into adjacent tissue.

2. The lesion is composed of sclerotic bands of fibrous tissue entrapping fat in vague lobules with fat necrosis, lymphoplasmacytic infiltrate, and lymphocytic phlebitis or venulitis.

3. The lesion may show focal actin and calponin immunoreactivity, but there is no specific immunoprofile for this lesion; it is negative for nuclear β-catenin, ALK, desmin, keratin, and S-100.

4. Sclerosing mesenteritis may represent a manifestation of IgG4 systemic sclerosing diseases and is responsive to steroid therapy.

plasma cells.[39] Nonspecific CD117 reactivity has been reported. The lesions are negative for ALK and nuclear β-catenin.[40]

Differential Diagnosis

The differential diagnosis includes other spindle cell lesions centered in the mesentery, including mesenteric fibromatosis and IMT. Involvement of

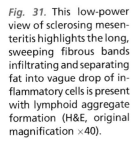

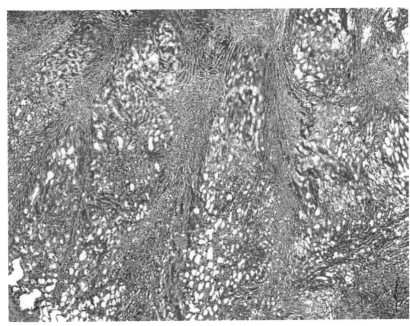

Fig. 31. This low-power view of sclerosing mesenteritis highlights the long, sweeping fibrous bands infiltrating and separating fat into vague drop of inflammatory cells is present with lymphoid aggregate formation (H&E, original magnification ×40).

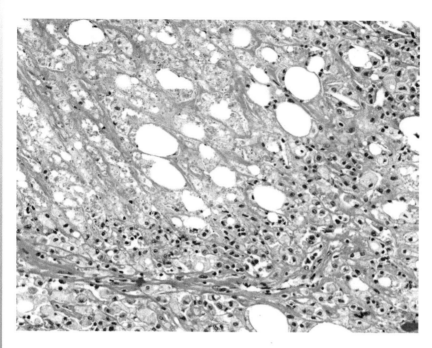

Fig. 32. Fat necrosis is a characteristic feature of sclerosing mesenteritis (H&E, original magnification ×200).

the mesentery by a liposarcoma should also be considered. Mesenteric fibromatosis has minimal to no inflammatory cells and is composed of long, sweeping fascicles of fibroblasts without significant fat entrapment. In addition, mesenteric fibromatosis exhibits nuclear reactivity for β-catenin. IMT does have a prominent inflammatory component but is composed of spindle cells arranged in a storiform pattern without fat entrapment. Additionally, IMTs may show ALK expression.

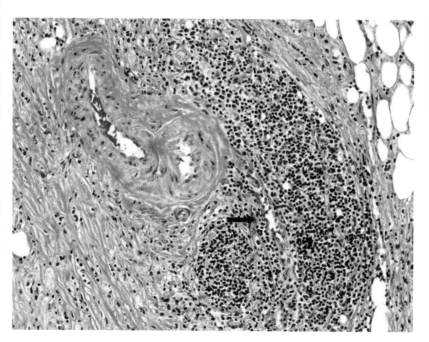

Fig. 33. Lymphocytic phlebitis is frequently seen in sclerosing mesenteritis. Note the damaged vein (*arrow*) adjacent to an uninvolved artery (H&E, original magnification ×200).

Differential Diagnosis
SCLEROSING MESENTERITIS

1. Mesenteric fibromatosis: this lesion lacks the inflammatory backdrop and fat entrapment with fat necrosis. In addition, it expresses nuclear β-catenin on immunohistochemistry.

2. Inflammatory myofibroblastic tumor: This lesion shows a cellular spindle cell population arranged in whorls without significant fat entrapment or fat necrosis. In addition, it may express ALK.

Prognosis and Therapy

The overall prognosis for sclerosing mesenteritis is favorable because approximately half of patients require no treatment. Treatment may consist of medical therapy, surgical therapy, or surgical therapy followed by medical therapy.[41] Approximately 60% of patients who receive tamoxifen in combination with prednisone show improvement.[42] Some patients may experience a prolonged and debilitating course, and, occasionally, patients die as a result of the lesion or complications of treatment.

Diagnostic Algorithm

The mesenteric location of this spindle cell lesion yields a limited differential diagnosis, as discussed previously. Because this lesion does not have a specific immunoprofile, immunohistochemistry is primarily used to exclude other lesions rather than confirm the diagnosis of sclerosing mesenteritis. A small panel, including β-catenin and ALK, differentiates the lesion from mesenteric fibromatosis and IMT, respectively. Recognition of the histologic pattern of bands of infiltrating sclerotic tissue with fat entrapment, fat necrosis, a lymphoplasmacytic backdrop, and lymphocytic phlebitis or venulitis is the key to diagnosis.

Pitfalls
SCLEROSING MESENTERITIS

! Given the inflammation, sclerosis, and fat necrosis, sclerosing mesenteritis may be mistaken for a reactive fibrosing process, especially if a patient has a history of abdominal trauma or surgery. It is important to recognize this entity, because it can be treated with steroids and most patients show improvement with medical or surgical therapy.

MESENTERIC (INTRA-ABDOMINAL) FIBROMATOSIS

Gross Features

Mesenteric fibromatosis presents as a large infiltrative mass centered on the mesentery. It has a firm, white, gritty cut surface.

Light Microscopic Features

This lesion is poorly circumscribed, with infiltrative margins, and is composed of spindled myofibroblasts and abundant collagen (**Fig. 34**). The spindled cells are arranged in long, sweeping, intersecting fascicles that run in parallel with delicate but conspicuous small vessels (**Fig. 35**). The vessels are thin-walled and may appear compressed or gaping in a hemangiopericytoma-like pattern (**Fig. 36**). Keloid-like collagen and hyalinization may be prominent features. Focal areas of hemorrhage, lymphoid aggregates, and calcification or chondro-osseous metaplasia may be present. The myofibroblasts have smooth nuclear contours with inconspicuous nucleoli and are hypochromatic in comparison to the darker adjacent vessels. Mitotic figures may be present but are infrequent.

Other Diagnostic Techniques

The myofibroblasts in mesenteric fibromatosis may express smooth muscle actin and, less frequently, desmin by immunohistochemistry. These lesions typically express nuclear β-catenin reactivity (**Fig. 37**) as well as estrogen receptor-β labeling but are nonreactive for CD34.[43] Depending on the manufacturer of the antibody, CD117 may show spurious cytoplasmic reactivity but not true membranous staining.[44]

Key Features
MESENTERIC FIBROMATOSIS

1. When intrabdominal, fibromatosis is typically centered on the mesentery and presents as a large, infiltrative, firm, white mass.

2. Histologically, the lesion is composed of intersecting long sweeping fascicles with conspicuous small vessels that run in parallel to the myofibroblasts.

3. Nuclear reactivity for β-catenin immunohistochemistry is a useful diagnostic marker.

4. Persistence and recurrence after surgical resection is common, especially in patients with familial disease (Gardner syndrome).

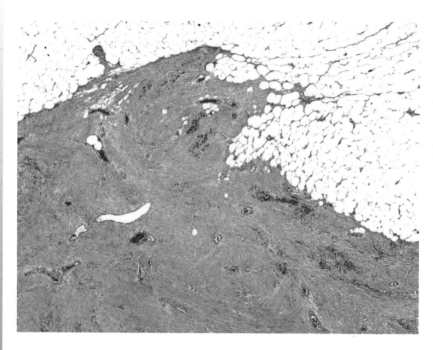

Fig. 34. Mesenteric fibromatosis has an infiltrative margin, which may focally entrap adjacent adipose tissue, but extensive fat entrapment with fat necrosis is not a prominent feature, as seen in sclerosing mesenteritis (H&E, original magnification ×40).

Differential Diagnosis

The differential diagnosis includes other spindle cell lesions centered on the mesentery, including sclerosing mesenteritis and IMT, as well as smooth muscle tumors and GIST. Sclerosing mesenteritis characteristically shows fat entrapment and fat necrosis in an inflammatory backdrop, features not seen in mesenteric fibromatosis. In addition, sclerosing mesenteritis lacks nuclear β-catenin reactivity. IMTs share with mesenteric fibromatosis the anatomic predilection for the mesentery but histologically show a more prominent lymphoplasmacytic component in addition

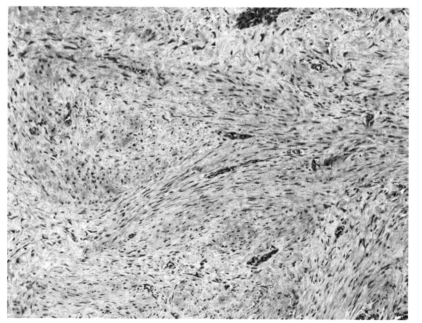

Fig. 35. Mesenteric fibromatosis is composed of intersecting long, sweeping fascicles with conspicuous small vessels that run in parallel with the myofibroblasts. Note how the vessels appear hyperchromatic in comparison to the lighter myofibroblasts, a feature helpful in excluding malignancy (H&E, original magnification ×100).

Fig. 36. Some examples of mesenteric fibromatosis may show gaping hemangiopericytoma-like vessels rather than the compressed, linear vessels seen in the previous example. Note the bland cytologic features of the myofibroblasts (H&E, original magnification ×200).

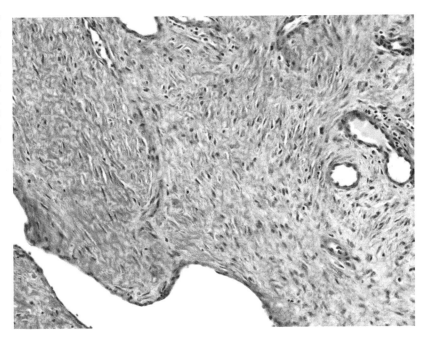

to whorling spindled cells and reactivity for ALK immunohistochemistry. Smooth muscle tumors enter the differential diagnosis as they express actin but differ from mesenteric fibromatosis in their reactivity for desmin and their lack of nuclear staining for β-catenin. GIST may present a diagnostic pitfall, because spurious cytoplasmic expression of CD117 in mesenteric fibromatosis has been demonstrated in antibodies provided by certain manufacturers. Because GIST is responsive to tyrosine kinase inhibitor therapy, it is important to distinguish this lesion from mesenteric fibromatosis. If in doubt, additional staining for β-catenin is of diagnostic value, because this should be negative in GIST.

Prognosis and Therapy

Mesenteric fibromatosis may be locally aggressive, causing constriction of adjacent organs and bowel obstruction. The lesion does not metastasize but is prone to local persistence and recurrence, especially in familial cases; this is seen in

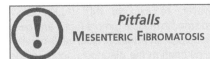

△△ Differential Diagnosis
MESENTERIC FIBROMATOSIS

1. Sclerosing mesenteritis: this tumor characteristically shows fat entrapment and fat necrosis in an inflammatory backdrop. In addition, this lesion lacks nuclear β-catenin reactivity.

2. Inflammatory myofibroblastic tumor: although this tumor is also centered on the mesentery, it shows a much more prominent lymphoplasmacytic component in addition to whorling spindled cells and reactivity for ALK immunohistochemistry.

3. Smooth muscle tumors: these lesions have perpendicularly intersecting fascicles of smooth muscle that are reactive for both actin and desmin and lack nuclear reactivity for β-catenin.

4. GIST: this lesion shows true membranous staining for CD117 and lacks nuclear reactivity for β-catenin.

⊘ Pitfalls
MESENTERIC FIBROMATOSIS

! Spurious cytoplasmic expression of CD117 in mesenteric fibromatosis has been shown in antibodies provided by certain manufacturers; this may lead to misdiagnosis as GIST. Because mesenteric fibromatosis is not responsive to tyrosine kinase inhibitor therapy used for GIST, it is important to distinguish these two lesions. Nuclear reactivity for β-catenin should confirm the diagnosis of mesenteric fibromatosis.

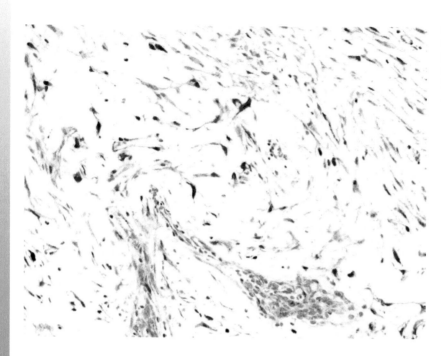

Fig. 37. Mesenteric fibromatosis has nuclear reactivity for β-catenin immunohistochemistry in the myofibroblasts (original magnification ×200).

up to 90% of patients with Gardner syndrome and in 10% to 15% of sporadic cases.[45,46] Gardner syndrome is an autosomal dominant familial disease with a female predilection, consists of numerous colorectal adenomatous polyps, osteomas, cutaneous cysts, soft tissue masses, and is related to familial adenomatous polyposis (FAP). Seven percent to 12% of patients with Gardner syndrome develop mesenteric fibromatosis. Surgical resection is the mainstay of therapy, and repeat excision may be required in recurrent cases.

Diagnostic Algorithm

As with other lesions, identifying the mesenteric location of the lesion's epicenter is the first step in diagnosis. Routine histology should be sufficient in most cases because the histologic features are characteristic. A panel of immunohistochemical stains, however, to exclude IMT (ALK), GIST (CD117), and smooth muscle tumors (actin and desmin) may be helpful. In addition, nuclear β-catenin reactivity helps confirm the diagnosis and exclude other lesions, such as sclerosing mesenteritis.

INFLAMMATORY MYOFIBROBLASTIC TUMOR (INFLAMMATORY FIBROSARCOMA)

Gross Features

IMTs are found in the mesentery or omentum as large, solid, infiltrative masses and are sometimes multilobulated. The cut surface is firm and white.

Light Microscopic Features

These tumors are composed of myofibroblasts and fibroblasts arranged in a storiform or fascicular pattern with inconspicuous vessels. The cells are spindled to stellate and typically show nuclear atypia with prominent nucleoli, but marked pleomorphism is not typical (**Figs. 38** and **39**). Although the lymphoplasmacytic inflammatory backdrop is

---

Key Features
INFLAMMATORY MYOFIBROBLASTIC TUMOR

1. IMTs are centered in the mesentery or omentum.

2. The lesions consist of spindled and stellate myofibroblasts and fibroblasts arranged in a storiform or fascicular pattern with a prominent backdrop of lymphoplasmacytic inflammation.

3. Nuclear atypia is characteristic, but marked pleomorphism is uncommon.

4. Approximately half of IMTs harbor mutations in the ALK gene and express ALK reactivity on immunohistochemistry.

5. These lesions are of intermediate biologic potential, may be locally aggressive, and exist along a spectrum with inflammatory fibrosarcoma.

Fig. 38. This IMT arose in the mesentery of the colon and extended inward to involve the submucosa. Note the prominent inflammatory backdrop with lymphoid aggregates (H&E, original magnification ×40).

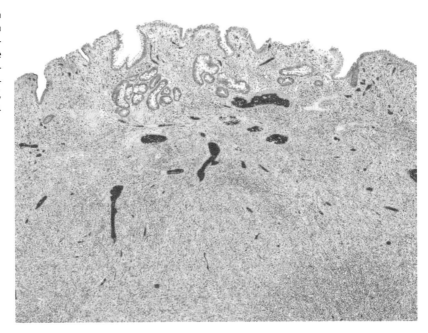

characteristic of this lesion, the degree of inflammation is variable among tumors, with some showing only sparse inflammation. Histiocytes and variable numbers of neutrophils and eosinophils may be admixed but are not a prominent feature. Occasional calcification and ossification may be present.

Other Diagnostic Techniques

Gene fusions involving the ALK1 gene at chromosome 2p23 have been described in these lesions. By immunohistochemistry, approximately 55% of cases label for ALK immunohistochemistry.[47,48] The lesions are also reactive for smooth muscle actin but not desmin. Cytokeratin staining is also

Fig. 39. This example of an IMT shows spindled to stellate myofibroblastic cells arranged in a storiform pattern with inconspicuous vessels and a prominent backdrop of lymphoplasmacytic cells (H&E, original magnification ×200).

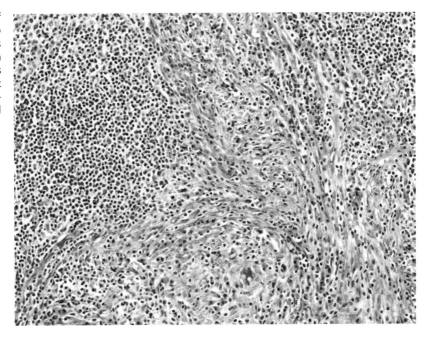

common in these tumors. Human herpesvirus 8 and Epstein-Barr virus expression have been reported in some cases but is not seen in cases with ALK1 positivity.[49]

Differential Diagnosis

The differential diagnosis includes other mesenteric spindle cell lesions, including calcifying fibrous tumor, sclerosing mesenteritis, and mesenteric fibromatosis, as well as other spindle cell lesions with a prominent inflammatory component, such as IFP and inflammatory leiomyosarcoma. Calcifying fibrous (pseudo) tumor was believed to be a burnt-out inflammatory myofibroblastic sarcoma because of its sclerotic background and inflammatory infiltrate, but this lesion is negative for ALK. Sclerosing mesenteritis shares similarities with IMT in that it is centered on the mesentery and may have a prominent lymphoplasmacytic backdrop. Histologically, however, sclerosing mesenteritis shows fat entrapment by bands of fibrous tissue that results in fat necrosis. In addition, sclerosing mesenteritis may show lymphocytic phlebitis or venulitis and is negative for ALK. Mesenteric (intra-abdominal) fibrosis is similarly centered on the mesentery, but it is composed of long, sweeping intersecting fascicles of myofibroblasts without a significant inflammatory component. Additionally, mesenteric fibrosis shows nuclear β-catenin and lacks ALK reactivity. IFP may enter the differential diagnosis due to its spindle cells and prominent background of inflammation. IFPs are centered in the submucosa, however, show prominent eosinophilic infiltration, have reactivity for CD34, and are nonreactive for ALK. Inflammatory leiomyosarcoma shows similarities to IMT in areas of inflammation, but it typically shows greater nuclear atypia and has at least focal areas of classic leiomyosarcoma. These lesions are reactive for both actin and desmin and are ALK negative.

Prognosis and Therapy

IMT is a neoplasm of intermediate biologic potential in the 2002 World Health Organization classification.[50] It is locally aggressive and frequently recurs (37%) but rarely metastasizes. It exists along a spectrum with inflammatory fibrosarcoma, and early reports were described as such; a few cases undergo sarcomatous transformation.[48] ALK-positive lesions have a better prognosis than those that are negative.[51] Patients experience B symptoms including fever, growth retardation, anemia, and weight loss, which are relieved by resection of the tumor. Treatment is limited to surgical resection.

Diagnostic Algorithm

Recognizing the mesenteric location of this lesion is the first step to correct diagnosis. Although immunohistochemistry is useful in lesions that express ALK, approximately half of these lesions are ALK negative. For this subset, it is necessary to rely on morphologic features, including the storiform or fascicular arrangement of mildly atypical spindle and stellate cells in a background of lymphoplasmacytic inflammation. Other immunohistochemical stains may aid in excluding other

---

△△ **Differential Diagnosis**
INFLAMMATORY MYOFIBROBLASTIC TUMOR

1. Calcifying fibrous tumor: once thought to be burnt-out IMTs, these lesions do not show ALK reactivity and are typically markedly sclerotic and have low cellularity.

2. Sclerosing mesenteritis: this lesion shows fibrous bands entrapping fat into vague lobules, fat necrosis, and lymphocytic phlebitis or venulitis, features not seen in IMTs.

3. Mesenteric fibromatosis: this lesion lacks the inflammatory backdrop seen in IMTs. In addition, it shows nuclear reactivity for β-catenin.

4. IFP: centered in the submucosa, the inflammatory component of this lesion is predominantly eosinophils. It lacks ALK expression but does label with CD34.

5. Inflammatory leiomyosarcoma: smooth muscle tumors are usually centered on the muscularis propria or muscularis mucosae. Perpendicularly intersecting fascicles of smooth muscle are usually present at least focally. This tumor is reactive with both actin and desmin and lacks reactivity for ALK.

 Pitfalls
INFLAMMATORY MYOFIBROBLASTIC TUMOR

! Approximately half of these lesions do not express ALK, so care must be taken not to place too much significance on this immunohistochemical stain. In lesions that lack ALK staining, exclusion of other lesions, such as inflammatory leiomyosarcoma by immunohistochemistry is prudent.

lesions, such as mesenteric fibromatosis (β-catenin), IFP (CD34), and inflammatory leiomyosarcoma (actin and desmin).

CLEAR AND GRANULAR LESIONS CENTERED ON THE MUSCULARIS PROPRIA

CLEAR CELL SARCOMA OF THE GASTROINTESTINAL TRACT (MALIGNANT MELANOMA OF SOFT PARTS)

Gross Features

CCS of the gastrointestinal tract is primarily found in the ileum, although tumors in the colon, pancreas, and stomach have also been reported. It is typically a lobulated gray-white mural-based mass, ranging in size from 2 cm to 6 cm.

Light Microscopic Features

CCS is composed of compact nests and fascicles of pale spindled or epithelioid cells surrounded by a delicate framework of fibrocollagenous tissue forming nests or packets reminiscent of a neuroendocrine organoid pattern. CCS may also grow in a more diffuse or sheet-like pattern, pseudoalveolar pattern, or myxoid/microcystic pattern or have a prominent chronic inflammatory infiltrate. The cells of CCS have lightly eosinophilic to amphophilic cytoplasm, with truly clear cells typically comprising only a minority of the neoplastic population (**Figs. 40** and **41**). The nuclei are uniform with prominent nucleoli, similar to melanoma.

> ### Key Features
> #### CLEAR CELL SARCOMA
>
> 1. The small bowel (ileum) muscularis propria is the most common site of CCS of the gastrointestinal tract.
>
> 2. Lesions are composed of infiltrating monotonous epithelioid to fusiform cells arranged in packets.
>
> 3. The cells are uniform with prominent macronucleoli and clear to lightly eosinophilic cytoplasm. Neoplastic multinucleated Touton giant cells may be present.
>
> 4. The immunohistochemical profile is identical to that of melanoma (positive for S-100, HMB-45, Melan-A, and microphthalmia-associated transcription factor [MITF]).
>
> 5. CCS behaves as a high-grade sarcoma with metastases to lymph nodes and liver.

Multinucleated Touton giant cells may be present. Pleomorphism, abundant mitoses, and necrosis are uncommon.

Other Diagnostic Techniques

CCS involving the gastrointestinal tract share identical morphologic, immunohistochemical, and ultrastructural features as their soft tissue counterparts. CCS shows an immunophenotype identical

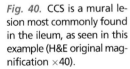

Fig. 40. CCS is a mural lesion most commonly found in the ileum, as seen in this example (H&E original magnification ×40).

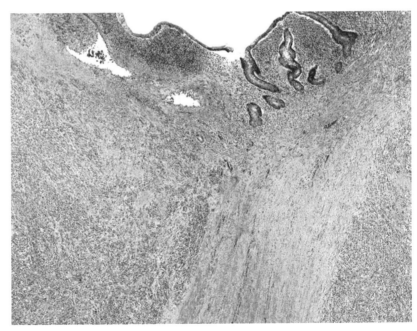

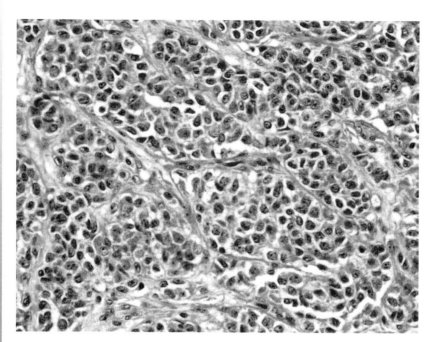

Fig. 41. CCSs are composed of epithelioid or spindled cells arranged in nests or packets. The cells are relatively uniform with prominent nucleoli. The cytoplasm is lightly eosinophilic or amphophilic, because clear cells comprise only a minority of the neoplastic population (H&E, original magnification ×400).

to that of conventional melanoma, with strong S-100 expression in 100% of cases and expression of the more-specific melanoma markers, HMB-45, Melan-A and MITF, in 97%, 71%, and 81% of cases, respectively.[52] The tumor shows variable expression for synaptophysin and CD56 and is negative for muscle markers and CD34. There is anomalous reactivity to cytokeratin and epithelial membrane antigen; care should be taken not to interpret this as a spindle cell carcinoma.

Regarding the genetics of CCS, more than 90% of cases are associated with a reciprocal translocation t(12;22)(q13;q12), resulting in the fusion of EWSR1 and ATF1, which may be detectable by polymerase chain reaction. EWS-CREB1 gene fusions have also been identified in several gastrointestinal and soft tissue CCS.[52]

Differential Diagnosis

The differential diagnosis of CCS centers on S-100 positive neoplasms found in the gastrointestinal tract, including malignant melanoma, schwannoma, and GCT. Melanoma is difficult to distinguish from CCS histologically but several features are helpful. CCS tends to occur in younger patients, with a female predilection and a preference for the muscularis propria of the small bowel. In addition, CCS has uniform cells and packeted organization and may contain Touton-type giant cells. Immunohistochemistry is not helpful in distinguishing melanoma from CCS, but molecular

genetic studies for the EWS-ATF1 or EWS-CREB1 fusion confirms the diagnosis of CCS. Schwannomas also reside in the muscularis propria and are strongly S-100 positive, but morphology should identify this lesion, because it is composed of palisading spindle cells rather than packeted epithelioid cells. In addition, schwannomas lack melanocytic markers. GCTs are typically submucosal in location, contain abundant coarsely granular cytoplasm, and lack melanocytic markers.

Differential Diagnosis
CLEAR CELL SARCOMA

1. Malignant melanoma: given the identical immunoprofile of these lesions, molecular testing for gene fusion of EWS-ATF1 or EWS-CREB1 may be necessary.

2. Schwannoma: this lesion is also centered on the muscularis propria but is composed of palisading spindled cells with a lymphoid cuff. Packeted arrangement of cells and expression of melanocytic markers are not features of schwannoma.

3. GCT: this lesion is centered on the submucosa. Although it expresses S-100 reactivity, GCTs do not express melanocytic markers.

Pitfalls
CLEAR CELL SARCOMA

! CCS expresses epithelial markers, including cytokeratin and EMA. Care should be taken not to mistake this for a spindle cell carcinoma. Additional immunohistochemistry for S-100 and melanocytic markers should aid in diagnosis.

Prognosis and Therapy

The prognosis of CCS is poor with a protracted clinical course, multiple local recurrences, and distant metastases.[53] Lymph node and liver are the most frequent location of metastatic disease from CCS of the gastrointestinal tract.[54] Up to 30% of patients present with metastases and the 5-year survival rate is approximately 50%. These lesions are not formally graded under either the French Federation of Cancer Centers or the National Cancer Institute soft tissue sarcoma grading schema but should be considered high grade for purposes of staging and therapy.[55] Treatment of CCS includes wide surgical excision and adjuvant radiotherapy with long-term follow-up.

Diagnostic Algorithm

The mural location of this clear cell tumor in the gastrointestinal tract should yield a limited differential diagnosis. The characteristic uniform cells and

packeted appearance, in conjunction with S-100 and melanocytic marker immunoreactivity, are the diagnostic hallmarks. Difficult cases, especially those in which melanoma is a consideration, may require molecular genetic testing for *EWS-ATF1* or *EWS-CREB1* fusion.

CLEAR AND GRANULAR TUMORS CENTERED IN THE SUBMUCOSA

GRANULAR CELL TUMOR

Gross Features

GCTs may be found anywhere along the gastrointestinal tract but are most commonly found in the esophagus, followed by the anus. They are poorly circumscribed submucosal-based lesions, measuring up to 5 cm, and sometimes form a polypoid mass that can be seen endoscopically (**Fig. 42**). The cut surface is yellow to white and firm.

Light Microscopic Features

These tumors are not encapsulated and are composed of plump polygonal to elongated eosinophilic cells with indistinct cell borders and abundant granular eosinophilic cytoplasm (**Fig. 43**). The nuclei are small, round to oval, and hyperchromatic. Overlying squamous mucosa may show pseudoepitheliomatous hyperplasia. A diagnosis of malignant GCT is made in the presence of three or more of the following atypical features: increased mitoses (>2 per 10 hpf), prominent

Fig. 42. This GCT in the cecum is centered in the submucosa and shows mucosal surface erosion (H&E, original magnification ×40).

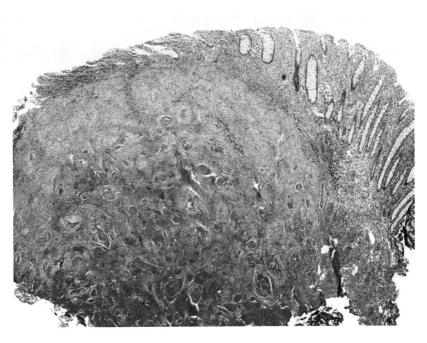

Key Features
GRANULAR CELL TUMOR

1. GCTs are submucosal-based lesions that may occur anywhere along the gastrointestinal tract, with esophagus the most common site, followed by anus.

2. The lesions are composed of sheets of plump cells with abundant granular cytoplasm and small hyperchromatic nuclei.

3. Pseudoepitheliomatous hyperplasia of the overlying mucosa is a common finding.

4. The lesions are periodic acid–Schiff positive after diastase digestion and are reactive for S-100 immunohistochemistry.

5. Malignant GCT is diagnosed when any three of the following are noted:

   a. >2 Mitoses per 10 hpf

   b. Prominent nucleoli

   c. High nuclear-to-cytoplasmic ratio

   d. Pleomorphism

   e. Necrosis

   f. Spindling of cells

nucleoli, increased nuclear-to-cytoplasmic ratio, pleomorphism, necrosis, or spindling of cells.[56]

Other Diagnostic Techniques

Ultrastructural examination shows that the abundant eosinophilic granules in the cytoplasm are composed of many lysosomes. These granules are periodic acid–Schiff positive and diastase resistant. The lesions are strongly and diffusely positive for S-100, CD68, carcinoembryonic antigen (CEA), inhibin, calretinen, and transcription factor E3 (TFE3) immunohistochemistry (Fig. 44) but lack muscle markers and melanocytic markers.[57,58]

Differential Diagnosis

The differential diagnosis includes other lesions of the gastrointestinal tract that show S-100 reactivity, including melanoma, CCS, and schwannoma. Melanoma and CCS label with more-specific melanocytic markers (HMB-45, Melan-A, MART-1, and MITF), which are nonreactive in GCT. In addition, CCSs have characteristic gene fusions of EWS-ATF1 or EWS-CREB1, although molecular testing is unlikely to be necessary for diagnosis. Schwannomas also share S-100 reactivity but are typically centered on the muscularis propria and composed of spindled rather than epithelioid cells, and they lack the abundant granular cytoplasm.

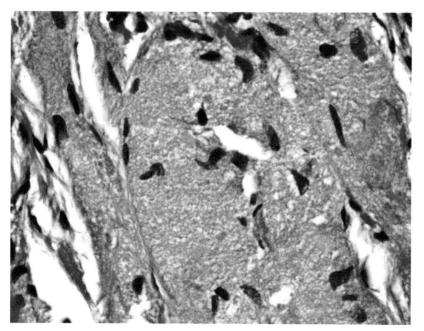

Fig. 43. The granular cells have indistinct cell borders with abundant cytoplasm containing numerous eosinophilic granules. The nuclei are small, round to oval, and hyperchromatic (H&E, original magnification ×1000 oil immersion).

Fig. 44. An S-100 immunohistochemical stain highlights a GCT undermining the squamous mucosa of the esophagus, the most common location for this tumor in the gastrointestinal tract (original magnification ×100).

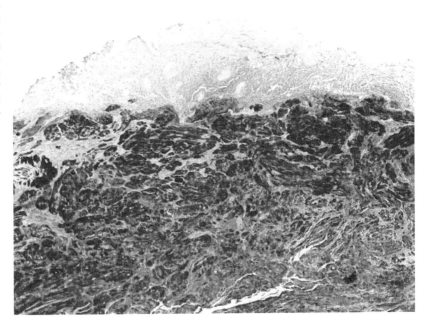

The presence of pseudoepitheliomatous hyperplasia in the overlying squamous mucosa may mimic squamous cell carcinoma, especially on small, superficial biopsies. This diagnostic pitfall may be avoided with adequate sampling and a properly oriented histologic section. Another diagnostic pitfall is the result of TFE immunoreactivity in GCT. This marker was initially believed specific for alveolar soft part sarcoma, which has a characteristic gene fusion *TFE3-ASPL*.

Additional staining for S-100 is negative in alveolar soft part sarcoma.

Prognosis

The majority of GCTs are benign and excision is curative. Recurrence or persistence of the lesion is seen in approximately 10% of cases. Malignant GCT is rare but may produce metastatic disease.[59]

Diagnostic Algorithm

After recognition of a submucosal-based lesion, most cases can be diagnosed on routine histology; the eosinophilic to amphophilic granular cytoplasm is characteristic. Confirmation with S-100 immunohistochemistry may be useful.

Differential Diagnosis
GRANULAR CELL TUMOR

1. Melanoma: this lesion shows diffuse strong S-100 reactivity like GCT but also labels with more-specific melanocytic markers (HMB-45, Melan-A, MART-1, and MITF), which are nonreactive in GCT.

2. Clear cell sarcoma: this lesion shows diffuse strong S-100 reactivity like GCT but also labels with more-specific melanocytic markers and harbors characteristic gene fusions of *EWS-ATF1 or EWS-CREB1*.

3. Schwannoma: this lesion also shares S-100 reactivity but is typically centered on the muscularis propria, has a prominent lymphoid cuff, and is composed of spindled cells that lack the abundant granular cytoplasm.

Pitfalls
GRANULAR CELL TUMOR

! Pseudoepitheliomatous hyperplasia in the overlying squamous mucosa may mimic squamous cell carcinoma, especially on small, superficial biopsies. This diagnostic pitfall may be avoided with adequate sampling and a properly oriented histologic section.

! GCTs are immunoreactive for TFE, a marker also found in alveolar soft part sarcoma. Additional staining for S-100 is negative in alveolar soft part sarcoma.

GANGLIOCYTIC PARAGANGLIOMA

Gross Features

Gangliocytic paragangliomas are exceptionally rare tumors that are nearly exclusively found in the gastrointestinal tract, most commonly in the duodenum or pylorus, although jejunal, colonic, and appendiceal tumors have been reported. The lesion is centered in the submucosa, has infiltrative borders, often with extension into the mucosa, and may form a luminal polypoid mass (**Fig. 45**). They range in size from 3 cm to 4 cm and have a tan-yellow cut surface.[60]

Light Microscopic Features

There are three constituent cell types comprising gangliocytic paraganglioma: Schwann cell-like spindle cells, ganglion cells with abundant granular cytoplasm, and epithelioid carcinoid-like cells that are arranged in nests. The cells may be present in varying proportions and may be well admixed or somewhat segregated such that superficial sampling on endoscopic biopsy may yield only one cell type (**Fig. 46**).

Other Diagnostic Techniques

Ultrastructural studies show that the Schwann-like spindle cells produce a discontinuous external lamina similar to schwannomas, the ganglion cells contain numerous lysosomes, and the carcinoid-like epithelial cells contain numerous dense-core secretory granules similar to true neuroendocrine cells.[61] Immunohistochemistry shows NSE is reactive in all three cell types. The Scwhann-like spindle cells show S-100 immunoreactivity, the ganglion cells show reactivity for synaptophysin and chromogranin, and the epithelioid cells may show

Key Features

GANGLIOCYTIC PARAGANGLIOMA

1. Gangliocytic paraganglioma is almost exclusively limited to the gastrointestinal tract, most commonly found in the duodenal submucosa.

2. This triphasic tumor is composed of varying proportions of Schwann-like spindle cells, ganglion cells, and nested epithelioid cells.

3. Immunohistochemistry labels each constituent cell type:

   a. Neuron-specific enolase (NSE) labels all three cell types.

   b. S-100 labels spindle cells.

   c. Synaptophysin and chromogranin labels ganglion cells.

   d. Somatostatin and keratin may label epithelioid cells.

4. The majority of these lesions are benign, but regional metastasis has been reported.

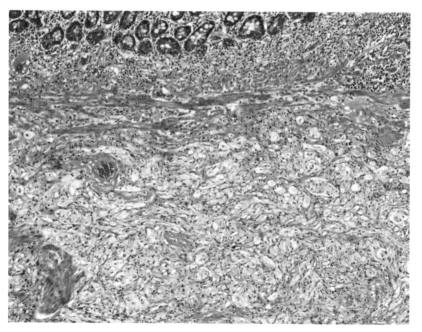

Fig. 45. This is an example of gangliocytic paraganglioma arising in the second part of the duodenum. The lesion is based in the submucosa with intact overlying mucosa (H&E, original magnification ×100).

Fig. 46. The three cell types of gangliocytic paraganglioma (Schwann-like spindle cells, ganglion cells, and epithelioid "carcinoid-like" cells) may be present in varying proportions, sometimes with one predominant cell type; this example shows principally ganglion cells with prominent nucleoli and abundant amphophilic granular cytoplasm (H&E, original magnification ×400).

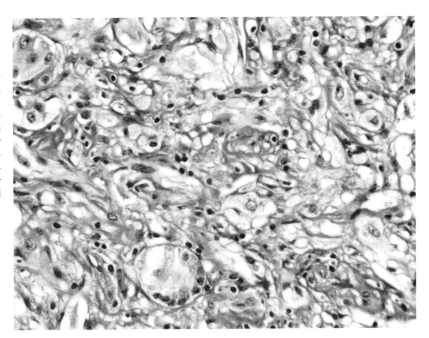

reactivity for somatostatin. A variety of hormones (somatostatin, human pancreatic polypeptide, gastrin, insulin, glucagon, gastrin, and vasoactive intestinal peptide) can be demonstrated in these lesions.[60,61] Keratin reactivity in the epithelioid cells may be present in up to 50% of cases.[62]

Differential Diagnosis

The triphasic morphology is exclusive to this tumor, and identification of each cell type unmistakably leads to the correct diagnosis. Because the tumor may have varying proportions of each cell type, however, the differential diagnosis encompasses spindle cell lesions and epithelioid lesions when either of these cell types predominates. For example, spindle cell predominant gangliocytic paragangliomas may be differentiated from schwannomas by location (schwannomas are typically centered on the muscularis propria) and by identification ganglion cells and epithelioid cells in gangliocytic paragangliomas. In the absence of more than one cell type, the lymphoid cuff and intralesional chronic inflammatory cells found in schwannomas are helpful diagnostic clues. Epithelioid predominant lesions should be distinguished from carcinoid tumors and carcinomas, a task that is complicated by the presence of neuroendocrine and hormone markers as well as keratin expression in up to 50% of cases. Finding the spindle cell and ganglion cell

Differential Diagnosis
GANGLIOCYTIC PARAGANGLIOMA

1. The following lesions enter the differential diagnosis when only one cell type is represented/sampled:

   a. Schwannoma: both schwannomas and the spindle cell component of gangliocytic paraganglioma are reactive for S-100. Schwannomas are typically centered on the muscularis propria and have a prominent lymphoid cuff and a sprinkling of intralesional chronic inflammatory cells.

   b. Carcinoid: carcinoid tumors resemble the epithelioid component of gangliocytic paragangliomas, because both show nested arrangement of epithelioid cells that may express keratin and synaptophysin immunoreactivity. Differentiating these tumors requires identification of the other constituent cells in gangliocytic paraganglioma.

   c. Carcinoma: although gangliocytic paragangliomas may show mild nuclear atypia, this is not as prominent a feature as seen in carcinomas.

   d. GIST: this tumor expresses CD117 and is nonreactive for S-100.

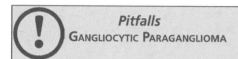

Pitfalls
GANGLIOCYTIC PARAGANGLIOMA

! Endoscopic mucosal biopsy may yield limited tissue without full representation of all three cell types. When only the epithelioid component is sampled, misdiagnosis of carcinoid tumor or carcinoma may occur due to the nested appearance and keratin reactivity of the epithelioid cells. This is of particular importance because treatment is markedly different.

Key Features
GANGLIONEUROMA

1. Isolated mucosal polyps represent sporadic ganglioneuromas and preferentially involve the distal colon.

2. The presence of numerous mucosal polyps (ganglioneuromatous polyposis) is associated with FAP.

3. Transmural diffuse lesions are associated with multiple endocrine neoplasia type 2B or neurofibromatosis type 1.

4. All lesions are composed of spindle cells interspersed with variable numbers of ganglion cells.

5. All lesions are benign.

component facilitates diagnosis. Small or superficial samples, such as in endoscopic mucosal biopsies, may not yield diagnostic material. Exclusion of GIST may be necessary in either spindle cell or epithelioid predominant lesions; GISTs have an epicenter in the muscularis propria and express CD117 but not S-100.

Prognosis and Therapy

Gangliocytic paragangliomas are generally benign but may cause gastric outlet obstruction or hemorrhage. Surgical excision is curative in the majority of cases. Metastatic disease occurs in up to 7% of cases, but no tumor-associated deaths have been reported.[63]

Diagnostic Algorithm

Adequate sampling and recognition of the three constituent cell types (Schwann-like spindle cells, ganglion cells, and epithelioid cells) of this submucosal-based lesion is sufficient for diagnosis.

CLEAR AND GRANULAR TUMORS CENTERED IN THE MUCOSA

GANGLIONEUROMA

Gross Features

Grossly, ganglioneuromas present in three distinct patterns that have clinical relevance. Solitary polyps of the colon are sporadic lesions and are often incidental findings on colonoscopy. In contrast, lesions that produce multiple exophytic polyps (ganglioneuromatous polyposis) is associated with FAP, and poorly demarcated transmural proliferations (gangliomneuromatosis) are associated with multiple endocrine neoplasia type 2B and neurofibromatosis type 1.[64,65]

Isolated polypoid ganglioneuromas are typically centered in the lamina propria of the distal colon, and measure 1 cm to 3 cm in diameter. The polyps in ganglioneuromatous polyposis are multiple (20–40), may be found in the mucosa or submucosa, and are found throughout the colon. Diffuse ganglioneuromatosis results in a poorly demarcated tan-white thickening that may be transmural.

Light Microscopic Features

Sporadic ganglioneuromas, ganglioneuromatous polyposis, and ganglioneuromatosis are all composed of a spindle cell population with interspersed ganglion cells. Sporadic ganglioneuromas and lesions of ganglioneuromatous polyposis are centered in the mucosa with expansion of the lamina propria and resulting crypt distortion caused by the neoplastic cells (**Fig. 47**). Submucosal extension of these lesions may be present, with involvement of the submucosal nerve plexus resulting in a plexiform pattern of growth (**Fig. 48**). The intramural or transmural lesions of diffuse ganglioneuromatosis are centered on the myenteric plexus and may extend into the lamina propria. All lesions are composed of fascicular or patternless spindle cells with elongated undulating nuclei and abundant fibrillary cytoplasm. This spindle cell background is interspersed with variable numbers of ganglion cells that have abundant eosinophilic to amphophilic granular cytoplasm and mild nuclear atypia.

Other Diagnostic Techniques

The ganglion cells express chromogranin, synaptophysin, NSE, and CD56. The spindle cells are S-100–reactive Schwann cells.[66]

Fig. 47. Ganglioneuromas cause lamina propria expansion by sheets of spindle cells with fibrillary cytoplasm and interspersed ganglion cells (H&E, original magnification ×400).

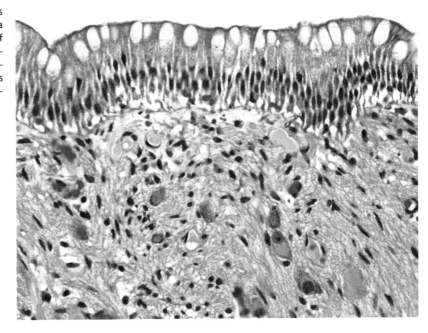

Differential Diagnosis

The differential diagnosis of ganglioneuroma includes gastrointestinal schwannomas, perineuriomas (benign fibroblastic polyp), and gangliocytic paragangliomas. The presence of ganglion cells excludes the first two tumors, although a small endoscopic biopsy may not demonstrate this diagnostic feature. Additional helpful features in schwannomas are the prominent lymphoid cuff, scattered backdrop of chronic inflammatory cells, and muscularis propria location. Perineuriomas expand the lamina propria similar to ganglioneuroma but stain with perineurial markers EMA, Glut1, and Claudin1 and also lack S-100 immunoreactivity. Differentiating ganglioneuromas from gangliocytic

Fig. 48. Sporadic ganglioneuromas are usually centered on the mucosa and expand the lamina propria, causing crypt distortion. Some examples may extend into the submucosa, involving the submucosal nerve plexus and take on a plexiform pattern, as in this case (H&E, original magnification ×40).

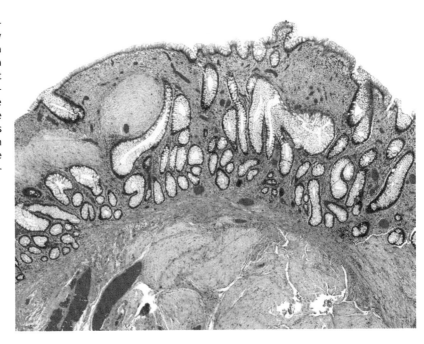

Differential Diagnosis
GANGLIONEUROMA

1. **Schwannoma:** this lesion typically arises in the muscularis propria, has a striking lymphoid cuff with a backdrop of intralesional chronic inflammatory cells, and lacks ganglion cells.

2. **Perineurioma (benign fibroblastic polyp):** although this lesion also expands the lamina propria with spindle cells, the cells are perineurial in nature and express EMA, Glut1, and Claudin1 and are nonreactive for S-100. Ganglion cells are not seen in perineurioma.

3. **Gangliocytic paraganglioma:** this lesion is triphasic, including spindle cells, ganglion cells, and nests of epithelioid cells that may be keratin positive.

paragangliomas requires the identification of nests of epithelioid cells that are seen in gangliocytic paragangliomas.

Prognosis

All forms of ganglioneuromas in the gastrointestinal tract are benign, but obstruction and hemorrhage may cause significant morbidity. Surgical excision is curative.

Diagnostic Algorithm

Diagnosis of this biphasic tumor requires adequate sampling such that the spindle cells and ganglion cells may be readily identified. Cases in which ganglion cells are sparse may benefit from NSE or synaptophysin immunostaining to aid in detection.

Pitfalls
GANGLIONEUROMA

! When ganglion cells are sparse, this lesion may be mistaken for schwannoma or perineurioma. Staining with NSE or synaptophysin may aid in detection of ganglion cells. Immunohistochemistry for S-100 and EMA also differentiates ganglioneuromas from perineuriomas.

REFERENCES

1. Miettinen M, Lasota J. Gastrointestinal stromal tumors: review on morphology, molecular pathology, prognosis, and differential diagnosis. Arch Pathol Lab Med 2006;130(10):1466–78.
2. Sarlomo-Rikala M, Kovatich AJ, Barusevicius A, et al. CD117: a sensitive marker for gastrointestinal stromal tumors that is more specific than CD34. Mod Pathol 1998;11(8):728–34.
3. Rubin BP, Heinrich MC, Corless CL. Gastrointestinal stromal tumour. Lancet 2007;369(9574):1731–41.
4. Miettinen M, Lasota J. Gastrointestinal stromal tumors—definition, clinical, histological, immunohistochemical, and molecular genetic features and differential diagnosis. Virchows Arch 2001;438(1):1–12.
5. Heinrich MC, Corless CL, Demetri GD, et al. Kinase mutations and imatinib response in patients with metastatic gastrointestinal stromal tumor. J Clin Oncol 2003;21(23):4342–9.
6. McWhinney SR, Pasini B, Stratakis CA. Familial gastrointestinal stromal tumors and germ-line mutations. N Engl J Med 2007;357(10):1054–6.
7. Medeiros F, Corless CL, Duensing A, et al. KIT-negative gastrointestinal stromal tumors: proof of concept and therapeutic implications. Am J Surg Pathol 2004;28(7):889–94.
8. Heinrich MC, Corless CL, Duensing A, et al. PDGFRA activating mutations in gastrointestinal stromal tumors. Science 2003;299(5607):708–10.
9. Hirota S, Isozaki K, Moriyama Y, et al. Gain-of-function mutations of c-kit in human gastrointestinal stromal tumors. Science 1998;279(5350):577–80.
10. Rubin BP, Singer S, Tsao C, et al. KIT activation is a ubiquitous feature of gastrointestinal stromal tumors. Cancer Res 2001;61(22):8118–21.
11. Lasota J, Corless CL, Heinrich MC, et al. Clinicopathologic profile of gastrointestinal stromal tumors (GISTs) with primary KIT exon 13 or exon 17 mutations: a multicenter study on 54 cases. Mod Pathol 2008;21(4):476–84.
12. Heinrich MC, Corless CL, Blanke CD, et al. Molecular correlates of imatinib resistance in gastrointestinal stromal tumors. J Clin Oncol 2006;24(29):4764–74.
13. Hornick JL, Fletcher CD. Immunohistochemical staining for KIT (CD117) in soft tissue sarcomas is very limited in distribution. Am J Clin Pathol 2002;117(2):188–93.
14. Miettinen M, Sobin LH, Sarlomo-Rikala M. Immunohistochemical spectrum of GISTs at different sites and their differential diagnosis with a reference to CD117 (KIT). Mod Pathol 2000;13(10):1134–42.
15. Miettinen M, Sobin LH, Lasota J. Gastrointestinal stromal tumors of the stomach: a clinicopathologic,

immunohistochemical, and molecular genetic study of 1765 cases with long-term follow-up. Am J Surg Pathol 2005;29(1):52–68.

16. Fletcher CD, Berman JJ, Corless C, et al. Diagnosis of gastrointestinal stromal tumors: a consensus approach. Hum Pathol 2002;33(5):459–65.

17. Miettinen M, Furlong M, Sarlomo-Rikala M, et al. Gastrointestinal stromal tumors, intramural leiomyomas, and leiomyosarcomas in the rectum and anus: a clinicopathologic, immunohistochemical, and molecular genetic study of 144 cases. Am J Surg Pathol 2001;25(9):1121–33.

18. Miettinen M, Shekitka KM, Sobin LH. Schwannomas in the colon and rectum: a clinicopathologic and immunohistochemical study of 20 cases. Am J Surg Pathol 2001;25(7):846–55.

19. Appelman HD, Helwig EB. Glomus tumors of the stomach. Cancer 1969;23(1):203–13.

20. Miettinen M, Paal E, Lasota J, et al. Gastrointestinal glomus tumors: a clinicopathologic, immunohistochemical, and molecular genetic study of 32 cases. Am J Surg Pathol 2002;26(3):301–11.

21. Fletcher CD, Kilpatrick SE, Mentzel T. The difficulty in predicting behavior of smooth-muscle tumors in deep soft tissue. Am J Surg Pathol 1995;19(1):116–7.

22. Miettinen M, Fetsch JF. Evaluation of biological potential of smooth muscle tumours. Histopathology 2006;48(1):97–105.

23. Weiss SW. Smooth muscle tumors of soft tissue. Adv Anat Pathol 2002;9(6):351–9.

24. Paal E, Miettinen M. Retroperitoneal leiomyomas: a clinicopathologic and immunohistochemical study of 56 cases with a comparison to retroperitoneal leiomyosarcomas. Am J Surg Pathol 2001;25(11):1355–63.

25. Miettinen M, Sarlomo-Rikala M, Sobin LH, et al. Esophageal stromal tumors: a clinicopathologic, immunohistochemical, and molecular genetic study of 17 cases and comparison with esophageal leiomyomas and leiomyosarcomas. Am J Surg Pathol 2000;24(2):211–22.

26. Miettinen M, Sarlomo-Rikala M, Sobin LH, et al. Gastrointestinal stromal tumors and leiomyosarcomas in the colon: a clinicopathologic, immunohistochemical, and molecular genetic study of 44 cases. Am J Surg Pathol 2000;24(10):1339–52.

27. Miettinen M, Sarlomo-Rikala M, Sobin LH. Mesenchymal tumors of muscularis mucosae of colon and rectum are benign leiomyomas that should be separated from gastrointestinal stromal tumors—a clinicopathologic and immunohistochemical study of eighty-eight cases. Mod Pathol 2001;14(10):950–6.

28. Ozolek JA, Sasatomi E, Swalsky PA, et al. Inflammatory fibroid polyps of the gastrointestinal tract: clinical, pathologic, and molecular characteristics.

Appl Immunohistochem Mol Morphol 2004;12(1):59–66.

29. Hasegawa T, Yang P, Kagawa N, et al. CD34 expression by inflammatory fibroid polyps of the stomach. Mod Pathol 1997;10(5):451–6.

30. Lasota J, Wang ZF, Sobin LH, et al. Gain-of-function PDGFRA mutations, earlier reported in gastrointestinal stromal tumors, are common in small intestinal inflammatory fibroid polyps. A study of 60 cases. Mod Pathol 2009;22(8):1049–56.

31. Schildhaus HU, Cavlar T, Binot E, et al. Inflammatory fibroid polyps harbour mutations in the platelet-derived growth factor receptor alpha (PDGFRA) gene. J Pathol 2008;216(2):176–82.

32. Groisman GM, Polak-Charcon S, Appelman HD. Fibroblastic polyp of the colon: clinicopathological analysis of 10 cases with emphasis on its common association with serrated crypts. Histopathology 2006;48(4):431–7.

33. Agaimy A, Stoehr R, Vieth M, et al. Benign serrated colorectal fibroblastic polyps/intramucosal perineuriomas are true mixed epithelial-stromal polyps (hybrid hyperplastic polyp/mucosal perineurioma) with frequent BRAF mutations. Am J Surg Pathol 2010;34(11):1663–71.

34. Eslami-Varzaneh F, Washington K, Robert ME, et al. Benign fibroblastic polyps of the colon: a histologic, immunohistochemical, and ultrastructural study. Am J Surg Pathol 2004;28(3):374–8.

35. Guler ML, Daniels JA, Abraham SC, et al. Expression of melanoma antigens in epithelioid gastrointestinal stromal tumors: a potential diagnostic pitfall. Arch Pathol Lab Med 2008;132(8):1302–6.

36. Agaimy A, Bihl MP, Tornillo L, et al. Calcifying fibrous tumor of the stomach: clinicopathologic and molecular study of seven cases with literature review and reappraisal of histogenesis. Am J Surg Pathol 2010;34(2):271–8.

37. Agaimy A, Wunsch PH, Hofstaedter F, et al. Minute gastric sclerosing stromal tumors (GIST tumorlets) are common in adults and frequently show c-KIT mutations. Am J Surg Pathol 2007;31(1):113–20.

38. Hill KA, Gonzalez-Crussi F, Chou PM. Calcifying fibrous pseudotumor versus inflammatory myofibroblastic tumor: a histological and immunohistochemical comparison. Mod Pathol 2001;14(8):784–90.

39. Chen TS, Montgomery EA. Are tumefactive lesions classified as sclerosing mesenteritis a subset of IgG4-related sclerosing disorders? J Clin Pathol 2008;61(10):1093–7.

40. Montgomery E, Torbenson MS, Kaushal M, et al. Beta-catenin immunohistochemistry separates mesenteric fibromatosis from gastrointestinal stromal tumor and sclerosing mesenteritis. Am J Surg Pathol 2002;26(10):1296–301.

41. Vlachos K, Archontovasilis F, Falidas E, et al. Sclerosing Mesenteritis: diverse clinical presentations

and dissimilar treatment options. A case series and review of the literature. Int Arch Med 2011;4(1):17.

42. Akram S, Pardi DS, Schaffner JA, et al. Sclerosing mesenteritis: clinical features, treatment, and outcome in ninety-two patients. Clin Gastroenterol Hepatol 2007;5(5):589–96 [quiz: 523–84].

43. Alman BA, Li C, Pajerski ME, et al. Increased beta-catenin protein and somatic APC mutations in sporadic aggressive fibromatoses (desmoid tumors). Am J Pathol 1997;151(2):329–34.

44. Miettinen M. Are desmoid tumors kit positive? Am J Surg Pathol 2001;25(4):549–50.

45. Burke AP, Sobin LH, Shekitka KM. Mesenteric fibromatosis. A follow-up study. Arch Pathol Lab Med 1990;114(8):832–5.

46. Burke AP, Sobin LH, Shekitka KM, et al. Intra-abdominal fibromatosis. A pathologic analysis of 130 tumors with comparison of clinical subgroups. Am J Surg Pathol 1990;14(4):335–41.

47. Coffin CM, Humphrey PA, Dehner LP. Extrapulmonary inflammatory myofibroblastic tumor: a clinical and pathological survey. Semin Diagn Pathol 1998; 15(2):85–101.

48. Hussong JW, Brown M, Perkins SL, et al. Comparison of DNA ploidy, histologic, and immunohistochemical findings with clinical outcome in inflammatory myofibroblastic tumors. Mod Pathol 1999;12(3):279–86.

49. Nishioka H, Shibuya M, Nakajima S, et al. A case of an intraventricular inflammatory pseudotumor presumably caused by Epstein-Barr virus infection. Surg Neurol 2009;71(6):685–8 [discussion: 688].

50. Coffin CM, Fletcher JA. Inflammatory myofibroblastic tumor. In: Fletcher CDM, Unni KK, Mertens F, editors. World Health Organization classification of tumors. Pathology and genetics of tumors of soft tissue and bone. Lyon: IARC Press; 2002. p. 91–3.

51. Coffin CM, Hornick JL, Fletcher CD. Inflammatory myofibroblastic tumor: comparison of clinicopathologic, histologic, and immunohistochemical features including ALK expression in atypical and aggressive cases. Am J Surg Pathol 2007;31(4):509–20.

52. Hisaoka M, Ishida T, Kuo TT, et al. Clear cell sarcoma of soft tissue: a clinicopathologic, immunohistochemical, and molecular analysis of 33 cases. Am J Surg Pathol 2008;32(3):452–60.

53. Enzinger FM. Clear-cell sarcoma of tendons and aponeuroses. An analysis of 21 cases. Cancer 1965;18:1163–74.

54. Kosemehmetoglu K, Folpe AL. Clear cell sarcoma of tendons and aponeuroses, and osteoclast-rich tumour of the gastrointestinal tract with features resembling clear cell sarcoma of soft parts: a review and update. J Clin Pathol 2010;63(5):416–23.

55. Fletcher CDM, Unni KK, Mertens F. World Health Organization, International Agency for Research on Cancer, International Academy of Pathology. Pathology and genetics of tumours of soft tissue and bone. Lyon (France): IARC Press; 2002.

56. Fanburg-Smith JC, Meis-Kindblom JM, Fante R, et al. Malignant granular cell tumor of soft tissue: diagnostic criteria and clinicopathologic correlation. Am J Surg Pathol 1998;22(7):779–94.

57. Lack EE, Worsham GF, Callihan MD, et al. Granular cell tumor: a clinicopathologic study of 110 patients. J Surg Oncol 1980;13(4):301–16.

58. Argani P, Lal P, Hutchinson B, et al. Aberrant nuclear immunoreactivity for TFE3 in neoplasms with TFE3 gene fusions: a sensitive and specific immunohistochemical assay. Am J Surg Pathol 2003;27(6):750–61.

59. Yoshizawa A, Ota H, Sakaguchi N, et al. Malignant granular cell tumor of the esophagus. Virchows Arch 2004;444(3):304–6.

60. Burke AP, Helwig EB. Gangliocytic paraganglioma. Am J Clin Pathol 1989;92(1):1–9.

61. Perrone T, Sibley RK, Rosai J. Duodenal gangliocytic paraganglioma. An immunohistochemical and ultrastructural study and a hypothesis concerning its origin. Am J Surg Pathol 1985;9(1):31–41.

62. Hironaka M, Fukayama M, Takayashiki N, et al. Pulmonary gangliocytic paraganglioma: case report and comparative immunohistochemical study of related neuroendocrine neoplasms. Am J Surg Pathol 2001;25(5):688–93.

63. Okubo Y, Wakayama M, Nemoto T, et al. Literature survey on epidemiology and pathology of gangliocytic paraganglioma. BMC Cancer 2011;11(1):187.

64. Thway K, Fisher C. Diffuse ganglioneuromatosis in small intestine associated with neurofibromatosis type 1. Ann Diagn Pathol 2009;13(1):50–4.

65. Shekitka KM, Sobin LH. Ganglioneuromas of the gastrointestinal tract. Relation to Von Recklinghausen disease and other multiple tumor syndromes. Am J Surg Pathol 1994;18(3):250–7.

66. d'Amore ES, Manivel JC, Pettinato G, et al. Intestinal ganglioneuromatosis: mucosal and transmural types. A clinicopathologic and immunohistochemical study of six cases. Hum Pathol 1991;22(3):276–86.

LIPOSARCOMAS

Aatur D. Singhi, MD, PhD[a],*, Elizabeth A. Montgomery, MD[b]

KEYWORDS

- Liposarcoma • Atypical lipomatous tumor/Well-differentiated liposarcoma • Dedifferentiated LPS
- Myxoid/Round cell LPS • Pleomorphic LPS • Mixed-type LPS

ABSTRACT

Liposarcoma is a common soft tissue sarcoma and represents a group of neoplasms, each with distinct clinical behavior and pathologic findings. Proper classification is critical for clinical management and prognostication. Until recently, immunohistochemistry played a limited role in diagnosis of these tumors. Increased understanding of the underlying genetic basis of disease has paved the way for development of improved tools for diagnosis and new forms of targeted therapy. This article summarizes the clinical, pathologic, and molecular findings of the main liposarcoma subtypes. Special attention to the differential diagnosis and difficulties the pathologist may face when interpreting these lesions is discussed.

OVERVIEW

Liposarcoma (LPS) is a malignant mesenchymal neoplasm demonstrating fat differentiation. It is one of the most common malignant soft tissue tumors, accounting for 20% of all adult sarcomas. Since the first histologic description by Rudolph Virchow in 1857,[1] the classification and nomenclature of LPS has gone through multiple revisions. The most recent World Health Organization classification of soft tissue tumors recognizes the following 5 categories[2]:

1. atypical lipomatous tumor/well-differentiated LPS, which includes the lipomalike, sclerosing, inflammatory, and spindle cell subtypes
2. dedifferentiated LPS
3. myxoid/round cell LPS
4. pleomorphic LPS
5. mixed-type LPS

With recent advances, however, it is becoming increasingly apparent that the so-called mixed-type LPS likely does not exist as a discrete entity, but rather a variety of unusual morphologic changes within one of the better-defined LPS subtypes. Regardless, each of the subtypes of LPS has distinct clinical, morphologic, and cytogenetic features. Consequently, distinguishing between the different types of LPS is more than of merely academic interest, but has important ramifications for determining metastatic potential, overall prognosis, and possible treatment strategies.

ATYPICAL LIPOMATOUS TUMOR/WELL-DIFFERENTIATED LIPOSARCOMA

OVERVIEW

Atypical lipomatous tumor (ALT)/well-differentiated liposarcoma (WDLPS), represents 40% to 45% of all LPS, and, thus, is the most common form of malignant adipocytic neoplasms. These tumors occur almost exclusively in adults with a peak incidence between the ages of 50 and 70 years and has a male predominance. Patients frequently present with a deep-seated, painless, slowly growing lesion. These tumors typically arise in the proximal lower extremities, especially the thigh, followed by the retroperitoneum, abdominal cavity, paratesticular region, and mediastinum. Less commonly involved sites include the head and neck and proximal upper extremities. Because of the anatomic location of the tumors,

[a] Department of Pathology, The Johns Hopkins Medical Institutions, 401 North Broadway, Weinberg 2247, Baltimore, MD 21231-2410, USA
[b] Department of Pathology, The Johns Hopkins Medical Institutions, 401 North Broadway, Weinberg 2242, Baltimore, MD 21231-2410, USA
* Corresponding author.
E-mail address: asinghi1@jhmi.edu

Surgical Pathology 4 (2011) 963–994
doi:10.1016/j.path.2011.08.011
1875-9181/11/$ – see front matter

Key Features
ATYPICAL LIPOMATOUS TUMOR/
WELL-DIFFERENTIATED LIPOSARCOMA

1. Four main histologic patterns are recognized: lipomalike, sclerosing, inflammatory, and spindle cell, which may overlap and coexist within the same lesion.

2. The lipomalike subtype is composed of atypical adipocytes and stromal cells that demonstrate marked variation in size and shape.

3. Sclerosing ALT/WDLPS contains scattered bizarre stromal cells with hyperchromatic nuclei set in a collagenous background.

4. A dense lymphoplasmacytic infiltrate, superimposed on lipomalike and/or sclerosing subtypes, characterizes inflammatory ALT/WDLPS.

5. The spindle cell subtype exhibits bland, neural-like spindle cells admixed with atypical, mainly univacuolated adipocytes.

6. ALT/WDLPS demonstrates supernumerary ring and/or giant chromosomes containing the q13-15 subregion of chromosome 12. Consequently, these tumors overexpress nuclear MDM2 and CDK4, which can be detected by immunohistochemistry.

patients often remain asymptomatic until the tumors reach a very large size.[3–5] Subcutaneous lesions also occur and are synonymously referred to as ALT or "atypical lipoma." ALTs are fundamentally the same tumor as their deep counterparts, indistinguishable by both histology and cytogenetics; however, the clinical behavior of these superficial tumors is sufficiently different that they are considered a separate group.[6,7]

GROSS FEATURES

On gross inspection, ALT/WDLPS is usually large, particularly when arising within the retroperitoneum and commonly exceeds 20 cm. The tumors are well circumscribed and demonstrate a lobular growth pattern. Their cut surface is soft and a paler yellow color as compared with the adjacent normal fat or a lipoma. In addition, the tumor often shows prominent, fibrous septal bands, imparting a firmer texture than that observed in lipomas. Larger lesions can have a more heterogeneous appearance, containing gelatinous or myxoid areas, fat necrosis, and focal hemorrhage.

MICROSCOPIC FEATURES

ALT/WDLPS can be subdivided into 4 main histologic patterns: lipomalike, sclerosing, inflammatory, and spindle cell. Multiple patterns may overlap and coexist within the same lesion. The distinction among these patterns is of limited clinical and prognostic importance, but their recognition will aid in the diagnosis. Common to all subtypes is the low to moderate cellularity, and relative lack of mitotic activity, consistent with a low-grade sarcoma.

The lipomalike ALT/WDLPS is the most common subtype, and is the predominant pattern in subcutaneous lesions and is at least focally present in deep-seated tumors. It is composed of a variable number of atypical adipocytes that exhibit marked variation in cell size and shape. The nuclei are enlarged, hyperchromatic, and prominent, even at low magnification (Figs. 1 and 2). In addition, there are often scattered atypical stromal cells embedded within fibrous septa (Fig. 3), as well as occasional floretlike multinucleated cells. Lipoblasts containing one or more cytoplasmic vacuoles and a hyperchromatic, scalloped nucleus may be present, particularly near fibrous septa, but are not required for the diagnosis (Fig. 4). Focal areas of fat necrosis and cellular infiltration by clusters of macrophages and lymphocytes are also common.

The sclerosing variant occurs most frequently in the retroperitoneum and paratesticular region. Microscopically, the tumor is dominated by a fibrillary collagenous background containing scattered bizarre stromal cells with hyperchromatic nuclei and rare lipoblasts (Figs. 5 and 6). Adipose tissue may be difficult to identify in some sections but should be present in at least some portion of the neoplasm.

Inflammatory ALT/WDLPS is seen in the retroperitoneum, head and neck, trunk, and thigh.[8,9] It is composed of a prominent lymphoplasmacytic infiltrate within a background of lipomalike and/or sclerosing ALT/WDLPS (Fig. 7). The inflammatory infiltrate can exhibit germinal center formation with clusters or sheets of plasma cells. In some instances, the inflammation can be exuberant, obscuring the adipocytic nature of the lesion (Fig. 8). The identification of atypical adipocytes, bizarre stromal cells, or lipoblasts are key diagnostic clues in establishing the diagnosis.

The spindle cell variant is rare and tends to occur in the subcutaneous tissues of the extremities, trunk, and the head and neck.[10] The spindle cells are bland, neural-like, and arranged in short, parallel fascicles. Atypical, univacuolar adipocytes

Fig. 1. Lipomalike ALT/WDLPS. (*A*) The tumor exhibits scattered atypical cells with enlarged hyperchromatic nuclei that are readily apparent at low magnification. (*B, C*) At higher magnification, the cells are identified as atypical adipocytes with variation in both size and shape. (Hematoxylin-eosin [H&E], original magnification *A*, ×40; *B*, ×100; *C*, ×400.)

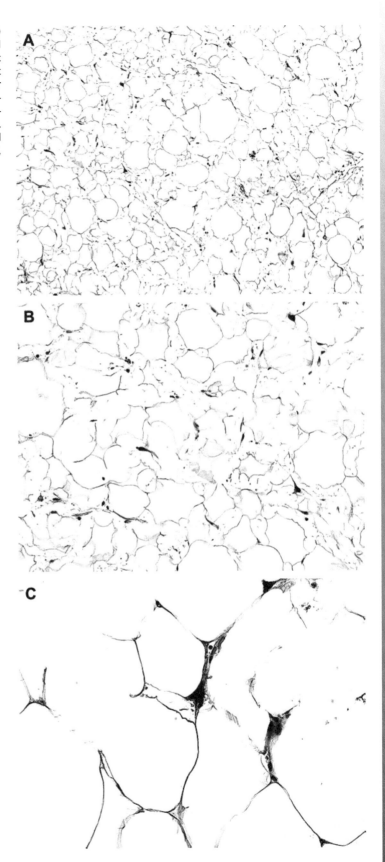

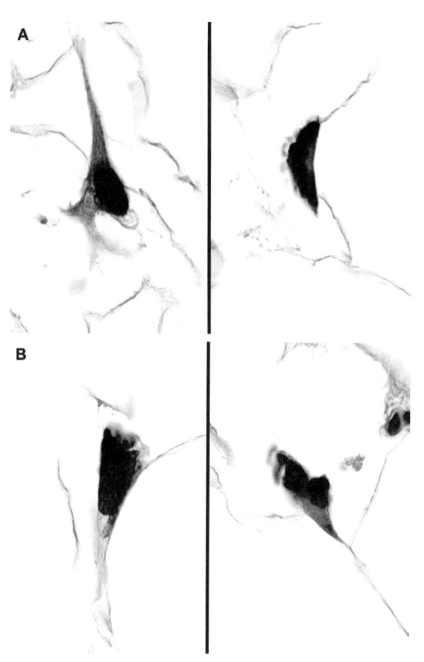

Fig. 2. Lipomalike ALT/ WDLPS. (*A, B*) Atypical adipocytes show a wide variety of appearances, common to which is nuclear enlargement and hyperchromasia (H&E, original magnification ×1000).

Fig. 3. Lipomalike ALT/WDLPS. Expanded fibrous tissue septa containing atypical stromal cells are a common finding (H&E, original magnification ×200).

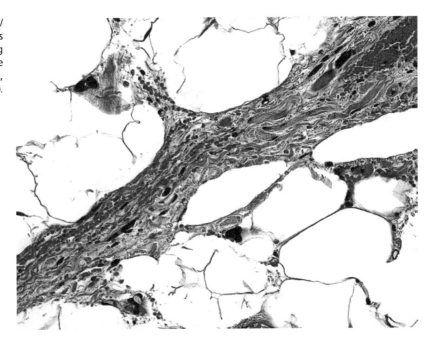

and prominent capillaries are interspersed among the spindle cells (**Fig. 9**).

Of note, in rare instances, heterologous differentiation within ALT/WDLPS can occur and includes smooth[11] and striated muscle, cartilage, and bone. This should not be mistaken for heterologous differentiation arising in a dedifferentiated liposarcoma.

Fig. 4. Lipomalike ALT/WDLPS. Although not required for the diagnosis, lipoblasts containing one or more vacuoles, and a hyperchromatic, scalloped nucleus may be seen (H&E, original magnification ×1000).

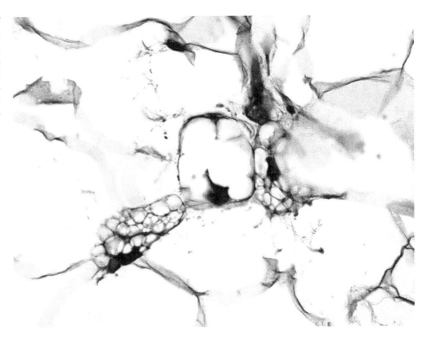

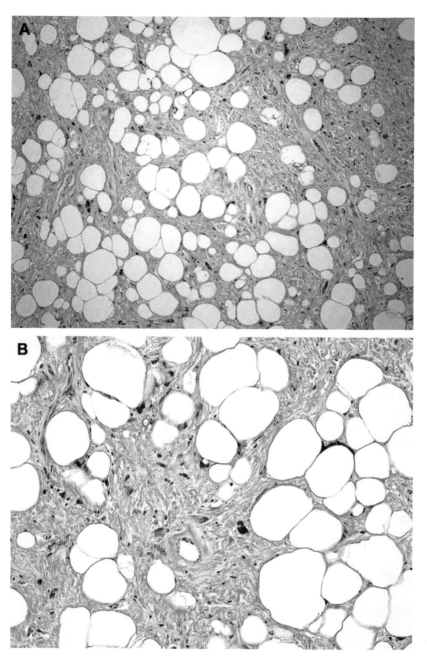

Fig. 5. Sclerosing ALT/WDLPS. (A, B) Atypical, mildly pleomorphic cells are embedded within a background of dense fibrillary, collagenous matrix and intervening mature adipocytes (H&E, original magnification A, ×200; B, ×400).

ANCILLARY STUDIES

Cytogenetically, ALT/WDLPS characteristically harbors supernumerary ring and/or giant chromosomes (Fig. 10). These chromosomes are composed of amplicons of the 12q13-15 chromosomal subregion, resulting in amplification of several genes, including MDM2 and CDK4 (Fig. 11A).[12,13] Immunohistochemical detection of the resulting overexpressed proteins is a reliable method to distinguish ALT/WDLPS from other soft tissue tumors (see Fig. 11B).[14]

Fig. 6. Sclerosing ALT/WDLPS. (A) In some cases, the fibrillary, collagenous stroma can be a dominating feature, obscuring the adipocytic nature of the neoplasm. (B) However, rare areas exhibiting lipogenic differentiation with atypical adipocytes can be invariably found and aid in the diagnosis (H&E, original magnification ×400).

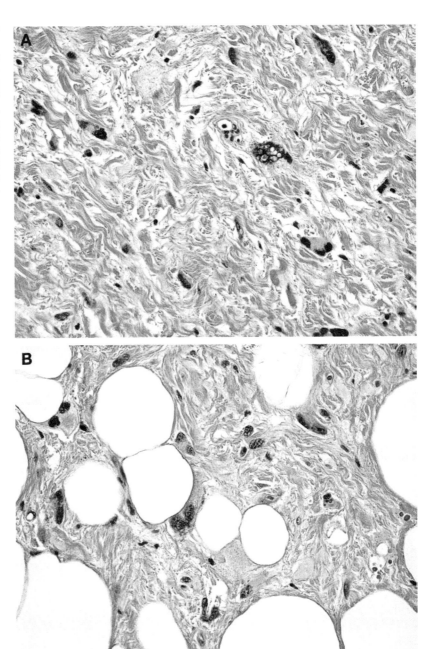

DIFFERENTIAL DIAGNOSIS

The differential diagnosis primarily includes soft tissue lipomas and its variants, especially spindle cell and pleomorphic lipoma, silicone granuloma, lymphedema in the morbidly obese, and sclerosing extramedullary hematopoietic tumor.

Although soft tissue lipomas tend to be small and superficial, larger lesions can occur and are typically deep-seated and intra-abdominal. Unlike ALT/WDLPS, lipomas are surrounded by a thin collagenous pseudocapsule and composed of mature adipocytes that lack cytologic atypia and hyperchromasia. A potential pitfall is a lipoma

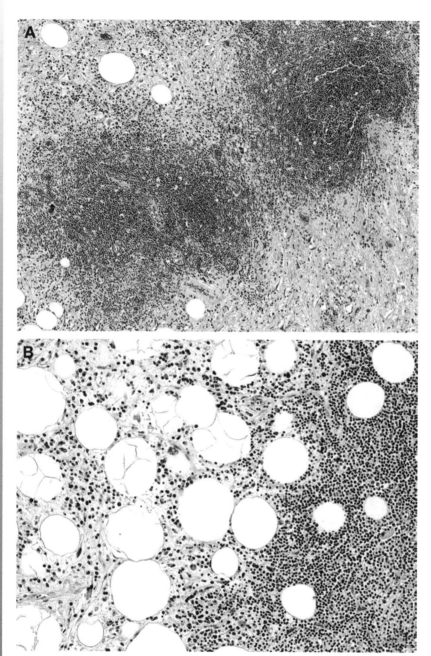

Fig. 7. Inflammatory ALT/ WDLPS. The neoplasm is composed of a prominent lymphoplasmacytic infiltrate set within a background of (*A*) sclerosing and/or (*B*) lipomalike ALT/ WDLPS. (H&E, original magnification *A*, ×100; *B*, ×200.)

with associated fat necrosis. It often involves large areas of tissue and is characterized by adipocyte shrinkage and dropout, mononuclear infiltrate, macrophages, and sometimes sclerosis. In some instances, the foamy macrophages may be mistaken for lipoblasts. A useful aid in distinguishing fat necrosis from ALT/WDLPS is to scan the lesion at low magnification. The atypical nuclei of the latter are hyperchromatic and stand out as compared with macrophages; however, with thick histologic sections, the nuclei of macrophages may overlap, giving the

Fig. 8. Inflammatory ALT/WDLPS. (A) The dense lymphoplasmacytic infiltrate can be exuberant, masking the atypical adipocytes within the lesion. (B) The identification of atypical adipocytes, bizarre stromal cells, or lipoblasts are key diagnostic clues. (H&E, original magnification A, ×200; B, ×400).

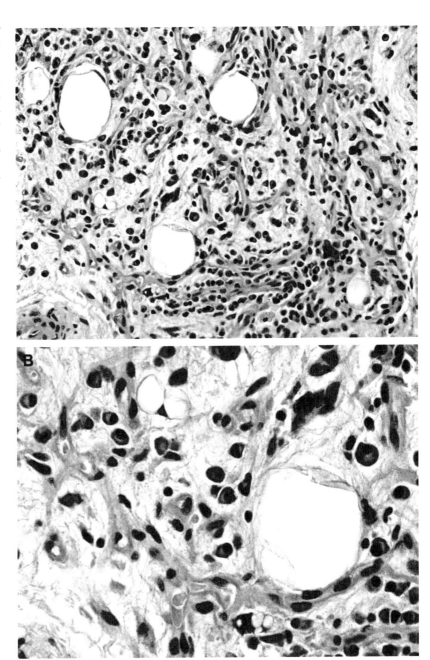

impression of hyperchromasia. In addition, "loch-kern" cells or adipocytes with artifactual intranuclear lipid invagination and nuclear enlargement (but not hyperchromasia) are more likely to be encountered in thicker sections. Therefore, thinly cut histologic sections are important when making such distinctions. In difficult cases, however, immunohistochemical stains for MDM2 or CDK4 can be useful.

Spindle cell and pleomorphic lipoma are morphologically and cytogenetically related lesions. They are composed of a mixture of bland spindle cells (spindle cell lipoma) and multinucleated floretlike giant cells (pleomorphic lipoma).

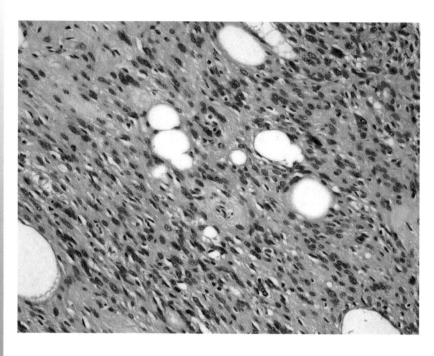

Fig. 9. Spindle cell ALT/WDLPS. Bland spindle cells arranged in short, parallel fascicles with interspersed, atypical adipocytes (H&E, original magnification ×200). (*Courtesy of* Drs C Fisher, K Thway, Department of Histopathology, Royal Marsden Hospital, London, UK; with permission.)

Although the pleomorphic cells are indistinguishable from those encountered in ALT/WDLPS, they lack MDM2 or CDK4 alterations, and feature a "ropelike" collagenous background.

The engulfing histiocytes, owing to leakage of synthetic compounds, such as silicone gel in mammary implants, are reminiscent of lipoblasts, especially because silicone gel does not consistently polarize. At scanning magnification, however, the nuclei of histiocytes differs from those of ALT/WDLPS in being small, uniform, and pale. Similar to fat necrosis, analysis of thicker

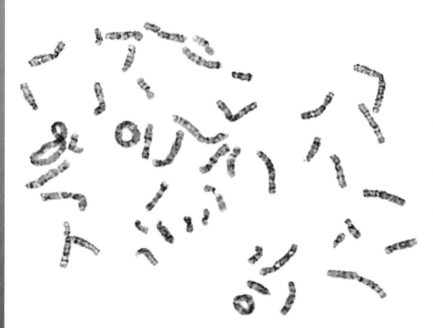

Fig. 10. ALT/WDLPS. Supernumerary ring and giant chromosomes containing amplicons of the q13-15 subregion of chromosome 12 are often found in Giemsa-stained metaphase spreads of ALT/WDLPS. (*Courtesy of* Dr PD Cin, C McLaughlin, Center for Advanced Molecular Diagnostics, Brigham and Women's Hospital, Boston, MA; with permission.)

Fig. 11. ALT/WDLPS. (*A*) Detection of *MDM2* amplification by FISH (MDM2 in red and chromosome 12 in green) and (*B*) nuclear protein overexpression by immunohistochemistry are useful ancillary diagnostic tools to distinguish ALT/WDLPS from their morphologic mimickers (*B*, MDM2 immunostain, original magnification ×400). (*FISH courtesy of Dr PD Cin, C McLaughlin, Center for Advanced Molecular Diagnostics, Brigham and Women's Hospital, Boston, MA; with permission.*)

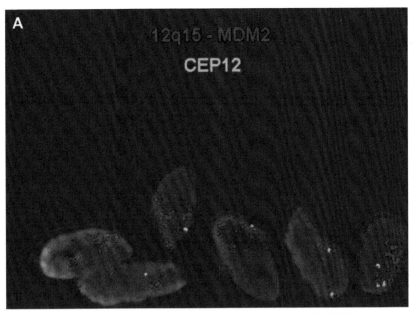

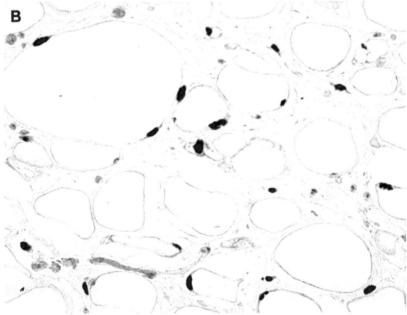

sections may prove challenging with overlapping histiocyte nuclei. In these cases, CD68 immunostaining can be helpful.

Localized massive lymphedema develops in the proximal extremities and is characterized by the presence of fibrous septa containing multinucleated fibroblastic cells. Careful examination of lymphedema will show the absence of atypical adipocytes, hyperchromatic stromal cells, and lipoblasts. Gross examination is also valuable, as in contrast to ALT/WDLPS, lymphedema lacks a discrete mass.

Patients with chronic myeloproliferative disorders occasionally develop tumorlike deposits of extramedullary hematopoiesis, termed sclerosing extramedullary hematopoietic tumor.[15] Their tendency to arise in the retroperitoneum, and display large hyperchromatic cells (megakaryocytes)

Differential Diagnosis
ATYPICAL LIPOMATOUS TUMOR/ WELL-DIFFERENTIATED LIPOSARCOMA

- Lipoma
- Spindle cell and pleomorphic lipoma
- Silicone granuloma
- Lymphedema in the morbidly obese
- Sclerosing extramedullary hematopoietic tumor

and fibrous bands, causes them to be mistaken for ALT/WDLPS. The distinction is aided by the presence of other hematopoietic elements, including erythroid and myeloid cells. Immunostaining of megakaryocytes with Factor VIII–related antigen or CD61 can also be helpful, especially in crushed needle biopsies.

PROGNOSIS

The prognosis and treatment of ALT/WDLPS is primarily dependent on its anatomic location. Subcutaneous lesions or ALT are adequately treated with wide surgical excision. Local recurrence is rare to nonexistent when clear margins

are achieved. In contrast, deep-seated WDLPS has a local recurrence of 43% in the limbs, 79% in the paratesticular region, and 91% in the retroperitoneum.[16] The rates of recurrence are most likely higher because of the inability to obtain negative margins and are responsible for a mortality rate of 14%.[16,17] In these cases, radiation and/or chemotherapy may be used as an adjunct to surgery.

ALT/WDLPS has no metastatic potential unless dedifferentiation occurs. The risk of dedifferentiation is also dependent on anatomic site with 5% in ALT and up to 28% in retroperitoneal WDLPS.[6,16,17] As is discussed in the next section, dedifferentiation is associated with increased overall mortality.

DEDIFFERENTIATED LIPOSARCOMA

OVERVIEW

Dedifferentiated liposarcoma (DDLPS) is defined as a malignant adipocytic neoplasm with transition from ALT/WDLPS to nonlipogenic sarcoma of variable histologic grade. It develops in the same age and gender predilection as patients with ALT/WDLPS. The retroperitoneum is the most common site of involvement, followed by the extremities,

Pitfalls
ATYPICAL LIPOMATOUS TUMOR/ WELL-DIFFERENTIATED LIPOSARCOMA

! The major pitfalls are mimickers of atypical adipocytes and stromal cells of ALT/WDLPS.

! Lochkern cells are typically found in thickly cut sections of adipose tissue and may be mistaken for atypical adipocytes. Although they exhibit intranuclear lipid invagination and nuclear enlargement, they lack hyperchromasia.

! Fat necrosis features adipocyte shrinkage and dropout, an inflammatory infiltrate, macrophages, and sclerosis.

! In some instances, the macrophages found in fat necrosis or in reaction to silicone may be mistaken for lipoblasts; however, hyperchromatic nuclei are absent.

! Multinucleated fibroblasts, as those present in lymphedema or even megakaryocytes in extramedullary hematopoiesis, can be confused with the atypical stromal cells of ALT/WDLPS.

Key Features
DEDIFFERENTIATED LIPOSARCOMA

1. DDLPS is characterized by the abrupt, gradual, or admixed transition from ALT/WDLPS to a nonlipogenic sarcoma.

2. The nonlipogenic component shows broad variation, but often overlaps with high-grade pleomorphic sarcoma or myxofibrosarcoma.

3. Low-grade dedifferentiation occurs in a minority of cases and is characterized by uniform spindle cells with mild nuclear atypia.

4. Heterologous differentiation, along skeletal muscle, smooth muscle, cartilage, bone, or vascular lineage can occur in approximately 10% of cases.

5. Rarely, meningothelial-like whorls may be identified and are often associated with metaplastic bone formation.

6. Retains the supernumerary ring and/or giant chromosomes of ALT/WDLPS, and consequently overexpresses MDM2 and CDK4.

Fig. 12. DDLPS. The transition from ALT/WDLPS *(left)* to a dedifferentiated nonlipogenic sarcoma *(right)* can be abrupt *(A)*, gradual *(B)*, or rarely, a diffuse admixture (H&E, original magnification ×100).

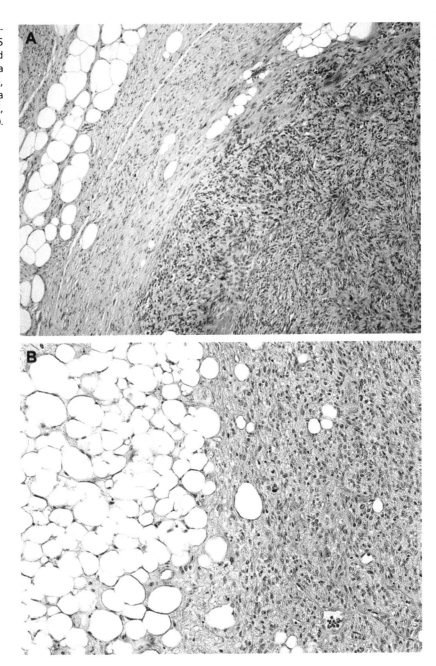

paratesticular region, and head and neck.[18,19] Dedifferentiation occurs in up to 10% of ALT/WDLPS cases, although there is a greater risk in deep-seated lesions as compared with the extremities.[7] In addition, it is more frequently found in the primary tumor (90%) than in local recurrences (10%).[5]

GROSS FEATURES

Grossly, dedifferentiation appears white to tan and firmer than the neighboring pale, yellow ALT/WDLPS. In addition, yellow to green zones of necrosis may be observed.

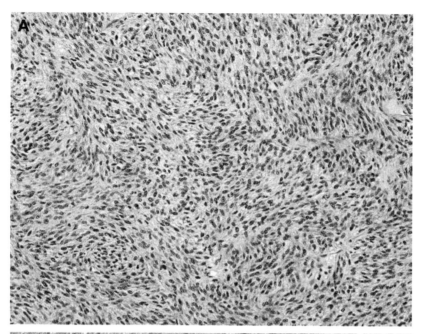

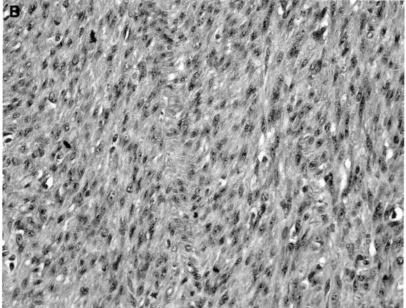

Fig. 13. DDLPS. The dedifferentiated component is that of high-grade sarcoma, often resembling malignant fibrous histiocytoma. The tumor cells demonstrate a variety of morphologic patterns, including storiform (*A*) and fascicular (*B*) arrangements. (H&E, original magnification *A*, ×200; *B*, ×400.)

MICROSCOPIC FEATURES

Histologically, the transition from ALT/WDLPS to nonlipogenic sarcoma is often abrupt; however, in rare cases, this may be gradual, or the 2 components may even be found as a diffuse admixture (Fig. 12). The extent of dedifferentiation can range from a minor to an overwhelming dominant component. In fact, there is no minimal amount of nonlipogenic sarcoma that must be present to be classified as DDLPS. The histologic patterns

Fig. 14. DDLPS. (*A, B*) The tumor cells tend to be characterized by a high degree of nuclear atypia including pleomorphism, multinucleation, and bizarre mitoses (H&E, original magnification ×400).

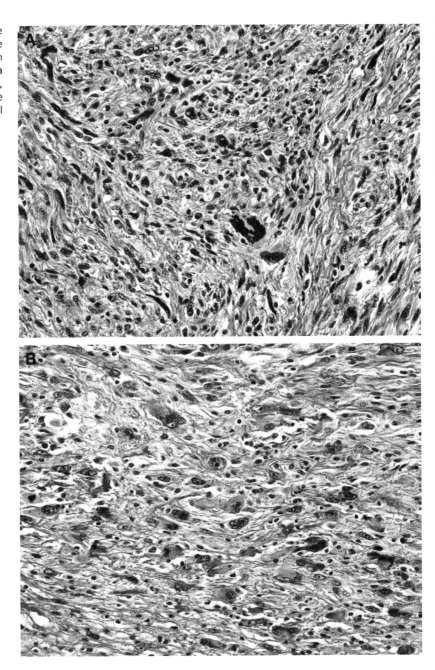

encountered are variable, but often overlap with high-grade pleomorphic sarcoma or myxofibrosarcoma (**Figs. 13–15**). A minority of DDLPS show low-grade dedifferentiation, characterized by uniform spindle cells with mild nuclear atypia and organized in a vaguely fascicular growth pattern (**Fig. 16**).[18,20] In such cases, necrosis is typically absent and the lesion exhibits lower cellularity than high-grade variants.

Approximately 10% of cases demonstrate heterologous differentiation, which is more often rhabdomyosarcomatous, osteosarcomatous/chondrosarcomatous (**Fig. 17**), leiomyosarcomatous (**Fig. 18**), or rarely, angiosarcomatous.[19] A

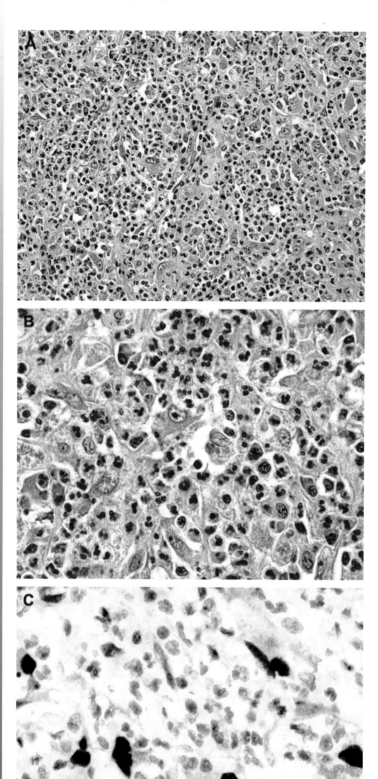

Fig. 15. DDLPS. (A, B) A subset of cases show a dense inflammatory infiltrate of neutrophils and eosinophils among scattered larger pleomorphic tumor cells with prominent nucleoli. In the past, such neoplasms were often classified as inflammatory malignant fibrous histiocytoma (H&E, original magnification A, ×200; B, ×400). (C) Nuclear immunoreactivity for MDM2 has proven to be helpful in establishing the correct diagnosis (C, MDM2 immunostain, original magnification ×400).

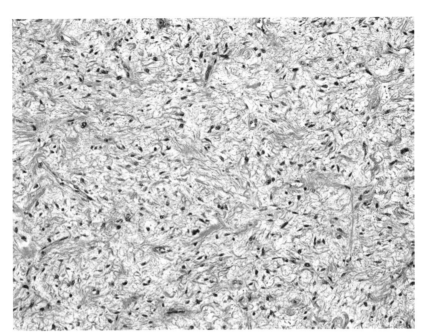

Fig. 16. DDLPS. A minority of cases show low-grade dedifferentiation similar to that of fibromatosis or low-grade fibrosarcoma. These tumors show uniform fibroblastic spindle cells with mild nuclear atypia (H&E, original magnification ×200).

small subset of cases may exhibit meningothelial-like whorls consisting of concentric perivascular proliferation of spindle to oval cells with minor atypia (**Fig. 19**). This pattern is usually in association with metaplastic bone formation and is actually of myofibroblastic, not meningothelial, differentiation.[21,22] Although it is important to recognize these patterns can occur in DDLPS so as to avoid misdiagnosing these lesions as a high-grade sarcoma, they do not appear to be prognostically significant.[23]

ANCILLARY STUDIES

Although DDLPS may demonstrate a complex cytogenetic profile, similar to those found in high-grade pleomorphic sarcomas, they are genetically related to ALT/WDLPS. Both DDLPS and ALT/WDLPS exhibit supernumerary ring and/or giant chromosomes containing 12q13-15 elements.[19] In addition, nuclear MDM2 and CDK4 overexpression can be detected by immunohistochemistry (see **Figs. 15**C and **17**B) and, thus, is a helpful aid in the differential diagnosis of DDLPS and other high-grade sarcomas.[23–25]

DIFFERENTIAL DIAGNOSIS

The diagnosis of DDLPS can be straightforward in cases where ALT/WDLPS is found adjacent to a high-grade sarcoma, but in cases with limited sampling and the presence of heterologous differentiation, distinguishing between DDLPS and high-grade sarcoma can be challenging. Thorough sampling and special attention to possible lipomatous elements can aid in the diagnosis of DDLPS. Correlation with radiologic studies are also often helpful in pinpointing a lipomatous component in an undifferentiated sarcoma. Furthermore, high-grade sarcomas arising in anatomic sites common to DDLPS, particularly the retroperitoneum, should prompt consideration of an adipocytic neoplasm. Previous studies have shown that retroperitoneal sarcomas originally diagnosed as malignant fibrous histiocytoma were found to be DDLPS on reevaluation.[26,27] In addition, MDM2 and CDK4 overexpression have proven to be useful in discriminating between DDLPS and other sarcomas.[25]

△△ ***Differential Diagnosis***
DEDIFFERENTIATED LIPOSARCOMA

- Other high-grade sarcomas
- Spindle cell ALT/WDLPS

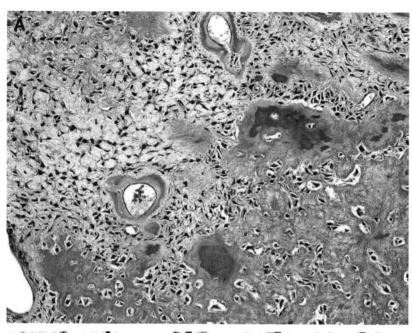

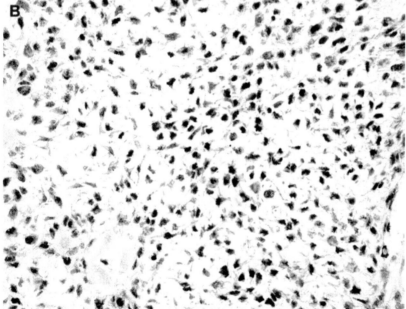

Fig. 17. DDLPS. In some cases, osteosarcomatous differentiation can occur (*A*) (H&E, original magnification ×200) and retains MDM2 nuclear immunostaining (*B*) (MDM2 immunostain, original magnification ×200).

Spindle cell ALT/WDLPS should also be included in the differential diagnosis, especially for low-grade DDLPS. Indeed, in cases of limited sampling and the appreciation that well-differentiated and dedifferentiated components may comingle, the histopathology of low-grade DDLPS can be indistinguishable from spindle cell ALT/WDLPS. However, low-grade DDLPS is considerably more cellular and atypical.

PROGNOSIS

DDLPS is more aggressive than ALT/WDLPS, but less than other high-grade pleomorphic sarcomas.

Fig. 18. DDLPS. Heterologous differentiation can take the form of smooth muscle. In this case, the neoplasm is arranged in perpendicular fascicles containing eosinophilic cytoplasm, perinuclear vacuoles, and pleomorphic nuclei with increased mitotic activity, reminiscent of a leiomyosarcoma (H&E, original magnification ×400).

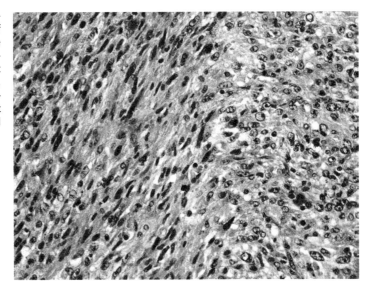

Fig. 19. DDLPS. (*A*) A rare finding is the presence of meningiothelial-like whorls found in nonlipogenic areas. (*B*) These typically consist of a concentric proliferation of spindle to oval cells (H&E, original magnification *A*, ×100; *B*, ×400).

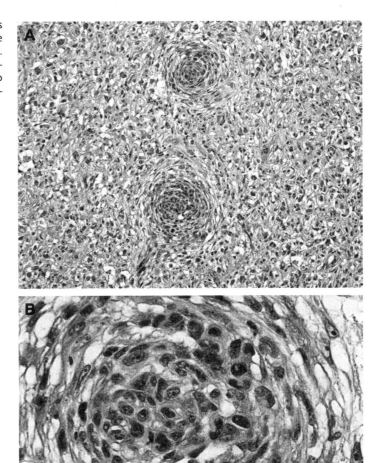

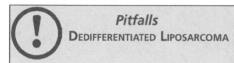

Pitfalls
DEDIFFERENTIATED LIPOSARCOMA

! If the lipogenic component is not abundant, DDLPS can be difficult to distinguish from other high-grade sarcomas. A thorough evaluation of the gross specimen with special attention to possible lipomatous areas is imperative; however, with limited material, such as needle biopsies, MDM2 immunostaining is useful.

! Heterologous differentiation can be challenging. DDLPS should always be considered in the differential diagnosis, especially when dealing with a high-grade sarcoma arising in anatomic sites common to DDLPS.

Key Features
MYXOID LIPOSARCOMA/ROUND CELL LIPOSARCOMA

1. MLPS is composed of small spindled to oval mesenchymal cells and scattered to numerous lipoblasts.

2. The background consists of a copious myxoid matrix and delicately, arborizing, thin-walled capillaries (referred to as "chicken-wire" or "crow's feet").

3. Progression to RCLPS is characterized by hypercellular cords, nests, or sheets of round cells with high nuclear to cytoplasmic ratio, nuclear overlap, and a prominent nucleolus.

4. Most cases show features of both MLPS and RCLPS, where the tumor is hypercellular, but the cells remain spindled, the vascular pattern is still discernible, and at least some myxoid stroma is present.

5. MLPS and RCLPS are characterized by the presence of t(12;16) and, less commonly, t(12;22) reciprocal translocations.

It has a strong tendency to recur locally with an overall rate of 41%.[18] As with ALT/WDLPS, anatomic location is the most important prognostic factor, with retroperitoneal lesions exhibiting essentially 100% local recurrence and invariably leading to death. Distant metastases, which most commonly affect the lungs, liver, and bone, are seen in 15% to 20% of cases; however, mortality is more related to uncontrolled local recurrences than to metastatic spread. The overall 5-year survival rate varies from 28% to 30%, but is probably much higher at 10 to 20 years. In addition, the extent of dedifferentiation does not seem to affect the clinical outcome.[18,28]

Standard treatment is wide surgical excision with negative margins. Adjuvant radiation and/or chemotherapy should also be considered, depending on the anatomic location. The recent development of specific small molecule MDM2 antagonists, such as Nutlin-3a, show promising results and could enhance conventional chemotherapy regimens.[29,30]

MYXOID AND ROUND CELL LIPOSARCOMA

OVERVIEW

Myxoid liposarcoma (MLPS) and its high-grade variant, round cell liposarcoma (RCLPS), are considered 2 ends of a histologic spectrum for the same neoplasm. These tumors are the second most common LPS and account for 30% to 40% of cases. They are also the most common form of LPS in children. MLPS/RCLPS typically presents in young to middle-aged adults with a peak incidence between 30 and 50 years and affects both sexes equally. It often arises as a large painless mass in the deep soft tissues of the extremities, particularly the thigh or popliteal fossa, and rarely, in the retroperitoneum or abdomen.[5,31,32]

GROSS FEATURES

MLPS/RCLPS is usually a large (>10 cm), well-circumscribed, lobular lesion. MLPS has a gelatinous, jellylike cut surface, whereas RCLPS has a gray-white, fleshy appearance. Multiple red-tinged foci are also present and correspond to areas of high vascularity.

MICROSCOPIC FEATURES

At low magnification, MLPS has a nodular growth pattern of bland fusiform to oval mesenchymal cells. The cells are arranged in cords and clusters with increased cellularity at the periphery of tumor lobules. The background consists of a copious myxoid matrix and numerous delicately branching, thin-walled capillaries (**Fig. 20**). The organization of the vessels is often referred to as a "chicken-wire" or "crow's feet" configuration. Scattered to numerous, small lipoblasts are present, and tend to cluster around vessels and at the periphery of the lesion (**Fig. 21**). Frequently, there is pooling of stromal mucin, resulting in large cystic

Fig. 20. MLPS. (*A*) The tumor is arranged in a nodular growth pattern and composed of uniform spindle cells and small, vacuolated lipoblasts. (*B*) The presence of a rich myxoid matrix and prominent, plexiform capillary network are diagnostic hallmarks of this lesion (H&E, original magnification ×100).

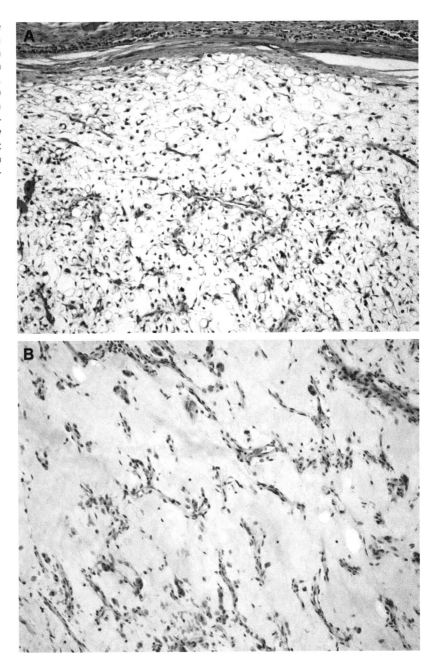

spaces, imparting a lymphangiomalike appearance (Fig. 22). Chondroid differentiation has also been described.

On the other end of the histologic spectrum, RCLPS is characterized by a marked increase in cellularity with a perivascular distribution. The tumor forms cords, nests, or solid sheets of round cells that exhibit a high nuclear to cytoplasmic ratio, nuclear overlap, and a prominent nucleolus (Fig. 23). In these areas, the mitotic index is generally increased, and the vascular pattern can be difficult to recognize secondary to the overgrowth of round cells. Usually small foci of MLPS can be identified to aid in the diagnosis (Fig. 24); however, the threshold as to when an MLPS becomes an RCLPS is not well defined.

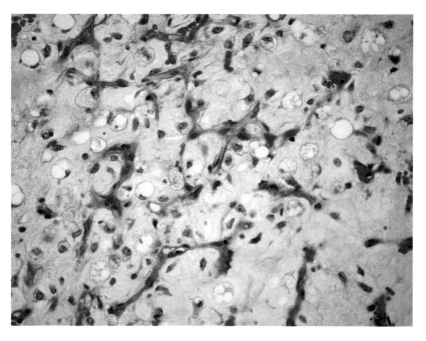

Fig. 21. MLPS. Numerous univacuolated and multi-vacuolated lipoblasts tend to cluster around delicate, arborizing, thin-walled capillaries. The organization of the vessels is often referred to as a "chicken-wire" or "crow's feet" configuration (H&E, original magnification ×200).

Most tumors show both myxoid and round cell features, which have been termed "transitional" by Smith and colleagues.[33] Transitional refers to those areas that are hypercellular as compared with MLPS, but the cells remain spindled, the characteristic vascular pattern is still discernible, and the cells are separated by at least some myxoid stroma (Fig. 25).

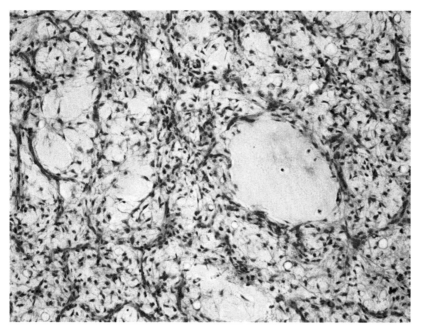

Fig. 22. MLPS. A frequent feature is pooling of extracellular mucin resulting in large cystic spaces and imparts a lymphangiomalike histologic pattern (H&E, original magnification ×100).

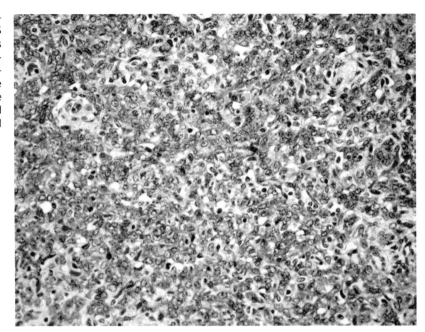

Fig. 23. RCLPS. As compared with MLPS, RCLPS is characterized by nests or solid sheets of primitive round cells. The vascular pattern can be difficult to recognize owing to the increased cellularity (H&E, original magnification ×100).

A small subset of MLPS occurring in children has either a spindle cell pattern (spindle cell MLPS) or a component of pleomorphic cells (pleomorphic MLS). These lesions are thought to represent low-grade and high-grade variants of MLS, respectively.[34]

ANCILLARY STUDIES

The hallmark of MLPS/RCLPS is the presence of 1 of 2 distinctive karyotypic alterations: a t(12;16) translocation that fuses the genes *DDIT3* (*CHOP*) and *FUS*[35] (**Fig. 26**), or a t(12;22) translocation that fuses *DDIT3* and *EWS*.[36] These translocations lead to the formation of fusion transcripts that can be detected by reverse transcriptase–polymerase chain reaction[37]; however, there is breakpoint heterogeneity at the t(12;16) translocation that may complicate the assay.[38] Therefore, this necessitates the use of multiple primers to detect fusion transcripts. Fluorescent in situ hybridization (FISH) studies for *DDIT3* may be a more efficient approach, which detects both t(12;16) and t(12;22) translocations (**Fig. 27**).

DIFFERENTIAL DIAGNOSIS

The differential diagnosis includes chondroid lipoma, lipoblastoma, and other myxoid sarcomas. Like MLPS, chondroid lipoma often arises in young adults as a well-circumscribed extremity mass, but it is often superficial and small. Histologically, it is composed of mature adipocytes and multivacuolated lipoblasts. Although the background of chondroid lipoma is characteristically chondromyxoid, MLPS can on occasion demonstrate chondroid differentiation; however, chondroid lipoma lacks the distinct delicate branching vascular pattern present in MLPS and is usually less cellular.

Both lipoblastoma and MLPS are lobular neoplasms, containing lipoblasts and spindled cells within a myxoid stroma and prominent capillary network. Although the neoplastic cells of lipoblastoma lack hypercellularity and nuclear atypia, such features are at least focally present in MLPS. Lipoblastoma is also more lobulated than most cases of MLPS.[39] Another helpful feature is the clinical setting of these lesions: most lipoblastomas occur before the age of 8, whereas MLPS is

 Differential Diagnosis
MYXOID LIPOSARCOMA/
ROUND CELL LIPOSARCOMA

- Chondroid lipoma
- Lipoblastoma
- Low-grade myxofibrosarcoma
- Extraskeletal myxoid chondrosarcoma

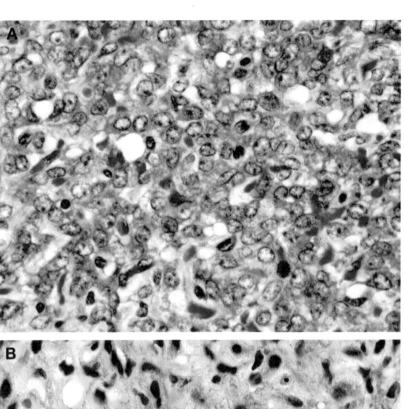

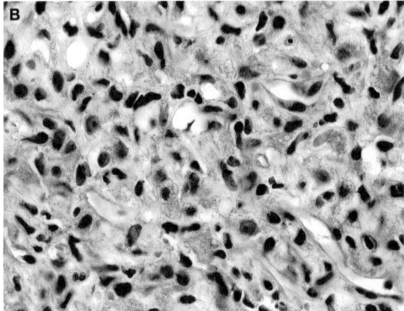

Fig. 24. RCLPS. (*A*) The round cells exhibit a high nuclear to cytoplasmic ratio, nuclear overlap, and a prominent nucleolus. The overgrowth of these cells can obscure the myxoid stroma and rich vascular network. (*B*) Usually small foci of MLPS containing rare lipoblasts and branching capillaries can be identified to aid in the diagnosis, however (H&E, original magnification ×400).

exceedingly rare in this age group. Finally, lipoblastomas are often characterized by structural rearrangements of 8q11-14 and lack the t(12;16) or t(12;22) translocation in MLPS.[40]

Low-grade myxofibrosarcoma and extraskeletal myxoid chrondrosarcoma are 2 entities that can be confused with MLPS/RCLPS. Low-grade myxofibrosarcoma exhibits atypical stromal cells

embedded within a myxoid matrix. In some cases, the tumor cells contain cytoplasmic vacuoles filled with mucin, resembling lipoblasts. In addition, prominent, curvilinear vessels are associated with this lesion, but the vessels are often thick-walled and appear coarse as compared with the delicate, thin-walled capillaries of MLPS. Extraskeletal myxoid chondrosarcoma is similarly

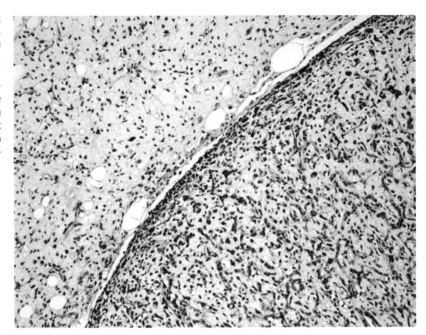

Fig. 25. MLPS/RCLPS. Most MLPS/RCLPS show a transition from MLPS *(top left)* to RCLPS *(bottom right),* termed "transitional areas." These areas exhibit increased cellularity, the presence of a plexiform vascular pattern, and at least some myxoid stroma (H&E, original magnification ×100).

myxoid with enhanced cellularity at the periphery of tumor lobules. The tumor cells are oval to round, but have an eosinophilic rim of cytoplasm, and are arranged as cords and rounded clusters in a hypovascular background. Lipoblasts are noticeably absent within the tumor.

PROGNOSIS

Pure MLPS is considered low grade and associated with a 5-year survival ranging from 80% to 100%. Despite the favorable clinical outcome, 19% to 35% of cases may metastasize.[32,33,41] Tumors with a round cell component of either at least 5%[33] or 25%,[32] depending on the study, have a poorer 5-year survival and higher risk of metastasis. Other unfavorable prognostic factors include a patient older than 45 years and the presence of tumor necrosis.[32]

Although MLPS/RCLPS can metastasize to the usual sites, such as the lungs and bone, it has the peculiar tendency to metastasize to other

Fig. 26. MLPS/RCLPS. A partial karyotype demonstrates the presence of t(12;16), found in more than 90% of cases. The translocation leads to the fusion of *DDIT3* and *FUS* genes at 12q13 and 16p11, respectively. (*FISH courtesy of* Dr PD Cin, C McLaughlin, Center for Advanced Molecular Diagnostics, Brigham and Women's Hospital, Boston, MA; with permission.)

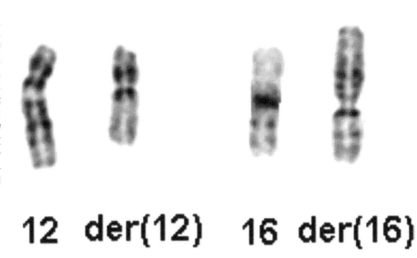

12 der{12} 16 der{16}

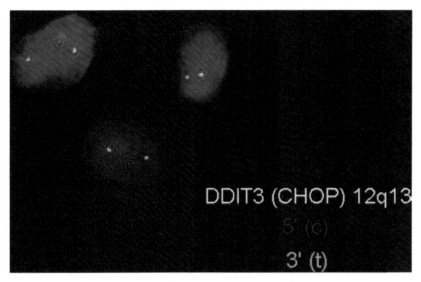

DDIT3 (CHOP) 12q13

5' (c)

3' (t)

Fig. 27. MLPS/RCLPS. The hallmark of MLPS/RCLPS is the presence of either t(12;16) or rarely, t(12;22) translocation that fuses *DDIT3* and *FUS*, or *DDIT3* and *EWS*, respectively. FISH assays using a dual-color break-apart probe for *DDIT3* is a practical method to detect both translocations. (*FISH courtesy of Dr PD Cin, C McLaughlin, Center for Advanced Molecular Diagnostics, Brigham and Women's Hospital, Boston, MA; with permission.*)

soft tissue locations, including the retroperitoneum, opposite extremity, and axilla. This raises the question of multifocal synchronous or metachronous spread versus metastatic disease. Analysis of *FUS-DDIT3* and *EWS-DDIT3* genomic rearrangements has established the monoclonal origin in such cases, confirming metastases rather than multiple independent tumors.[42]

The primary mode of therapy typically involves wide surgical excision. In high-grade lesions, adjuvant therapy may be warranted.[43] Chemotherapy agents, such as doxorubicin plus ifosamide or, more recently, trabectedin (ET-743) have proven to be effective in treating locally advanced and metastatic disease.[44]

PLEOMORPHIC LIPOSARCOMA

OVERVIEW

Pleomorphic liposarcoma (PLPS) is the rarest subtype, constituting fewer than 5% of all cases of LPS. Most cases arise in adults older than 50 with a slight male predominance. Patients typically present with a firm, painless mass that tends to occur intramuscularly in the extremities, particularly

---

> ⚠ **Pitfalls**
> **MYXOID LIPOSARCOMA/**
> **ROUND CELL LIPOSARCOMA**
>
> ! The myxoid stroma is common to several soft tissue tumors. Therefore, it is important to recognize the other diagnostic features of these tumors, including primitive mesenchymal cells, lipoblasts, and arborizing capillaries.
>
> ! The round cell component may exhibit overgrowth, so as to mask the myxoid stroma and vascular network. This is particularly troublesome in limited specimens. With thorough sampling, low-grade areas can be identified, but in difficult cases, detection of t(12;16) and t(12;22) translocations should aid in the diagnosis.

> **Key Features**
> **PLEOMORPHIC LIPOSARCOMA**
>
> 1. High-grade sarcoma associated with sparse to numerous multivacuolated, bizarre lipoblasts.
>
> 2. Three main histologic patterns with the most common composed of high-grade pleomorphic or spindle cell sarcoma with scattered lipoblasts.
>
> 3. The second subtype consists of high-grade pleomorphic sarcoma with solid, cohesive sheets of epithelioid areas and variable number of lipoblasts.
>
> 4. An intermediate-grade to high-grade sarcoma with prominent myxoid areas, resembling myxofibrosarcoma, except for the presence of lipoblasts, characterizes the third subtype.
>
> 5. Eosinophilic hyaline globules are a common finding.

Fig. 28. PLPS. (*A, B*) Most cases consist of high-grade pleomorphic cells associated with scattered atypical adipocytes and bizarre, multivacuolated lipoblasts (H&E, original magnification ×400).

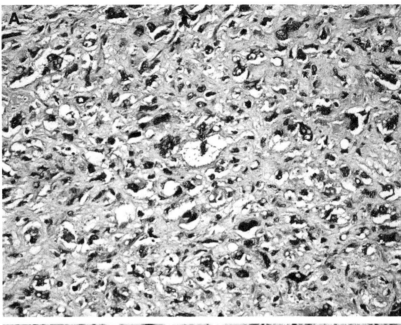

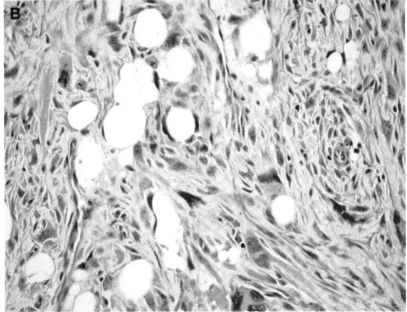

the thigh, followed by the trunk and abdomen.[45–47] Rare cases have been reported in subcutaneous tissues and dermis.[48]

GROSS FEATURES

On gross inspection, PLPS is often large and typically exceeds 10 cm. It is a firm, nodular mass with a white to yellow, fleshy cut surface. Variable

amounts of tumor necrosis and hemorrhage may be present.

MICROSCOPIC FEATURES

PLPS is a high-grade sarcoma, characterized by the presence of markedly pleomorphic lipoblasts. The lipoblasts are frequently enlarged, multivacuolated, and contain bizarre, hyperchromatic, scalloped nuclei. A prominent nucleolus is often

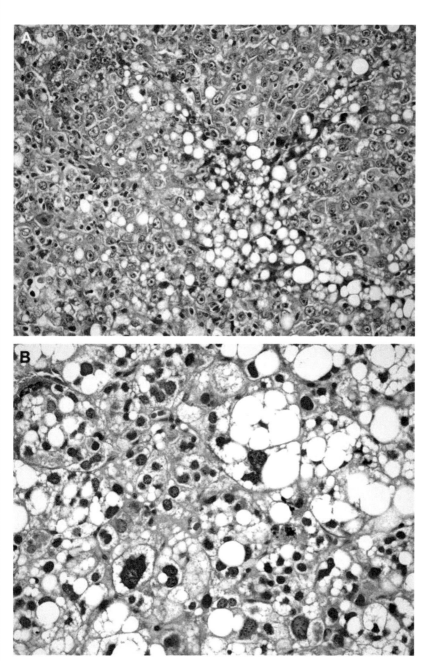

Fig. 29. PLPS. (*A*) In some examples, the tumor shows zones of epithelioid cells with prominent nucleoli and eosinophilic cytoplasm. (*B*) A variable number of markedly pleomorphic, multivacuolated lipoblasts are found intervening between these areas. (H&E, original magnification *A*, ×200; *B*, ×400.)

present; however, in some cases, the number of lipoblasts can be sparse and, therefore, careful examination of an optimally sampled neoplasm is prudent. PLPS can be subdivided into 3 histologic patterns that may coexist in the same lesion. The most common subtype is predominantly high-grade pleomorphic or spindle cell sarcoma with scattered lipoblasts (**Fig. 28**). The second subtype consists of high-grade pleomorphic sarcoma with solid, cohesive sheets of epithelioid areas and a variable amount of lipoblasts (**Fig. 29**). The last subtype is an intermediate-grade to high-grade sarcoma with prominent myxoid areas, resembling myxofibrosarcoma, except for the presence of lipoblasts (**Fig. 30**). The mitotic rate is usually high with numerous atypical forms. In addition, the

Fig. 30. PLPS. (*A*) Rare cases are composed of an intermediate-grade to high-grade sarcoma with prominent myxoid areas. (*B*) The presence of adipocytic differentiation and pleomorphic lipoblasts distinguish this lesion from myxofibrosarcoma (H&E, original magnification ×200).

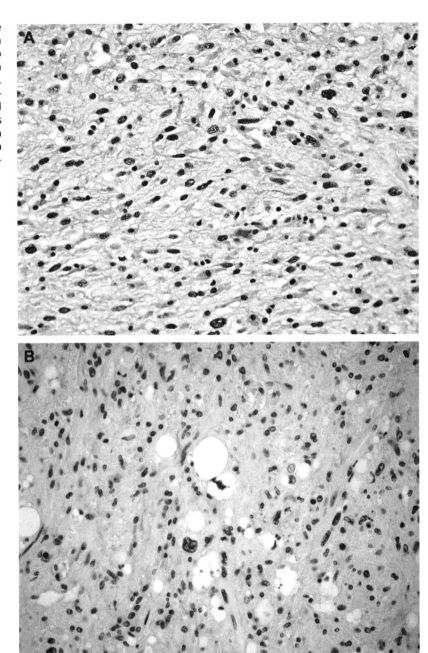

presence of eosinophilic globules is a frequent finding, although of no diagnostic significance.

ANCILLARY STUDIES

PLPS exhibits a complex karyotype with numerous heterogeneous structural aberrations and polyploidy in some cases. The most frequent alterations are gains in chromosomal subregions 20q, 5 p, 17 p, 1q, and 9q.[49] Of note, the 12q13-15 amplification, typically seen in ALT/WDLPS and DDLPS, is absent in PLPS[50]; however, gene expression analysis has shown that the epithelioid variant of PLPS shares the t(12;16) translocation found in MLPS/RCLPS.[51]

DIFFERENTIAL DIAGNOSIS

Because of its wide morphologic spectrum, PLPS may be confused with other high-grade pleomorphic

---

△△ Differential Diagnosis
PLEOMORPHIC LIPOSARCOMA

- Other high-grade pleomorphic sarcomas
- DDLPS
- Carcinoma
- Melanoma

Pitfalls
PLEOMORPHIC LIPOSARCOMA

! Pleomorphic lipoblasts can be sparse, and adequate tumor sampling is important in distinguishing PLPS from other high-grade pleomorphic sarcomas and DDLPS.

! Epithelioid areas can resemble other epithelioid neoplasms and melanoma, both of which lack lipoblasts.

---

sarcomas, DDLPS, carcinoma, and melanoma. As previously emphasized, adequate tumor sampling plays a critical role is differentiating PLPS from other high-grade pleomorphic sarcomas. Although a panel of immunohistochemical markers and even ultrastructural evaluation may be useful, the recognition of pleomorphic lipoblasts represents the most important diagnostic clue of PLPS and permits distinction from other sarcoma subtypes.

Because well-differentiated and dedifferentiated components in DDLPS can in rare instances be found as an admixture, the histopathology of DDLPS may be indistinguishable from PLPS. In the case of DDLPS, however, clinicoradiologic correlation, more extensive sampling, and/or review of the patient's history usually reveals evidence of evolution from ALT/WDLPS. Furthermore, the dedifferentiated component is typically nonlipogenic. Cytogenetic studies may also be useful, considering DDLPS retains the ring and marker chromosomes of ALT/WDLPS. In contrast, PLPS frequently has a highly abnormal and complex karyotype.[50] Thus, PLPS is MDM2 negative.

The epithelioid areas of PLPS can resemble other epithelioid malignancies, including poorly differentiated carcinoma, renal cell carcinoma, adrenal cortical carcinoma, and melanoma. The finding that up to 50% of epithelioid PLPS shows immunoreactivity for cytokeratins, further compounds this issue.[52,53] But the epithelioid morphology is generally well demarcated and adjacent to more conventional PLPS with scattered pleomorphic lipoblasts, which would be absent in carcinomas.

PROGNOSIS

PLPS is an aggressive neoplasm, where standard treatment is wide surgical excision combined with adjuvant therapy. Despite treatment, 30% to 50% of patients will develop distant metastases, usually to the lungs, bone, retroperitoneum, and trunk. In addition, epithelioid morphology is associated with increased risk of recurrence and metastasis. The 5-year survival is poor and ranges from 29% to 63% in reported studies. Tumors smaller than 5 cm, and those located superficially and in the extremities seem to have a better prognosis.[45–47]

REFERENCES

1. Virchow R. Ein Fall von bösartigen zum Theil in der Form des Neurons auftretenden Fettgeschwulsten. Arch A Pathol Anat Phys 1857;11:281–8.
2. Fletcher CDM, Unni KK, Mertens F. Pathology and genetics of tumours of soft tissue and bone. Lyon (France): IARC Press; 2002.
3. Dei Tos AP, Pedetour F. Atypical lipomatous tumors/ well-differentiated liposarcoma. In: Fletcher CD, Unni KK, Mertens F, editors. Pathology and genetics of tumours of soft tissue and bone. Lyon (France): IARC Press; 2002. p. 35–7.
4. Enzinger FM, Winslow DJ. Liposarcoma. A study of 103 cases. Virchows Arch Pathol Anat Physiol Klin Med 1962;335:367–88.
5. Weiss SW, Goldblum JR. Liposarcoma. In: Weiss SW, Goldblum JR, editors, Enzinger and Weiss's soft tissue tumors, vol. 5. St Louis (MO): Mosby; 2008. p. 477–516.
6. Azumi N, Curtis J, Kempson RL, et al. Atypical and malignant neoplasms showing lipomatous differentiation. A study of 111 cases. Am J Surg Pathol 1987;11(3):161–83.
7. Evans HL. Atypical lipomatous tumor, its variants, and its combined forms: a study of 61 cases, with a minimum follow-up of 10 years. Am J Surg Pathol 2007;31(1):1–14.
8. Argani P, Facchetti F, Inghirami G, et al. Lymphocyte-rich well-differentiated liposarcoma: report of nine cases. Am J Surg Pathol 1997;21(8):884–95.
9. Kraus MD, Guillou L, Fletcher CD. Well-differentiated inflammatory liposarcoma: an uncommon and easily overlooked variant of a common sarcoma. Am J Surg Pathol 1997;21(5):518–27.

10. Dei Tos AP, Mentzel T, Newman PL, et al. Spindle cell liposarcoma, a hitherto unrecognized variant of liposarcoma. Analysis of six cases. Am J Surg Pathol 1994;18(9):913–21.

11. Evans HL. Smooth muscle in atypical lipomatous tumors. A report of three cases. Am J Surg Pathol 1990;14(8):714–8.

12. Dal Cin P, Kools P, Sciot R, et al. Cytogenetic and fluorescence in situ hybridization investigation of ring chromosomes characterizing a specific pathologic subgroup of adipose tissue tumors. Cancer Genet Cytogenet 1993;68(2):85–90.

13. Wolf M, Aaltonen LA, Szymanska J, et al. Complexity of 12q13-22 amplicon in liposarcoma: microsatellite repeat analysis. Genes Chromosomes Cancer 1997; 18(1):66–70.

14. Sirvent N, Coindre JM, Maire G, et al. Detection of MDM2-CDK4 amplification by fluorescence in situ hybridization in 200 paraffin-embedded tumor samples: utility in diagnosing adipocytic lesions and comparison with immunohistochemistry and real-time PCR. Am J Surg Pathol 2007;31(10):1476–89.

15. Remstein ED, Kurtin PJ, Nascimento AG. Sclerosing extramedullary hematopoietic tumor in chronic myeloproliferative disorders. Am J Surg Pathol 2000;24(1):51–5.

16. Weiss SW, Rao VK. Well-differentiated liposarcoma (atypical lipoma) of deep soft tissue of the extremities, retroperitoneum, and miscellaneous sites. A follow-up study of 92 cases with analysis of the incidence of "dedifferentiation". Am J Surg Pathol 1992; 16(11):1051–8.

17. Lucas DR, Nascimento AG, Sanjay BK, et al. Well-differentiated liposarcoma. The Mayo Clinic experience with 58 cases. Am J Clin Pathol 1994;102(5): 677–83.

18. Henricks WH, Chu YC, Goldblum JR, et al. Dedifferentiated liposarcoma: a clinicopathological analysis of 155 cases with a proposal for an expanded definition of dedifferentiation. Am J Surg Pathol 1997; 21(3):271–81.

19. Dei Tos AP, Pedetour F. Dedifferentiated liposarcoma. In: Fletcher CD, Unni KK, Mertens F, editors. Pathology and genetics of tumours of soft tissue and bone. Lyon (France): IARC Press; 2002.

20. Elgar F, Goldblum JR. Well-differentiated liposarcoma of the retroperitoneum: a clinicopathologic analysis of 20 cases, with particular attention to the extent of low-grade dedifferentiation. Mod Pathol 1997;10(2):113–20.

21. Nascimento AG, Kurtin PJ, Guillou L, et al. Dedifferentiated liposarcoma: a report of nine cases with a peculiar neurallike whorling pattern associated with metaplastic bone formation. Am J Surg Pathol 1998;22(8):945–55.

22. Thway K, Robertson D, Thway Y, et al. Dedifferentiated liposarcoma with meningothelial-like whorls, metaplastic bone formation, and CDK4, MDM2, and p16 expression: a morphologic and immunohistochemical study. Am J Surg Pathol 2011;35(3): 356–63.

23. Binh MB, Guillou L, Hostein I, et al. Dedifferentiated liposarcomas with divergent myosarcomatous differentiation developed in the internal trunk: a study of 27 cases and comparison to conventional dedifferentiated liposarcomas and leiomyosarcomas. Am J Surg Pathol 2007;31(10):1557–66.

24. Aleixo PB, Hartmann AA, Menezes IC, et al. Can MDM2 and CDK4 make the diagnosis of well differentiated/dedifferentiated liposarcoma? An immunohistochemical study on 129 soft tissue tumours. J Clin Pathol 2009;62(12):1127–35.

25. Binh MB, Sastre-Garau X, Guillou L, et al. MDM2 and CDK4 immunostainings are useful adjuncts in diagnosing well-differentiated and dedifferentiated liposarcoma subtypes: a comparative analysis of 559 soft tissue neoplasms with genetic data. Am J Surg Pathol 2005;29(10):1340–7.

26. Coindre JM, Mariani O, Chibon F, et al. Most malignant fibrous histiocytomas developed in the retroperitoneum are dedifferentiated liposarcomas: a review of 25 cases initially diagnosed as malignant fibrous histiocytoma. Mod Pathol 2003;16(3): 256–62.

27. Coindre JM, Hostein I, Maire G, et al. Inflammatory malignant fibrous histiocytomas and dedifferentiated liposarcomas: histological review, genomic profile, and MDM2 and CDK4 status favour a single entity. J Pathol 2004;203(3):822–30.

28. McCormick D, Mentzel T, Beham A, et al. Dedifferentiated liposarcoma. Clinicopathologic analysis of 32 cases suggesting a better prognostic subgroup among pleomorphic sarcomas. Am J Surg Pathol 1994;18(12):1213–23.

29. Muller CR, Paulsen EB, Noordhuis P, et al. Potential for treatment of liposarcomas with the MDM2 antagonist Nutlin-3A. Int J Cancer 2007;121(1): 199–205.

30. Ambrosini G, Sambol EB, Carvajal D, et al. Mouse double minute antagonist Nutlin-3a enhances chemotherapy-induced apoptosis in cancer cells with mutant p53 by activating E2F1. Oncogene 2007;26(24):3473–81.

31. Antonescu CR, Ladanyi M. Myxoid liposarcoma. In: Fletcher CD, Unni KK, Mertens F, editors. Pathology and genetics of tumours of soft tissue and bone. Lyon (France): IARC Press; 2002. p. 40–3.

32. Kilpatrick SE, Doyon J, Choong PF, et al. The clinicopathologic spectrum of myxoid and round cell liposarcoma. A study of 95 cases. Cancer 1996;77(8): 1450–8.

33. Smith TA, Easley KA, Goldblum JR. Myxoid/round cell liposarcoma of the extremities. A clinicopathologic study of 29 cases with particular attention to

extent of round cell liposarcoma. Am J Surg Pathol 1996;20(2):171–80.

34. Alaggio R, Coffin CM, Weiss SW, et al. Liposarcomas in young patients: a study of 82 cases occurring in patients younger than 22 years of age. Am J Surg Pathol 2009;33(5):645–58.

35. Crozat A, Aman P, Mandahl N, et al. Fusion of CHOP to a novel RNA-binding protein in human myxoid liposarcoma. Nature 1993;363(6430):640–4.

36. Dal Cin P, Sciot R, Panagopoulos I, et al. Additional evidence of a variant translocation t(12;22) with EWS/CHOP fusion in myxoid liposarcoma: clinicopathological features. J Pathol 1997;182(4): 437–41.

37. Hisaoka M, Tsuji S, Morimitsu Y, et al. Detection of TLS/FUS-CHOP fusion transcripts in myxoid and round cell liposarcomas by nested reverse transcription-polymerase chain reaction using archival paraffin-embedded tissues. Diagn Mol Pathol 1998;7(2):96–101.

38. Kuroda M, Ishida T, Horiuchi H, et al. Chimeric TLS/FUS-CHOP gene expression and the heterogeneity of its junction in human myxoid and round cell liposarcoma. Am J Pathol 1995;147(5):1221–7.

39. Chung EB, Enzinger FM. Benign lipoblastomatosis. An analysis of 35 cases. Cancer 1973;32(2): 482–92.

40. Dal Cin P, Sciot R, De Wever I, et al. New discriminative chromosomal marker in adipose tissue tumors. The chromosome 8q11-q13 region in lipoblastoma. Cancer Genet Cytogenet 1994;78(2):232–5.

41. Spillane AJ, Fisher C, Thomas JM. Myxoid liposarcoma—the frequency and the natural history of nonpulmonary soft tissue metastases. Ann Surg Oncol 1999;6(4):389–94.

42. Antonescu CR, Elahi A, Healey JH, et al. Monoclonality of multifocal myxoid liposarcoma: confirmation by analysis of TLS-CHOP or EWS-CHOP rearrangements. Clin Cancer Res 2000;6(7):2788–93.

43. Engstrom K, Bergh P, Cederlund CG, et al. Irradiation of myxoid/round cell liposarcoma induces volume reduction and lipoma-like morphology. Acta Oncol 2007;46(6):838–45.

44. Grosso F, Jones RL, Demetri GD, et al. Efficacy of trabectedin (ecteinascidin-743) in advanced pretreated myxoid liposarcomas: a retrospective study. Lancet Oncol 2007;8(7):595–602.

45. Hornick JL, Bosenberg MW, Mentzel T, et al. Pleomorphic liposarcoma: clinicopathologic analysis of 57 cases. Am J Surg Pathol 2004;28(10):1257–67.

46. Downes KA, Goldblum JR, Montgomery EA, et al. Pleomorphic liposarcoma: a clinicopathologic analysis of 19 cases. Mod Pathol 2001;14(3):179–84.

47. Gebhard S, Coindre JM, Michels JJ, et al. Pleomorphic liposarcoma: clinicopathologic, immunohistochemical, and follow-up analysis of 63 cases: a study from the French Federation of Cancer Centers Sarcoma Group. Am J Surg Pathol 2002;26(5):601–16.

48. Dei Tos AP, Mentzel T, Fletcher CD. Primary liposarcoma of the skin: a rare neoplasm with unusual high grade features. Am J Dermatopathol 1998;20(4): 332–8.

49. Mertens F, Fletcher CD, Dal Cin P, et al. Cytogenetic analysis of 46 pleomorphic soft tissue sarcomas and correlation with morphologic and clinical features: a report of the CHAMP Study Group. Chromosomes and MorPhology. Genes Chromosomes Cancer 1998;22(1):16–25.

50. Fritz B, Schubert F, Wrobel G, et al. Microarray-based copy number and expression profiling in dedifferentiated and pleomorphic liposarcoma. Cancer Res 2002;62(11):2993–8.

51. De Cecco L, Gariboldi M, Reid JF, et al. Gene expression profile identifies a rare epithelioid variant case of pleomorphic liposarcoma carrying FUS-CHOP transcript. Histopathology 2005;46(3):334–41.

52. Huang HY, Antonescu CR. Epithelioid variant of pleomorphic liposarcoma: a comparative immunohistochemical and ultrastructural analysis of six cases with emphasis on overlapping features with epithelial malignancies. Ultrastruct Pathol 2002; 26(5):299–308.

53. Miettinen M, Enzinger FM. Epithelioid variant of pleomorphic liposarcoma: a study of 12 cases of a distinctive variant of high-grade liposarcoma. Mod Pathol 1999;12(7):722–8.

Index

Note: Page numbers of article titles are in **boldface** type.

Surgical Pathology 4 (2011) 995–1003
doi:10.1016/S1875-9181(11)00181-4
1875-9181/11/$ – see front matter © 2011 Elsevier Inc. All rights reserved.

Moving?

Make sure your subscription moves with you!

To notify us of your new address, find your **Clinics Account Number** (located on your mailing label above your name), and contact customer service at:

Email: journalscustomerservice-usa@elsevier.com

800-654-2452 (subscribers in the U.S. & Canada)
314-447-8871 (subscribers outside of the U.S. & Canada)

Fax number: 314-447-8029

Elsevier Health Sciences Division
Subscription Customer Service
3251 Riverport Lane
Maryland Heights, MO 63043

*To ensure uninterrupted delivery of your subscription, please notify us at least 4 weeks in advance of move.

Printed and bound by CPI Group (UK) Ltd, Croydon, CR0 4YY

03/10/2024

01040350-0004